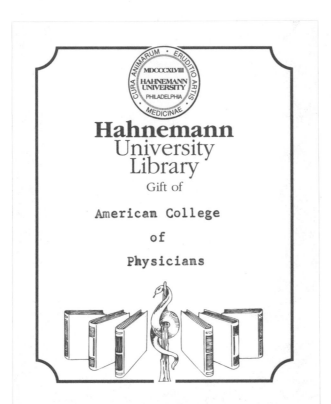

The Bristol-Myers Squibb Symposium on Pain Research

Hyperalgesia and Allodynia

The Bristol-Myers Squibb Symposium on Pain Research Series

Pain and Central Nervous System Disease: The Central Pain Syndromes
Kenneth L. Casey, Editor, 304 pp., 1991

Hyperalgesia and Allodynia
William D. Willis, Jr., Editor, 416 pp., 1992

The Bristol-Myers Squibb Symposium on Pain Research

Hyperalgesia and Allodynia

Editor

William D. Willis, Jr., M.D., Ph.D.

Department of Anatomy and Neurosciences
and Marine Biomedical Institute
University of Texas Medical Branch
Galveston, Texas

Raven Press ✺ New York

Raven Press, Ltd., 1185 Avenue of the Americas, New York, New York 10036

Made in the United States of America

Library of Congress Cataloging-in-Publication Data
Bristol-Myers Squibb Symposium on Pain Research (2nd : 1991 : Galveston, Tex.)
   Hyperalgesia and allodynia : the Bristol-Myers Squibb Symposium on Pain Research / editor, William D. Willis, Jr.
      p.   cm. — (The Bristol-Myers Squibb Symposium on Pain Research series)
   Includes bibliographical references and index.
   ISBN 0-88167-897-X
   1. Hyperalgesia—Congresses. 2. Allodynia—Congresses. I. Willis, William D., 1934–   . II. Title. III. Series: Bristol-Myers Squibb Symposium on Pain Research. Bristol-Myers Squibb Symposium on Pain Research series.
   [DNLM: 1. Hyperalgesia—congresses. 2. Nociceptors—congresses. 3. Pain—physiopathology—congresses. 4. Pain—therapy—congresses.
WL 704 B861h   1991]
RB 127.B75   1991
616'.0472—dc20
DNLM/DLC
for Library of Congress   92-6601
                                                                      CIP

9 8 7 6 5 4 3 2 1

Contents

Characteristics and Mechanisms of Primary Hyperalgesia

Mechanisms of Secondary Hyperalgesia

Role of Central Changes in Hyperalgesia

Contributing Authors

Nadine Attal, M.D. *Unité de Physiopharmacologie du Système Nerveux, U161, INSERM, 2 rue d'Alésia, 75014 Paris, France*

Allan I. Basbaum, Ph.D. *Departments of Anatomy and Physiology, Keck Center for Integrative Neurosciences, University of California, Box 0452, San Francisco, California 94143*

Gary J. Bennett, Ph.D. *Neurobiology and Anesthesiology Branch, National Institute of Dental Research, National Institutes of Health, Building 30, Room B20, 9000 Rockville Pike, Bethesda, Maryland 20892*

Jean-Michel Benoist, M.D. *Unité de Physiopharmacologie du Système Nerveux, U161, INSERM, 2 rue d'Alésia, 75014 Paris, France*

Jean-Marie Besson, D.Sc. *Unité de Physiopharmacologie du Système Nerveux, U161, INSERM, 2 rue d'Alésia, 75014 Paris, France*

Jörgen Boivie, M.D. *Department of Neurology, University Hospital, S-581 85 Linköping, Sweden*

John J. Bonica, M.D., D.Sc., FFARCS *Department of Anesthesiology, RN-10, Multidisciplinary Pain Center, University of Washington School of Medicine, Seattle, Washington 98195*

Elizabeth Bullitt, M.D. *Division of Neurosurgery, Department of Physiology, CB #7060, University of North Carolina, Chapel Hill, North Carolina 27599*

James N. Campbell, M.D. *Department of Neurosurgery, Applied Physics Laboratory, Johns Hopkins University School of Medicine, 600 N. Wolfe Street, Meyer 7-113, Baltimore, Maryland 21205*

Kenneth L. Casey, M.D. *Departments of Neurology and Physiology, The University of Michigan, Ann Arbor, Michigan 48109 and Neurology Service, Veterans Affairs Medical Center, 2215 Fuller Road, Ann Arbor, Michigan 48105*

Shu-Ing Chi, Ph.D. *Department of Anatomy, and Keck Center for Integrative Neurosciences, University of California, San Francisco, California 94143*

Karen D. Davis, Ph.D. *Department of Neurosurgery, Johns Hopkins University School of Medicine, 600 N. Wolfe Street, Meyer 7-113, Baltimore, Maryland 21205*

Ronald Dubner, D.D.S., Ph.D. *Neurobiology and Anesthesiology Branch, National Institute of Dental Research, National Institutes of Health, Building 30, Room B20, 9000 Rockville Pike, Bethesda, Maryland 20892*

Howard L. Fields, M.D., Ph.D. *Department of Neurology, University of California Medical School, Room 794, Box 0114, San Francisco, California 94143*

Kathleen M. Foley, M.D. *Department of Neurology, Memorial Sloan-Kettering Cancer Center, 1275 York Avenue, New York, New York 10021*

G. F. Gebhart, Ph.D. *Department of Pharmacology, University of Iowa College of Medicine, 2-471 Bowen Science Building, Iowa City, Iowa 52242-1109*

Gisèle Guilbaud, M.D. *Unité de Physiopharmacologie du Système Nerveux, U161, INSERM, 2 rue d'Alésia, 75014 Paris, France*

Jane E. Haley, Ph.D. *Department of Pharmacology, Graduate Program in Neuroscience, University of Minnesota, 3-249 Millard Hall, 435 Delaware Street SE, Minneapolis, Minnesota 55455*

H. O. Handwerker, M.D. *Institut für Physiologie und Biokybernetik, Universität Erlangen-Nürnberg, Universitätsstrasse 17, D-8520 Erlangen, Germany*

U. Hanesch, M.D. *Institute of Physiology, University of Würzburg, Röntgenring 9, D-8700 Würzburg, Germany*

Per Hansson, M.D., D.M.Sc., D.D.S. *Department of Neurology, Karolinska Hospital, Box 605 00, S-10401 Stockholm, Sweden*

Philip H. Heller, M.D. *Department of Oral and Maxillofacial Surgery, Division of Neurosciences, University of California, San Francisco, California 94143-0724*

B. Heppelmann, M.D. *Institute of Physiology, University of Würzburg, Röntgenring 9, D-8700 Würzburg, Germany*

Valérie Kayser, M.D. *Unité de Physiopharmacologie du Système Nerveux, U161, INSERM, 2 rue d'Alésia, 75014 Paris, France*

Jennifer M. A. Laird, Ph.D. *Neurobiology and Anesthesiology Branch, National Institute of Dental Research, National Institutes of Health, Building 30, Room B20, 9000 Rockville Pike, Bethesda, Maryland 20892*

Robert H. LaMotte, Ph.D. *Department of Anesthesiology and Section of Neurobiology, Yale University School of Medicine, 333 Cedar Street, New Haven, Connecticut 06510*

Jon D. Levine, M.D., Ph.D. *Departments of Medicine, Anatomy, and Oral and Maxillofacial Surgery, Divisions of Neurosciences and Rheumatology, U-426, Box 0724, University of California, San Francisco, California 94143*

John C. Liebeskind, Ph.D. *Department of Psychology, University of California, Los Angeles, 1285 Franz Hall, 405 Hilgard Avenue, Los Angeles, California 90024*

Ulf Lindblom, M.D. *Department of Neurology, Karolinska Hospital, Box 605 00, S-10401 Stockholm, Sweden*

K. Messlinger, M.D. *Institute of Physiology, University of Würzburg, Röntgenring 9, D-8700 Würzburg, Germany*

Richard A. Meyer, M.D. *Department of Neurosurgery, Applied Physics Laboratory, Johns Hopkins University School of Medicine, 600 N. Wolfe Street, Meyer 7-113, Baltimore, Maryland 21205*

Robert R. Myers, Ph.D. *Department of Anesthesiology, T-018, University of California, San Diego, La Jolla, California 92093*

José Ochoa, D.Sc., M.D., Ph.D. *Departments of Neurology and Neurosurgery, Good Samaritan Hospital and Medical Center, Oregon Health Sciences University, 1040 N.W. 22nd, Suite N460, Portland, Oregon 97210*

Edward R. Perl, M.D. *Department of Physiology, University of North Carolina at Chapel Hill, Chapel Hill, North Carolina 27599*

Srinivasa Raja, M.D. *Department of Anesthesiology, Johns Hopkins University School of Medicine, 600 N. Wolfe Street, Meyer 7-113, Baltimore, Maryland 21205*

P. W. Reeh, M.D. *Institut für Physiologie und Biokybernetik, Universität Erlangen-Nürnberg, Universitätsstrasse 17, D-8520 Erlangen, Germany*

Mary Ann Ruda, Ph.D. *Neurobiology and Anesthesiology Branch, National Institute of Dental Research, National Institutes of Health, Building 30, Room B20, 9000 Rockville Pike, Bethesda, Maryland 20892*

A. Rustioni, M.D. *Department of Cell Biology and Anatomy, University of North Carolina, Chapel Hill, North Carolina 27599*

Hans-Georg Schaible, M.D. *Institute of Physiology, University of Würzburg, Röntgenring 9, D-8700 Würzburg, Germany*

R. F. Schmidt, M.D., Ph.D. *Institute of Physiology, University of Würzburg, Röntgenring 9, D-8700 Würzberg, Germany*

Yetunde O. Taiwo, Ph.D. *Department of Oral and Maxillofacial Surgery, University of California, San Francisco, California 94143-0724*

Erik Torebjörk, M.D., Ph.D. *Department of Clinical Neurophysiology, University Hospital, S-75185 Uppsala, Sweden*

Edgar T. Walters, Ph.D. *Department of Physiology and Cell Biology, University of Texas Medical School at Houston, P.O. Box 20708, Houston, Texas 77225*

R. J. Weinberg, Ph.D. *Department of Cell Biology and Anatomy, University of North Carolina, Chapel Hill, North Carolina 27599*

George L. Wilcox, Ph.D. *Department of Pharmacology, Graduate Program in Neuroscience, University of Minnesota, 3-249 Millard Hall, 435 Delaware Street SE, Minneapolis, Minnesota 55455*

William D. Willis, Jr., M.D., Ph.D.   *Department of Anatomy and Neurosciences, Marine Biomedical Institute, University of Texas Medical Branch, 200 University Blvd., Suite 608, Galveston, Texas 77550-2772*

Clifford J. Woolf, M.D.   *Department of Anatomy and Developmental Biology, University College London, Gower Street, London WC1E 6BT, England*

Tony L. Yaksh, Ph.D.   *Department of Anesthesiology, T-018, University of California, San Diego, La Jolla, California 92093*

Tatsuo Yamamoto, M.D.   *Department of Anesthesiology, T-018, University of California, San Diego, La Jolla, California 92093*

Editor's Foreword

The Second Annual Bristol-Myers Squibb Symposium on Pain Research was held in Galveston, Texas, on May 20–24, 1991. This unique forum brought together the world's most renowned scientific experts to review and discuss growing knowledge about the symposium topic — hyperalgesia.

The notion that nerve fibers change their sensitivity due to pain was first hypothesized over 75 years ago. Since that time, research has made great progress in understanding underlying mechanisms of primary and secondary hyperalgesia, which are characterized by lowered pain threshold, increased sensitivity to suprathreshold stimuli, and spontaneous pain.

From the numerous fine papers presented at this year's symposium, we can see clearly that the recent accelerated rate of growth of knowledge about hyperalgesia has brought scientific research to the threshold of major breakthroughs in therapy.

Special recognition is owed to William D. Willis, Jr., M.D., Ph.D., Ashbel Smith, Professor and Chairman of Anatomy and Neurosciences, Professor of Physiology and Biophysics, and Director of the Marine Biomedical Institute at The University of Texas Medical Branch at Galveston. As course director, Dr. Willis' outstanding leadership and organizational qualities contributed greatly to the symposium's success.

On behalf of Bristol-Myers Squibb, I wish to express my sincere gratitude to Dr. Willis, his committee, the participants, and the University for bringing this program to fruition. I know that this gratitude is shared by all those who attended and will read these historic proceedings.

George A. Blewitt, M.D.
Series Editor

Foreword

According to the National Chronic Pain Outreach Association, pain affects nearly 90 million Americans and costs the U.S. economy an estimated $90 billion a year in direct expenses, lost workdays, and compensation. Pain is considered to be the most frequent cause of suffering and disability.

Over the past two decades, however, great progress has been made in understanding the mechanisms of pain. Researchers predict the 1990s will be an exciting decade for advances in this growing field.

The Second Bristol-Myers Squibb Symposium on Pain Research was devoted to a review of current knowledge about the mechanisms of hyperalgesia. Held in Galveston in May, 1991, the symposium was organized by the Department of Anatomy and Neurosciences of The University of Texas Medical Branch at Galveston. The chairman was William D. Willis, Jr., M.D., Ph.D., a leader in hyperalgesia research.

Bristol-Myers Squibb has committed $2.75 million in unrestricted funding to date in support of basic pain research. In addition to sponsoring an annual symposium, we underwrite the annual Bristol-Myers Squibb Award for Distinguished Achievement in Pain Research, and the Bristol-Myers Squibb Unrestricted Pain Research Grants Program, five-year commitments of no-strings-attached grants for the study of pain.

We are proud to have sponsored this opportunity for the international scientific community to come together to exchange valuable information. We look forward to next year's symposium and to the expanding role that pain research will continue to play in improving our quality of life.

Richard L. Gelb
Chairman of the Board
Bristol-Myers Squibb Company

Acknowledgment

The publication of this book and the symposium on which it is based have been made possible through the generosity of the Bristol-Myers Squibb Company.

Hyperalgesia and Allodynia,
edited by W. D. Willis, Jr.
Raven Press, Ltd., New York © 1992.

1

Hyperalgesia and Allodynia

Summary and Overview

William D. Willis, Jr.

*Department of Anatomy and Neurosciences, Marine Biomedical Institute,
University of Texas Medical Branch, Galveston, Texas 77550-2772*

The second Bristol-Myers Squibb Symposium on Pain Research was held in May 1991, in Galveston, Texas, on the topic of hyperalgesia and allodynia. The plan of the symposium was to bring together from around the world leading experts on hyperalgesia as expressed either in animal models or human subjects. The sessions were sequenced so that peripheral mechanisms were considered first, followed by central mechanisms, and then clinical applications and future directions. This volume consists largely of chapters based on the presentations. In addition, the set of chapters corresponding to each session is preceded by an overview written by the session chairman and followed by an edited transcript of the discussion.

HISTORICAL BACKGROUND

Although the phenomenon of hyperalgesia has been recognized clinically for centuries, the term was first used by Gowers in the late 19th century (see Bonica, Chapter 3). The relationship of hyperalgesia to referred pain was established by investigators of the same era, such as Sturge, Ross, Head, and MacKenzie, as was its occurrence in central pain states, as shown by such investigators as Déjérine and Roussy, Head and Holmes, and Riddoch. Studies of the mechanisms of hyperalgesia have been facilitated by the distinction made between primary and secondary hyperalgesia by Lewis (2) and then by Hardy et al. (1). Lewis used the term "erythralgia" for the condition later named primary hyperalgesia by Hardy et al. and the terms "diffuse hyperalgesia" and "nocifensor tenderness" for secondary hyperalgesia. Erythralgia is not an ideal descriptor, since hyperalgesia can occur without erythema (2).

Hardy et al. (1) defined hyperalgesia as "a state of increased pain sensation induced by either noxious or ordinarily non-noxious stimulation of peripheral tissue." Primary hyperalgesia is "that occurring at the site of injury" and secondary hyperalgesia is "that associated with the injury but occurring in apparently undamaged tissue." Primary hyperalgesia is characterized by increased sensitivity to both thermal and mechanical stimuli, whereas secondary hyperalgesia involves an increased sensitivity only to mechanical stimuli (1,2).

A further distinction has been made between hyperalgesia and allodynia in the taxonomy adopted in 1982 by the International Association for the Study of Pain (Bonica, Chapter 3). Hyperalgesia is defined in the taxonomy as an increase in the pain produced by a stimulus that is normally painful, and allodynia is pain produced by a stimulus that is not normally painful (3). Hyperalgesia and allodynia can also be produced by damage to peripheral nerves or the central nervous system.

Following tissue damage, primary hyperalgesia occurs in the region of injury, whereas secondary hyperalgesia is distributed in the surrounding undamaged area or, in the case of referred pain, in a distant region. Primary hyperalgesia results from injury to the skin, mucous membranes, or deep somatic structures. For example, in Fig. 1.1, the hatched areas show the distribution of primary hyperalgesia at the sites of damage made by a small punctate burn and a larger patch-like burn. Erythema may spread beyond the area of primary hyperalgesia (LaMotte, Chapter 16). The decrease in pain threshold and increase in pain evoked by a constant painful stimulus are illustrated diagrammatically in Fig. 1.2. Secondary hyperalgesia develops in an area surrounding the region of damage (Fig. 1.1, left).

The duration and spatial distribution of secondary hyperalgesia depend on the severity and time course of the injury. During prolonged, minimally painful stimulation, an area of secondary hyperalgesia spreads progressively from the site of damage, and when the painful stimulation is halted, the area of secondary hyperalgesia retracts and disappears within minutes (Fig. 1.3). With more severe injuries, the secondary hyperalgesia lasts for periods of hours or even days (2).

Both primary and secondary hyperalgesia depend on activity established in nerve fibers supplying the damaged area, since local anesthesia prevents the development

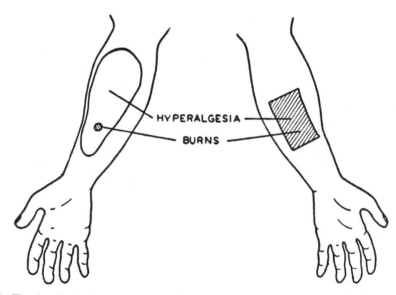

FIG. 1.1. The *hatched areas* show the distribution of primary hyperalgesia after mild burns. On the left, the distribution of secondary hyperalgesia is also shown by the oval line. (From ref. 1.)

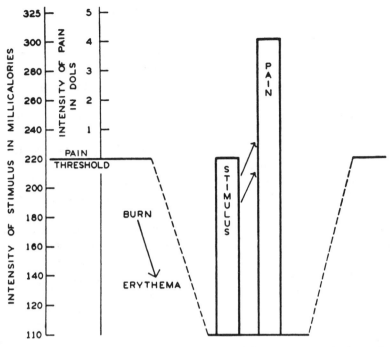

FIG. 1.2. The changes in pain threshold and pain sensibility in an area of primary hyperalgesia. (From ref. 1.)

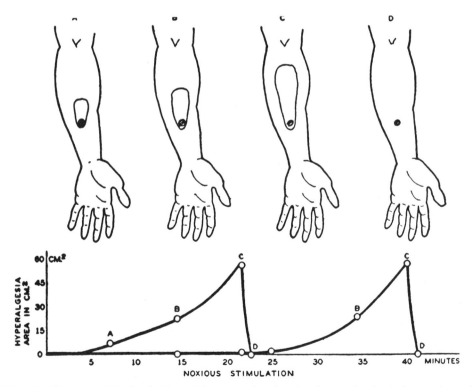

FIG. 1.3. The spread in distribution of the area of secondary hyperalgesia during prolonged, minimally painful thermal stimulation of the skin. The graph shows the area of secondary hyperalgesia at different time points. Note that with such weak stimulation, the secondary hyperalgesia outlasts the stimulation by only minutes. (From ref. 1.)

of either form of hyperalgesia. For example, Fig. 1.4 shows that the primary and secondary hyperalgesia caused by a cutaneous burn can be delayed by injection of procaine into the area to be burned. Both types of hyperalgesia appear after the anesthetic wears off.

Lewis (2) attributed primary hyperalgesia to the release of chemical factors from damaged tissue and their acting on nociceptive nerve endings. To explain the spread of secondary hyperalgesia, he proposed the release of a pain-provoking chemical agent from the terminals of a hypothetical set of nocifensor nerve fibers innervating both the damaged and undamaged areas by way of an axon reflex. This chemical substance would act on other nerve endings, making them more sensitive to stimulation, thus causing tenderness.

Hardy et al. (1) agreed with the notion that primary hyperalgesia may be produced by the local release of chemical substances following damage. However, they proposed that secondary hyperalgesia is due to an increase in excitability in the central nervous system due to neural input caused by the initial damage. Figure 1.5 shows diagrammatically how the spread of activity in the dorsal horn of the spinal cord might cause an increased excitability of interneurons and also of spinothalamic tract cells to stimuli originating from receptors in the area of developing secondary hyperalgesia. This idea was presaged by Mitchell's similar proposal in 1872 and by the ideas of other authors of the late 19th century (Bonica, Chapter 3).

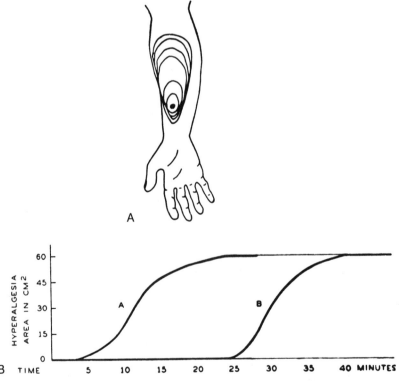

FIG. 1.4. Time course of development of secondary hyperalgesia. **A:** Normal time course is shown following injury. **B:** Time course is seen to be delayed by injection of procaine into the skin prior to injury. (From ref. 1.)

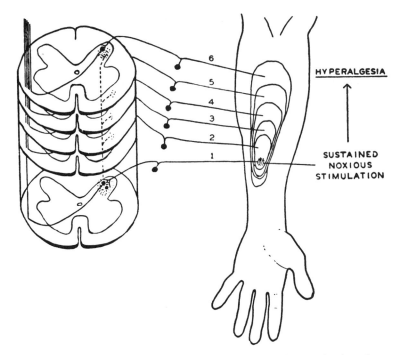

FIG. 1.5. Diagram showing how sensitization of central neurons in circuits whose output is transmitted by spinothalamic tract cells might lead to secondary hyperalgesia. (From ref. 1.)

As mentioned earlier, hyperalgesia can be produced not only by tissue damage, but also by injuries to nervous tissue, in either the peripheral or central nervous system (2). Early work on neuropathic pain includes that of Mitchell, Déjérine and Roussy, Head and Holmes, and Riddoch (Bonica, Chapter 3). A particularly important issue in the case of neuropathic pain due to peripheral nerve injuries is the contribution of the sympathetic nervous system to what is now called "sympathetically maintained pain" (Perl, Chapter 5; Campbell et al., Chapter 12; Ochoa, Chapter 13). Sympathetic block is thought to be effective in alleviating neuropathic pain and preventing its persistence if the block is done early in the course of the affliction (Bonica, Chapter 3). However, for some reason sympathetic block becomes ineffective if delayed. The mechanism for the association of sympathetic activity and neuropathic pain is not yet understood nor is the reason for the changed effectiveness of sympathetic block with time. Animal models are now becoming available for the study of neuropathic pain due to peripheral nerve damage (Bennett and Laird, Chapter 26), and experimental studies are being done that demonstrate changes in sensitivity of nociceptors to catecholamines after peripheral nerve injury (Perl, Chapter 5; Campbell et al., Chapter 12), suggesting that answers to these questions may be forthcoming in the near future. Experimental studies should also contribute to a better understanding of the neuropathic pains associated with herpes zoster, diabetes, and other conditions as well. Satisfactory models of pain due to central nervous system damage are not yet available but would be important for the experimental examination of the mechanisms of central neuropathic pain.

SENSITIZATION OF NOCICEPTORS

A very important characteristic of nociceptors is that they can be sensitized following damage. Sensitization of nociceptors occurs even in such primitive organisms as the marine mollusc *Aplysia,* in which it can be shown to depend on the activation of second messenger systems (Walters, Chapter 4). Sensitization was first observed in mammalian nociceptors following heat stimulation and can now be studied in *in vitro* preparations, where it can be induced even in the absence of blood constituents (Perl, Chapter 5). Sensitization appears to be triggered by release of a complex of chemical agents from damaged cells.

A particularly striking example of sensitization of nociceptors is provided by the change in responsiveness of joint receptors during the development of experimental arthritis (Hanesch et al., Chapter 6). Some joint nociceptors are unresponsive to innocuous or noxious joint movements under normal circumstances ("sleeping nociceptors") but are "awakened" or sensitized by inflammation.

A variety of chemical substances, including bradykinin, prostaglandins, histamine, and serotonin, can serve as mediators of inflammatory pain ("inflammatory soup"), and a lowered pH makes an important additional contribution (Handwerker and Reeh, Chapter 7). Silent nociceptors are found in skin as well as in joints, and these can become sensitized during inflammation. Chemical mediators of hyperalgesia may act directly on nociceptors or indirectly through other cells, such as neutrophils (Levine et al., Chapter 8). An example of the latter is leukotriene B_4, a neutrophil attractant that causes hyperalgesia, apparently by releasing chemical substances such as 8R,15S-diHETE. Directly acting hyperalgesics often produce their effects by way of second messenger systems.

SENSITIZED NOCICEPTORS AND PRIMARY HYPERALGESIA

Recordings from nociceptors quite similar to those in animals can be made in human subjects using microneurography (Torebjörk, Chapter 11). Sensitization of human C nociceptors can be produced experimentally and appears to be responsible for primary hyperalgesia in at least some clinical circumstances, since the hyperalgesia remains after conduction in A fibers is blocked.

Following injury to a peripheral nerve, a different kind of sensitization comes into play. The axons of C nociceptors develop sensitivity to catecholamines (Perl, Chapter 5), which may result in sympathetically maintained pain (Campbell et al., Chapter 12), if nociceptive afferent fibers develop abnormal responses to norepinephrine released from sympathetic terminals. The enhanced responses to norepinephrine appear to be due to the upregulation of alpha-adrenergic receptors on nociceptor terminals (Perl, Chapter 5; Campbell et al., Chapter 12). There may be a species difference in the type of alpha receptor that is upregulated in nociceptors following damage. The alpha-2 receptor is the one that changes in animal experiments (Perl, Chapter 5), whereas the alpha-1 subtype is involved in human patients (Campbell et al., Chapter 12).

Hyperalgesia can be to warm, cold, or mechanical stimuli, and there can be either static or dynamic mechanical hyperalgesia (Ochoa, Chapter 13). Burning sensation is triggered by activity in C nociceptors, whereas sharp pain is due to input conducted in A fibers. A burning sensation is characteristic of the ABC syndrome (angry backfiring C-nociceptor syndrome), a condition in which the skin is hot, apparently due to the release of vasoactive chemical substances from C nociceptors. Interestingly, hyperalgesia in these patients can be eliminated for both thermal and mechanical stimuli by cooling the skin. Another syndrome involving thermal hyperalgesia is the "triple cold syndrome," in which there is cold hyperalgesia, cold hypesthesia, and cold skin; the associated pain is burning in quality, and this syndrome also depends on C-fiber input.

CENTRAL CHANGES IN SECONDARY HYPERALGESIA

Primary and secondary hyperalgesia can be produced in humans by intradermal injection of capsaicin (LaMotte, Chapter 16). The experiments support the hypothesis that the development of secondary hyperalgesia depends initially on neural activity originating in the area of injury and carried by chemosensitive afferent fibers. They also indicate that this activity sensitizes central neurons. Intraneural microstimulation in a human peripheral nerve shows that mechanoreceptor afferent fibers can elicit pain in the area of secondary hyperalgesia produced by intradermal injection of capsaicin in human experimental subjects; consistent with this, secondary hyperalgesia is not present when A fibers are blocked (Torebjörk, Chaper 11). Apparently, sensitized central neurons mediating pain can be activated by A mechanoreceptors during secondary hyperalgesia.

In parallel experiments on primates, only heat and/or chemically sensitive nociceptors respond to nearby capsaicin injections, and no types of cutaneous afferents are affected in the area of secondary hyperalgesia (LaMotte, Chapter 16). Primate spinothalamic neurons show increased responsiveness to noxious heat pulses in the area of primary but not in the area of secondary hyperalgesia and to innocuous and noxious mechanical stimuli in the area of secondary hyperalgesia. Therefore, the increased responsiveness of central neurons to mechanical stimulation in secondary hyperalgesia can be directly demonstrated by recordings from spinothalamic cells.

Similarly, the injection of carrageenan into the rat hindpaw causes a lowered nociceptive threshold for stimulation of the injected paw as well as of the noninjected paws (Guilbaud et al., Chapter 17). There is also an increased responsiveness of neurons in the ventral posterior lateral thalamic nucleus to stimulation of the original receptive field, as well as an expansion of the receptive field to include all four extremities (Guilbaud et al., Chapter 17). Clearly, such changes in receptive fields must be due to a central action. Similar changes occur in rats following the establishment of a mononeuropathy by loose ligatures on the sciatic nerve.

During the development of acute arthritis in cats caused by injection of a mixture of kaolin and carrageenan into the knee joint, the responsiveness of spinal cord projection neurons to stimulation not only of the knee but also of the cutaneous receptive field increases; sometimes the receptive field becomes bilateral (Schaible, Chapter 18). These changes are less apparent when the spinal cord is intact, indicating that descending inhibitory controls limit the development of secondary hyperalgesia. N-methyl-D-aspartate (NMDA) receptors appear to be involved in the central changes, since the enhanced excitability of many spinal cord neurons was reversed by NMDA antagonists, such as D-2-amino-5-phosphonovalerate or ketamine. An involvement of peptides is suggested by observations of intraspinal release of substance P and also neurokinin A during the development of arthritis, using antibody microprobes.

In behavioral studies on rats, intrathecal naloxone is found to produce hyperalgesia, but not allodynia (Woolf, Chapter 19). High doses of intrathecal morphine also produce hyperalgesia but with allodynia. Tissue damage also results in enhanced nociceptive responses and responses to normally innocuous stimuli. These changes are produced by input over C fibers but result from sensitization of central neurons. The receptive fields of dorsal horn neurons increase when C fibers are activated. This can be explained on the basis of an increase in excitability of central neurons, allowing previously subthreshold inputs to exceed threshold. Direct evidence for such changes in the excitability of central neurons comes from experiments on slices of rat spinal cord in which intracellular recordings showed a prolonged depolarization that is due at least in part to an action of excitatory amino acids on NMDA receptors.

Hyperalgesia is associated with the mononeuropathy produced by loose ligatures placed around the sciatic nerve in rats (Yaksh et al., Chapter 20). This results in demyelination with relative preservation of unmyelinated afferent fibers distal to the ligatures. Axon transport would be blocked by compression of the nerve. However, blocking axon transport with colchicine did not cause hyperalgesia and in fact prevented the development of hyperalgesia, provided that the colchicine is applied central to the site of compression. The hyperalgesia is reduced by NMDA antagonists.

MECHANISMS OF CENTRAL CHANGES PRODUCED BY PERIPHERAL DAMAGE

As many as 70% of dorsal root ganglion cells in rats contain glutamate immunoreactivity (Rustioni and Weinberg, Chapter 23). Most of these are small, and 25% of the glutamate-containing cells are also immunoreactive for substance P. Glutamate and substance P also coexist in synapses of primary afferent fibers in the dorsal horn, including synapses that are likely to belong to C afferent fibers. Most small dorsal root ganglion cells also contain aspartate immunoreactivity, as do their terminals in the dorsal horn. An interesting possibility is independent release of glutamate, aspartate, and substance P, which then could act, respectively, on AMPA, NMDA, and NK-1 receptors. Evidence for separate release zones for amino acids and peptides is that exocytosis of large dense core vesicles takes place away from the synaptic active zone. Furthermore, anterogradely transported wheat germ agglutinin conjugated horseradish peroxidase may spill into the extracellular space outside the synaptic cleft, suggesting that glycoproteins also escape from synaptic endings away from the active zone.

Sensitization of central neurons can be due to a number of changes, including increased release of excitatory neurotransmitters from primary afferent terminals and increased responsiveness of postsynaptic neurons (Haley and Wilcox, Chapter 24). Substance P appears to be involved in the mechanism of hyperalgesia. In addition to exciting dorsal horn neurons, substance P potentiates the excitatory effects of NMDA. In behavioral studies, intrathecally administered substance P, as well as NK-1 and NK-2 receptor agonists, causes nociceptive behavior in mice. Other peptides, such as calcitonin gene-related peptide (CGRP), somatostatin, and bombesin, may also play a role in hyperalgesia. Other excitatory agents that may be involved include the excitatory amino acids. This has been investigated with selective agonists and antagonists. NMDA receptors appear to be particularly important for "windup" and other neural responses to nociceptive inputs. Non-NMDA receptors may "prime" NMDA receptors by depolarizing the cells, relieving the Mg^{2+} block of the NMDA receptors. NMDA receptors may also be influenced by actions at the metabotropic glutamate receptor and by peptides through second messenger systems.

Transection of the sciatic nerve in rats causes the expression of c-fos in many neurons of the spinal cord (Basbaum et al., Chapter 25). A similar change is likely after partial nerve injury as well. The action of c-fos is unclear, but the c-fos gene can be regarded as a third messenger that regulates many other genes. The distribution of affected cells provides a convenient way to follow changes produced by noxious stimuli or injury. After sciatic nerve ligation, c–fos-labeled neurons are found in the dorsal horn for a month after surgery. Since c-fos has a half-life of hours, this suggests continued input from the neuroma and a chronic pain state. The number of labeled cells is affected by local anesthetic. The increase in c-fos expression that follows formalin injection into a hindpaw is reduced by MK 801, an NMDA receptor antagonist, indicating that c-fos expression is mediated in part through NMDA receptors. Another possible action of excitatory amino acids is excitotoxicity. If inhibitory interneurons are killed by massive release of glutamate, a hyperalgesic state may be produced. Damage to the sciatic nerve in rats by loose ligation causes many myelinated primary afferent fibers to develop spontaneous discharges within a few days and unmyelinated fibers show a similar effect after a week or more (Bennett and Laird, Chapter 26). A number of "dark neurons" appear in the dorsal horn. These may represent degenerating inhibitory interneurons. More are seen if neuropathy is combined with strychnine. Another change is a reduction in the size of the negative dorsal root potential, indicating decreased presynaptic inhibition. It may be that this loss of inhibition is produced by the degeneration of inhibitory interneurons.

Inflammation caused by injection of complete Freund's adjuvant or carrageenan into the hindpaw of rats results in hyperalgesia (Ruda and Dubner, Chapter 27). Changes in projection neurons of the superficial dorsal horn include enlargement of the receptive fields and increased spontaneous activity. These appear to be due to altered sensory processing in the dorsal horn. Accompanying these behavioral and physiological changes is an increase in mRNA coding for dynorphin precursor proteins in dorsal horn neurons. mRNA for c-fos also increases in neurons with a similar localization, and in some cases it has been possible to double label for both mRNAs. There is also an increase in mRNA for preproenkephalin, and this too could sometimes be double labeled with mRNA for c-fos. It is possible that the gene for c-fos is coupled with those for the opioids. These changes were not as prominent after neonatal capsaicin treatment, which causes a loss of substance P and CGRP-immunoreactive primary afferent fibers. Local application of dynorphin or the kappa agonist U-50,488H to the spinal cord increases the sizes of the receptive fields of many neurons in the superficial dorsal horn. Other cells show decreases. Thus, kappa agonists can facilitate or inhibit the activity of dorsal horn neurons. DAMGO, a mu opioid agonist, and DPDPE, a delta agonist, given intrathecally to rats reduce the hyperalgesia, apparently through a central action, as does the alpha-adrenergic agonist clonidine.

DIAGNOSIS AND THERAPY

Hyperalgesia and allodynia can be demonstrated in patients with neuropathic pain by using suitable methods of stimulation and pain assessment (Hansson and Lindblom, Chapter 30). The threshold for pain may be unchanged, decreased, or increased in neuropathic pain. Furthermore, the slope of the curve relating the magnitude of a painful stimulus to the amount of pain evoked can be unchanged, increased, or decreased. It is suggested that the definition of hyperalgesia should be altered to "a lowered pain threshold due to sensitization of nociceptive afferents or an increased rate of growth of pain intensity as a function of graded nociceptive stimulation." The term allodynia should be reserved for "pain evoked by stimuli activating non-nociceptive afferents." Allodynia by this definition is common in neurogenic pain patients, and it would apply to the secondary hyperalgesia that develops around acute tissue lesions.

Therapy for hyperalgesia is often unsatisfactory (Bullitt, Chapter 31). The reflex sympathetic dystrophies include causalgia, which is due to nerve injury, and reflex sympathetic dystrophy, which is caused by tissue damage. It is thought that early chemical or surgical sympathectomy can prevent the development of reflex sympathetic dystrophy. If this fails or treatment is delayed, other therapies are rather ineffective. Postherpetic neuralgia is also difficult to treat. The most effective current therapy is amitriptyline, a tricyclic antidepressant. There is little that can be done for central pain due to damage to the central nervous system, although experimental procedures, such as dorsal root entry zone lesions or deep brain stimulation, have been tried in extreme cases.

For the hyperalgesia and allodynia caused by central nervous system lesions, one cannot distinguish between primary and secondary hyperalgesia (Boivie, Chapter 32). Hyperalgesia and allodynia can be associated with a variety of central nervous system lesions, including syringomyelia and syringobulbia, multiple sclerosis, trauma, and cerebrovascular disease. Central pain develops in some cases when a lesion interrupts the spinothalamocortical pathway at any level, including the spinal cord, brain stem, thalamus, or subcortical region. Some, but not all, of these central pain patients have hyperalgesia and allodynia. The hyperalgesia can be to mechanical and thermal stimuli, allodynia most commonly to cold. Mechanical allodynia, when present, is usually caused by transient stimuli.

FUTURE DIRECTIONS

Future work on the hyperalgesia and allodynia produced by cutaneous injury or nerve damage should provide the information needed on which to base improvements in the treatment of conditions that cause these symptoms (Besson, Chapter 33). Future advances will depend on improved knowledge of nociceptors, better approaches to understanding the chemical substances in "inflammatory soup," as well as the elucidation of peripheral versus central mechanisms of hyperalgesia. Some of the challenges in hyperalgesia research include (a) the neurochemistry and pharmacology of different kinds of nociceptors; (b) the nature of the transduction mechanism in nociceptors; (c) the characteristics of human nociceptors in joints, muscles, and viscera; (d) the isolation of factors that affect experiments, such as the complications of the *in vivo* environment and the problem of relevance of *in vitro* preparations; (e) the nature of the microenvironment around fine nerve terminals; (f) the central mechanisms of hyperalgesia; and (g) the availability of animal models that mimic the clinical situation better. Future work should include human psychophysical studies of experimental models and well-defined clinical syndromes. Mechanical, cooling, heating, and chemical stimuli should all be tried, and the characteristics of human muscular, articular, and visceral nociceptors should be determined. Imaging techniques should be used to demonstrate central effects during hyperalgesia. Animal studies are needed to define the mechanisms of nociceptor sensitization. Monoclonal antibodies should be used to identify subpopulations. Peripheral release of activators and sensitizers should be measured. Better antagonists are needed, and cooperative interactions should be studied with combinations of antagonists and antibodies. Putative analgesics should be tried in models of hyperalgesia rather than in normal animals. In the central nervous systems of animals, the central changes produced during hyperalgesia due to cutaneous injury or neuropathy should be examined. Possible changes in ascending pathways should be studied during hyperalgesia. The possibility of sleeping central nervous system neurons should be investigated. Changes in descending controls during hyperalgesia should be defined. In behavioral studies, as many tests as possible should be used to define each model. There is a problem in relating clinical signs to pain in animals. Simple tests of analgesia should be used, in addition to intrathecal and intracerebroventricular injections. The role of c-fos and other proto-oncogenes needs to be determined, but this is a promising approach for studying physiological and pharmacological aspects of hyperalgesia.

REFERENCES

1. Hardy, J. D., Wolff, H. G., and Goodell, H. (1952/1967): *Pain sensations and reactions.* Williams & Wilkins, New York. (Reprinted by Hafner Publishing, New York, 1967.)
2. Lewis, T. (1942): *Pain.* Macmillan, London.
3. Mersky, H., ed. (1986): Classification of chronic pain: description of chronic pain syndromes and definition of pain terms. *Pain,* suppl. 3;S1.

Hyperalgesia and Allodynia,
edited by W. D. Willis, Jr.
Raven Press, Ltd., New York © 1992.

2

Nociceptors and Their Sensitization

Overview

Kenneth L. Casey

*Departments of Neurology and Physiology, The University of Michigan,
Ann Arbor, Michigan 48109; Neurology Service, Veterans Affairs Medical Center,
Ann Arbor, Michigan 48105*

John Bonica introduces the subject of this volume by providing an extensive historical review of the description by early clinicians of the phenomena we now call hyperalgesia, hyperpathia, allodynia, and referred pain. The observation common to all these terms is that a somatic stimulus produces an abnormally intense painful experience. This presents a serious therapeutic challenge to health care providers and is the source of much unnecessary discomfort, suffering, and prolonged convalescence among patients.

Over the past decade, attention has increasingly focused on the systematic identification of different forms of these pathologic pain phenomena. It is hoped that this will help to guide basic and clinical research and lead to a better understanding of the many abnormal pain states. For example, allodynia (pain produced by normally painless stimuli) and hyperalgesia (abnormally intense pain produced by normally painful stimuli) do not always occur together and may have distinctly different underlying pathophysiologies in different disease states. There is evidence that, in some instances, allodynia is caused by increased central nervous system responses to the normal activation of non-nociceptive tactile afferents. In other conditions, however, allodynia could be attributed to a sensitization process by which some nociceptors acquire abnormally low thresholds. Nociceptive sensitization could explain both allodynia and hyperalgesia in those cases in which both are present.

The mechanisms that produce hyperalgesia have probably evolved over many millennia. Hyperalgesia may have survival value because it amplifies protective reflexes and promotes immobilization of the injury. Edgar Walters observes that specialized nociceptive systems are found in many invertebrate species and that plastic changes in nociceptive systems can be induced by noxious stimuli. Immediately following injurious stimulation of the marine mollusc *Aplysia,* for example, the activated nociceptors excite modulatory interneurons that induce in the central neuropil a state of hyperexcitability lasting several seconds. After the escape response, *Aplysia* becomes nearly motionless but displays exaggerated withdrawal reflexes and a lowered threshold for escape responses. These behavioral patterns, which can last for weeks, can be attributed to a long-lasting synaptic facilitation and an increased excitability of the soma of nociceptive neurons; in addition, the mechanosensory thresholds of peripheral nociceptive terminals are lowered and their receptive fields are enlarged. Thus, neuronal cellular injury induces in these invertebrates both short- and long-term specific changes in the excitability of nociceptive neurons. Walters presents evidence that Ca^{2+} and cyclic AMP are particularly important in generating the plastic changes in nociceptive systems following injury. In the short term, Ca^{2+} enhances cyclic AMP production, leading to decreased K^+ conductance, increased neuronal excitability, and transmitter release. For the long-term changes, there is evidence that Ca^{2+} and cyclic AMP both facilitate the phosphorylation and activation of a protein that binds to DNA, perhaps regulating the expression of genes that control membrane structure and function.

Are the molecular mechanisms observed in *Aplysia* responsible, at least in part, for the sensitization of nociceptors in mammals? There is insufficient evidence at hand to answer this question. However, a series of critical experiments by Edward Perl and associates has provided important evidence on the factors involved in nociceptor sensitization. In the *in vitro* innervated rabbit ear preparation, nociceptor sensitization has the same characteristics as those seen in the intact *in vivo* preparation. The significance of this observation is that the *in vitro* tissues are perfused with an oxygenated serum that lacks the cellular and other normal constituents of whole blood. Using the same preparation, Perl and colleagues also showed that various nonsteroidal anti-inflammatory compounds impaired the sensitization of some nociceptors but had no effect on about one-half of those tested. Substance P and substance P antagonists also had no apparent effect on nociceptor sensitization. These observations reveal significant differences among nociceptors and provide important guides in the search for the mediators of sensitization.

Equally notable are the results of experiments by Perl and colleagues on the role of sympathetic efferents in producing pain following nerve damage. In the *in vivo* rabbit ear preparation, they were able to show that electrical stimulation of sympathetic efferent fibers or intraarterial injection of norepinephrine directly excited some nociceptive afferents and enhanced the sensitization of others in the partially damaged cutaneous sensory nerve. Antagonists of alpha-2 adrenergic receptors reversibly blocked these effects. The importance of these observations in understanding the pathophysiology of causalgia and other sympathetically maintained pains is obvious.

Nociceptor sensitization is not limited to cutaneous nerves, as shown by Robert Schmidt and co-workers using the cat knee joint model to study subcutaneous or deep nociceptive afferents. The joint capsule is densely innervated by finely beaded axons that are thought to be the terminals of nociceptive afferents. Schmidt and colleagues have shown that, in the normal joint, nearly 30% of all afferent fibers and 50% of all nociceptors are mechanically insensitive. When the joint is inflamed, however, approximately 75% to 80% of all fibers and 80% of the nociceptors become active and highly responsive to mechanical stimulation. In this model, nociceptor sensitization and activation can be produced or enhanced by prostaglandin E2 and by phorbol esters that activate cyclic AMP. The "awakening" of silent nociceptors by the inflammatory response to injury is perhaps an extreme example of nociceptor sensitization but is probably a common natural occurrence.

Handwerker and Reeh present evidence for the existence of silent nociceptors in normal mammalian skin. On the speculation that these and other cutaneous nociceptors would be sensitized by specific components of the inflammatory process, they have used an *in vitro* skin–nerve preparation that can be exposed to solutions containing various components of the inflammatory reaction. It is found that some nociceptors can be sensitized by bradykinin, histamine, serotonin, substance P, or combinations of these compounds. Of particular importance, however, is the pH of the bathing solution. If the pH is lowered from 7.0 to 4.3, there is a marked increase in the sensitization of afferents and in the capacity of other substances to produce or enhance the sensitization process. These studies have thus identified a critical variable that must be considered in future studies of sensitization and hyperalgesia.

Finally, however, we must acknowledge the evidence that hyperalgesia and allodynia, as clinical phenomena, may be produced by several independent or interdependent mechanisms. Some of these may act by the direct sensitization of nociceptors, but others may require intermediate modulators that act on specific classes of nociceptive terminals or produce central, long-term changes in the excitation of nociceptive pathways. In a series of studies that include the use of rodent behavioral models of hyperalgesia and recordings from cultured neurons, Levine and colleagues have shown that a specific product of activated neutrophils, 8R-15S-diHETE, produces hyperalgesia within 1 min of intradermal injection; prostaglandins E2 (PGE2), I1 (PGI1), and adenosine have similar rapid effects. Bradykinin and norepinephrine, however, appear to produce hyperalgesia indirectly because their action is delayed and requires the presence of postganglionic sympathetic neurons that produce PGE2 and PGI2. The hyperalgesia produced by all these methods appears to depend on an elevated intracellular cyclic AMP and, probably, Ca^{2+} level.

The critical role of Ca^{2+} and cyclic AMP brings us back to the *Aplysia* model of Edgar Walters and reminds us of how the elements of important protective mechanisms are preserved and elaborated on during the course of evolution. Unfortunately, these complex processes can become deranged to produce the distressing and maladaptive condition of chronic hyperalgesia.

Hyperalgesia and Allodynia,
edited by W. D. Willis, Jr.
Raven Press, Ltd., New York © 1992.

3

Clinical Importance of Hyperalgesia

John J. Bonica

Department of Anesthesiology, Multidisciplinary Pain Center,
University of Washington School of Medicine, Seattle, Washington 98195

The objective of this introductory chapter is to emphasize the critical importance of hyperalgesia as a clinical problem and thus, it is hoped, set the stage for this volume devoted primarily to the discussion of mechanisms. This critical importance is due to several considerations: (a) Hyperalgesia and hyperesthesia are concomitant symptoms and signs of disease or injury to skin, subcutaneous tissue, mucous membranes, and deep somatic tissue, of many visceral diseases, and of lesions of the peripheral or central nervous system or both. Consequently, they have been and continue to be useful diagnostic aids and a measure of the efficacy of therapy that has been employed. (b) With many conditions such as causalgia, the hyperalgesia and allodynia markedly increase the pain and suffering of the patient. (c) The area of hyperalgesia associated with visceral disease and certain somatic structures has been used to suggest the nerve supply of these structures, and subsequently the segmental supply of viscera was confirmed by paravertebral block with local anesthetic or by rhizotomy in patients with visceral pain. (d) Hyperalgesia often accompanies referred pain caused by disease or disorders of the viscera or deep somatic structures. Consequently, study of the hyperalgesia and how it is modified by local infiltration has elucidated the mechanisms of referred pain. (e) Recent studies of the mechanism of hyperalgesia have led to a much better understanding of the anatomy and characteristics of nociceptors and other peripheral nerves and alterations in the central nervous system. (f) The information derived from such studies has prompted the development of more effective therapeutic strategies of pain associated with these various pain syndromes.

To duly emphasize these and other important aspects of hyperalgesia as a clinical problem, this chapter consists of: (a) current definitions and characteristics of hyperalgesia and its occurrence with various painful disorders; (b) a brief historical overview of the study of this phenomenon and its usefulness in clinical practice; (c) a discussion of the association of secondary hyperalgesia and referred pain and the related phenomena that occur with injury to deep somatic and visceral structures with emphasis on the commonality of mechanisms among these various responses to injury; (d) a brief discussion of the influence of subcutaneous infiltration of local anesthetics into the area of secondary hyperalgesia and referred pain as a research and therapeutic measure; (e) a summary of the responses to tissue injury that produce pain, hyperalgesia, and associated phenomena; and (f) a discussion of the clinical implications of these various pathophysiologic processes and the use of various modalities in the prevention and therapy of postoperative and posttraumatic pain and the pain of childbirth. Although the focus is on hyperalgesia, I will also discuss the more global problem of pain.

DEFINITION, TYPES, AND CHARACTERISTICS OF HYPERALGESIA

Although it would seem superfluous to mention and define the types and characteristics of hyperalgesia, I believe it is important at the outset to establish precisely what is discussed in this volume. Until a decade ago, hyperalgesia was traditionally defined as a state of increased pain sensation due to either noxious or non-noxious stimulation of peripheral tissue (28). It has also been known that hyperalgesia occurs in both superficial and deep tissue in areas with pain thresholds that are normal, lowered, or raised. During the past six decades it has also been recognized that hyperalgesia can occur at the site of injury or disease and hence is called *primary hyperalgesia,* and/or it can occur at a remote site where it is associated with referred pain and hence is called *secondary hyperalgesia* (28,52). Studies during the past several decades have shown that primary hyperalgesia is characterized by a lowered threshold to mechanical and thermal stimuli, increased sensibility to suprathreshold stimuli, and spontaneous pain (15). Secondary hyperalgesia is characterized by a lowered threshold to mechanical but not to thermal stimuli and is associated with either localized or referred pain.

The taxonomy adopted by the International Association for the Study of Pain (IASP), published in 1986, revised the definitions with the term *hyperalgesia* reserved for increased (painful) responses to a stimulus that is normally painful, and the term *allodynia* is used for pain due to stimuli that do not normally provoke pain. Hyperalgesia can be provoked by mechanical, heat, or cold noxious stimulation, and similarly there can be tactile and/or thermal allodynia. Although a number of clinicians/scientists have adopted and used the IASP definitions, the single traditional term is still used by others, including some outstanding investigators of this field (15). It is hoped that in the future the IASP definition will be adopted by all workers in the field of pain research and treatment and used universally.

Although most of the recent studies have focused on primary or secondary hyperalgesia caused by iatrogenic injury to the skin in human volunteers and animals, for more than a century several clinical categories of hyperalgesia have been recognized (28,52):

1. Hyperalgesia associated with injury to skin, e.g., sustained exposure to ultraviolet irradiation (sunburn), chemical, thermal, or electric burns, and freezing, scratching, or crushing of the skin.
2. Primary hyperalgesia of mucous membranes in the nose, mouth, pharynx, esophagus, stomach, intestine, and urinary bladder.
3. Primary hyperalgesia associated with herpes zoster and other inflammatory conditions of peripheral nerves or other causes of neuropathy.
4. Hyperalgesia associated with traumatic interruptions (usually incomplete) of a peripheral nerve, such as occurs in causalgia.
5. Hyperalgesia in the margin of an area supplied by a degenerating nerve or in the zone supplied by a regenerating nerve.
6. Secondary hyperalgesia associated with referred pain caused by a variety of visceral diseases. The pain and hyperalgesia may be located in the skin, subcutaneous tissue, muscles, and vertebrae.

7. Primary and secondary hyperalgesia associated with injury or disease of deep somatic structures.
8. Secondary hyperalgesia associated with disease or lesions of the spinal cord, brain stem, or brain that constitute a characteristic of various central pain syndromes.
9. Diffuse, patchy secondary cutaneous hyperalgesia not infrequently seen with patients with influenza, typhoid fever, smallpox, acute rheumatisms, and a variety of other systemic disorders (31).
10. Hyperalgesia associated with certain psychologic and psychiatric disorders, which is characterized by a glove- or stocking-type of distribution rather than that typical of interruption of long neural pathways (31).

This wide prevalence of hyperalgesia and allodynia in such a variety of diseases and injuries for reasons previously given makes this phenomenon one of the most important issues that require further intensive investigation.

HISTORICAL PERSPECTIVE

It is likely that cutaneous tenderness caused by non-noxious or noxious manual stimulation was used by ancient physicians in Egypt, India, China, and Greece as an aid in the diagnosis of painful disorders and in following the progress of certain therapeutic modalities. This technique was extensively used by the Hippocratic school in ancient Greece as well as by physicians in ancient Rome. Moreover, in ancient times and even today the area of cutaneous tenderness has been used as a site of application of mustard plasters and other modalities that produce counter-irritation (or what today is conceived to be stimulation of large fibers) in treating various painful disorders. Similarly, an ancient art that persists today of immersing an injured part in cold water or in hot baths to relieve pain produced its beneficial effects by decreasing thermal hyperalgesia and allodynia. Although I have not been able to find references, it is likely that tenderness associated with various painful conditions continued to be used by physicians in the Middle Ages and the Renaissance.

In the writings of the 17th and 18th centuries there are passing references to the association of cutaneous tenderness with visceral disease and nerve injuries. John Hunter (40) reported that after an attack of angina pectoris his left arm was so sensitive that he could not bear it to be touched. In 1813 Denmark (21) mentioned excessive burning pain and apparently severe cutaneous tenderness (hyperalgesia and allodynia) in a patient who had sustained a musket ball wound of the arm and from the description apparently had developed causalgia.

Sometime during this period the increased sensitivity of the skin associated with pain, which we now call hyperalgesia and allodynia, noted with various diseases became referred to as *hyperesthesia* or *hyperaesthesia*. The first such reference of the use of the term hyperesthesia is found in the book by Morgagni published in 1761 in which there is a case of a patient with basal pneumonia who manifested upper abdominal pain and a patch of hyperesthesia (70). Paolo Procacci *(personal communication)* quotes Professor Vasoli, expert in medical history and philosophy at the University of Florence, in suggesting that the relation of pain and hyperesthesia was recognized by a number of scientists of the German school of psychophysics such as Weber and Fechner during the mid-19th century.

In 1863 Hilton (37), in the first edition of his book *Rest and Pain,* emphasized hyperesthesia as an important sign associated with pain caused by various painful disorders. A year later Weir Mitchell and associates (68) emphasized the important role of severe hyperesthesia (allodynia) associated with burning pain as a phenomenon that greatly increased the suffering of patients with causalgia. In his book published in 1872 in which he first used the term causalgia, he discussed the association of hyperesthesia with various peripheral nerve injuries in great detail (67) and proposed the hypothesis that the pain and hyperalgesia were caused by two mechanisms: (a) a peripheral pathophysiologic process responsible for pain and hyperesthesia in the field of the injured nerve and (b) the development of abnormal neural activity in the spinal cord that spread and was responsible for the extension of pain beyond the territory of the injured nerve. A year later Letievant (50) of France in an extraordinary monograph on the treatment of peripheral nerve injuries discussed causalgia and the associated hyperesthesia in peripheral nerve injuries. Like Mitchell, Letievant presented the hypothesis that pain and hyperalgesia and allodynia were due to a peripheral and a spinal cord mechanism but added that intense and persistent nociceptive impulses reached the brain where they produced abnormal characteristics of the pain, perhaps partly due to psychologic factors.

In 1864 Martyn (61) mentioned the presence of cutaneous tenderness and pain in the breast region as a consequence of heart disease and speculated that these referred phenomena were due to "irritation" of spinal centers. Subsequently the phenomenon of hyperesthesia associated with referred pain caused by visceral disease or other disorders was discussed by Lange (47) in 1875–1876, by Sturge (86) in 1883, Ross (83) in 1887, and Head (30,31) and MacKenzie (58,59) in 1892–1893. Sturge (86), apparently unaware of Martyn's contribution, also suggested that the pain and tenderness in the left arm and fingers associated with heart disease were due to an "abnormal commotion" in the gray matter of the spinal cord, a concept subsequently accepted by Ross (83), Head (31), and MacKenzie (59).

In June 1892 Head (30) presented a summary of the exhaustive studies done during the preceding 3 years in his thesis at Cambridge University and published it in parts I and II of volume 16 of the journal *Brain* (31). By careful study he was able to determine the area of cutaneous tenderness caused by diseases of various abdominal and thoracic viscera and correlated these with the areas of herpetic eruptions to determine the nerve supply of the abdominal and thoracic viscera and also to develop a map of dermatomes.[1] In part II of the report he differentiated hyperesthesia

---

[1]Three decades later Kappis, Lawen, and Mandl used paravertebral block with procaine in patients with painful disorders caused by pathology of each specific viscus and noted if block of the segments suggested by Head provided complete pain relief. The results indicated that segments suggested by Head for each viscus were confirmed within ±1 or 2 segments. Subsequently the technique was used as a diagnostic procedure and still later as a temporary therapeutic measure using local anesthetics or for a prolonged period of time by injecting alcohol in patients with severe intractable angina pectoris and severe cancer pain. Still later I used the area of hyperalgesia to study the segmental nerve supply of the uterus involved in transmitting the pain associated with uterine contractions during the first stage of labor and the nerve supply of the human cervix by using discrete paravertebral block. This study, carried out in 275 parturients and gynecologic patients over a 20-year period, showed that during early labor the pain is transmitted via the T11 and T12 nerves but in late first stage pain also involves the two adjacent segments (T10 and L1). This study clearly showed that the human cervix is supplied with nociceptive fibers that enter the spinal cord via the same nerves as the body of the uterus and not via the middle three sacral segments, as stated in every major textbook of anatomy (10). Hansen and Schliack also used cutaneous hyperalgesia and the distribution of skin eruptions of herpes zoster to study the dermatomes and nerve supply of viscera.

from hyperalgesia and used the term hyperalgesia. However, it was Gowers (26) who first used the term hyperalgesia 7 years earlier. MacKenzie (58) carried out a concurrent and similarly exhaustive study of visceral pain and the associated sensory disturbances, including skin tenderness, which he called hyperesthesia, that was first reported in 1892 and in a more extensive form as part III of the same volume of *Brain* in which Head's articles had preceded (59). It is of interest to note that Head used the head of a pin, which did not produce pain when applied to normal skin, to determine the area of cutaneous tenderness, whereas MacKenzie used both the ball and point of a pin to determine cutaneous tenderness. In modern terms, Head was eliciting areas of allodynia, whereas MacKenzie studied both allodynia and hyperalgesia. Subsequently, Head continued to use the term hyperalgesia in most of his writing, including the article by him and Campbell on herpes zoster published in 1900 (33).

During the first four decades of this century the term hyperalgesia used to denote an increased pain response to noxious stimulation was differentiated from hyperesthesia, which was used for pain provoked by light pressure (now called allodynia). In the first book on pain published in this century (1906), Schmidt (85) devoted a chapter to the work of Head and MacKenzie on the association of hyperalgesia and visceral disease. In his textbook, first published in 1909, MacKenzie (60) devoted an entire chapter to hyperalgesia that develops in patients with visceral disease. Five years later Behan (4), in the first comprehensive textbook on pain published in the United States, discussed hyperalgesia with disease or lesions of virtually every organ or structure in the body including the tongue. Head's book *Studies in Neurology* (32) published in 1920 has a major section on hyperalgesia associated with various nerve injuries.

The phenomenon of hyperalgesia associated with the thalamic syndrome was included in a classic report by Déjérine and Roussy (20), and subsequently Head and Holmes (34), Holmes (38), and Riddoch (79) in their extensive reports on "central pain" emphasized hyperalgesia caused by various lesions of the spinal cord, brain stem, and brain. It is also of interest to note that Head and co-workers (35) used their provocative theory of "epicritic and protopathic sensibilities," which they proposed in 1905, to explain in part the mechanism of hyperalgesia.

During the 1930s and 1940s many scientists and clinicians studied the mechanism and possible site of pathophysiology as well as the characteristics of hyperalgesia. Limitations of space permit mention of only a few of them. Gellhorn and associates (25) carried several investigations, W. K. Livingston (56) included an extensive discussion of this topic in his book, Foerster (24) described hyperalgesia associated with rhizotomy, which he carried out to treat chronic pain in humans. Pollock and Davis (76) carried out extensive studies on the association of visceral disease and referred pain and the associated hyperalgesia, and Cohen (16) who, in his Lettsomian lectures, presented a very extensive discussion of the mechanisms of visceral pain and associated phenomena. These and others had hypothesized that primary hyperalgesia was due to "irritation" or "disturbance" of nerve endings of peripheral neurons, whereas secondary hyperalgesia was due to increased excitation of second order neurons and internuncial neurons in the spinal cord.

The first comprehensive and systematic study of the characteristics and mechanisms of pain and hyperalgesia was done by Lewis and Hess (53) in 1932–1933 and was subsequently continued by Lewis and others during the ensuing decade, all of which are summarized in Lewis's excellent book (52). As a result of their studies,

Lewis and associates were the first to note and report the differences between hyperalgesia associated with cutaneous lesions that were localized to the area of injury, which they called erythralgic hyperalgesia, and the hyperalgesia found in noninjured skin consequent to stimulating small cutaneous nerves, which they called diffuse hyperalgesia. Lewis (51) used his "nocifensor nerves" theory to explain the development of diffuse hyperalgesia. Lewis and co-workers (53,54) also studied cutaneous and deep hyperalgesia that was associated with referred pain caused by disease or disorders of deep somatic structures or viscera or nerve lesions. Although the occurrence of referred pain and cutaneous tenderness associated with disease of deep somatic structures had been noted by Head (31) and MacKenzie (59), Kellgren (44,45) and Lewis and Kellgren (54) were the first to carry out a comprehensive and systematic study on the distribution of pain and the associated hyperalgesia and allodynia provoked by noxious stimulation (achieved by injection of 6% saline) into deep somatic structures including the periosteum, muscles, interspinous ligaments, and joints. These revealed that muscles and ligaments produced pain and associated phenomena that were segmental in nature, although, as expected, the segments did not conform exactly to the segmental supply to the skin or the segmental supply of hyperalgesia due to visceral disease.

Contrary to recently published reports (15), the terms primary hyperalgesia and secondary hyperalgesia were not coined by Lewis but were first proposed in 1950 by Hardy et al. (27) in their report of the extensive study of the characteristics and mechanisms of hyperalgesia, which had been carried out a decade earlier. As mentioned above, Lewis used the term erythralgic hyperalgesia for primary hyperalgesia and the term diffuse hyperalgesia for secondary hyperalgesia. In their textbook published 2 years later, Hardy and associates (28) summarized their findings that led them to conclude that secondary hyperalgesia was the result of increased excitability in the network of internuncial neurons in the spinal cord that received convergent impulses from cutaneous and deep somatic tissues or from cutaneous tissue and viscera. They concluded that their formulation of secondary hyperalgesia as being due to central mechanisms was in a sense a restatement in modern physiologic terms of views expressed by Sturge, Ross, Head, MacKenzie, Livingston, and Cohen, among others. Because discussion of the findings of Lewis and associates and Hardy and co-workers regarding their studies and their conclusions about mechanisms will be presented by others, these are not included here except to stress that both groups used similar methodology for producing primary and secondary hyperalgesia and that the same methods have been used even in recent years.

The discovery that tissue damage and injury produce sensitization of peripheral nociceptors about two decades ago (6) led to an almost immediate acceptance that such hypersensitivity was the basis of primary hyperalgesia at the site of injury. However, the idea that secondary hyperalgesia was caused by increased excitability in the dorsal horn was discarded or ignored, and investigators continued to search for a peripheral mechanism (23). This was most surprising in view of the hypothesis suggested by many investigators over the past century and especially in view of the findings of Hardy and associates. Fortunately, in the 1980s studies by Woolf and Wall, Dubner and co-workers, LaMotte and collaborators, Campbell and associates, Guilbaud et al., Yaksh et al., and others who have contributed to this volume have provided impressive evidence that secondary hyperalgesia is primarily due to sensitization of cells in the spinal cord and other parts of the neuraxis. These studies will be presented in detail elsewhere in this volume.

SOME CHARACTERISTICS OF HYPERALGESIA AND ALLODYNIA ASSOCIATED WITH DISEASE OF THE VISCERA OR DEEP SOMATIC STRUCTURES

In view of the extensive literature on the study of primary and secondary hyperalgesia caused by cutaneous lesions, I will focus my comments on secondary hyperalgesia and allodynia associated with pain caused by disease of deep somatic structures or viscera and briefly comment on neuropathic pain.

Secondary Hyperalgesia and Allodynia and Referred Pain

The term "referred pain" is generally employed for pain localized not to the site of its cause but to an area that may be adjacent to or at a distance from such a site. Although Head (31) and MacKenzie (59) are usually given the credit for first using the term referred pain in their 1893 reports, three decades earlier Martyn (61) theorized that the pain felt in the chest region as a consequence of heart disease was "expressive of some distress in the heart that was due to irritation of spinal centers and the central impression is radiated and *referred* [italics represent author's] by the mind to the sensitive skin."

Deep somatic and/or visceral diseases are invariably manifested by referred pain and secondary hyperalgesia and allodynia in the dermatomes supplied by the same and often adjacent spinal segments that supply the deep structure or viscera. Invariably the referred pain and hyperalgesia are associated with reflex muscle spasm, deep tenderness and hyperalgesia, and autonomic responses that involve segmental and suprasegmental reflexes, which are discussed in a later section.

Characteristics of Referred Pain and Hyperalgesia

The distribution of referred pain and the secondary hyperalgesia and allodynia depends on the intensity and duration of the noxious stimuli. Early in the course of the disease when the stimulation is mild, the hyperalgesia and allodynia may be absent or present in only part of specific dermatomes. However, as the noxious stimulus and associated referred pain become more intense, they may cover all the dermatomes supplied by the primary spinal segments that supply the viscus or deep structure. With very intense stimulation as the pathophysiologic process progresses, the hyperalgesia covers the dermatomes supplied by the primary and adjacent nerve segments. This is probably due to spread of the sensitization of neurons in the spinal cord. Thus, I have noted that early in labor parturients have hyperalgesia and some allodynia, which are located in the dermatomes supplied by T11 and T12. However, as the intensity and frequency of the contractions progress to the latter part of the first stage and during the second stage, the referred pain from the contraction is more severe and the hyperalgesia is present in all of the dermatomes supplied by T10, T11, T12, and L1 and occasionally spills over to T9 and L2 (10) (Fig. 3.1).

The influence of the *intensity of the stimulus* on the spread of referred pain and the associated hyperalgesia and allodynia is also noted with diseases of deep somatic structures. This was well demonstrated by the studies of Kellgren (44), who showed that mild stimulation of the fourth, fifth, and sixth intercostal spaces each produced referred pain and hyperalgesia limited to each specific segment stimulated. However,

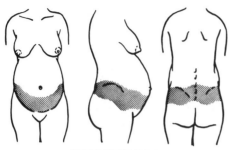

EARLY FIRST STAGE

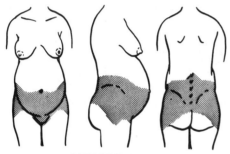

LATE FIRST STAGE

FIG. 3.1. The extent of analgesia during the early and late first stage of labor. Early, only two segments developed hyperalgesia, whereas later in labor when the uterine contractions are more intense, the extent of hyperalgesia and the distribution of the pain associated with uterine contractions are more extensive and involve T10–L1 inclusive.

a more intense stimulus by injection of the left fifth intercostal muscle provoked referred pain and hyperesthesia that was spread over the three segments (Fig. 3.2). This undoubtedly was due to the spread of sensitization in the spinal cord to the two adjacent segments.

The influence of the *duration of stimulus* on the spread of pain is often observed clinically and was shown experimentally by McAuliffe and co-workers (62), who noted that brief stimulation of the mucosa about the ostium of the maxillary sinus resulted in a localizable intranasal sensation of pain, whereas prolonged stimulation of the same area caused the pain to spread over the homolateral portion of the nose and cheek, along the zygoma, into the temporal region, and into the upper teeth. That is, the area of pain spread over most of the area of the distribution of the second division of the fifth cranial nerve and ultimately spread to involve adjacent portions supplied by the first and third divisions.

FIG. 3.2. The influence of intensity of the stimulus and spread of referred pain and hyperalgesia. Note that mild stimulation of the fourth (4), fifth (5), and sixth (6) intercostal spaces each produced referred pain and hyperalgesia limited to each specific segment stimulated. However, a more intense stimulus by injection of the left fifth intercostal muscle provoked referred pain and hyperesthesia that was spread over three segments. (Modified from ref. 44.)

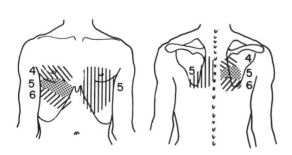

Another example of the influence of the duration and intensity of noxious stimulation on the character and duration of reflex spasm and the associated pain and hyperalgesia was reported by McLelland and Goodell (63), who noted that brief low-intensity electrical stimulation or overinflation of a balloon placed in the ureter caused localized pain and little or no muscle contraction, whereas prolonged or intense stimulation evoked a more complex phenomenon. Following intense prolonged stimulation, the muscles of the abdominal wall on the stimulated side remained contracted and after about half an hour the side began to ache. Within a few hours the pain became severe and lasted 6 hr, after which the pain subsided, but the deep tenderness in the muscle continued until the following day.

This phenomenal spread due to a prolonged intense stimulus is often seen clinically; not infrequently a localized pain due to minor injury that remains unrelieved becomes diffuse, poorly localizable, and referred to a part that is remote from the original site of injury.

Influence of Duration of Neuropathic Pain

The influence of the duration of noxious stimulus on the location and spread of pain, hyperalgesia, and allodynia, mentioned in regard to Kellgren's studies, is of great clinical importance, particularly in relation to efficacy of treatments. Many reports and personal observations of patients with causalgia indicate that sympathetic blockade, initiated within the first few days of the onset of the pain, hyperalgesia, and allodynia, which initially are usually located in the distal distribution of the injured nerve and repeated several times at appropriate intervals, will completely and eventually permanently relieve the burning pain, hyperalgesia, and allodynia. On the other hand, delay of this therapy until many weeks or some months have passed will result in: (a) spread of the pain, hyperalgesia, and allodynia to parts of the limb supplied by other nerves and may even spread to the contralateral side and (b) although sympathetic interruption with local anesthetic or guanethidine or another pharmacologic agent will relieve the burning pain, this is a temporary measure and sympathectomy will be required. Moreover, if effective therapy is delayed for many months or years, neither pharmacologic or surgical interruption nor other more drastic or neurosurgical procedures in the spinal cord and brain stem will relieve the pain.

Another example of the duration of the pathologic process on the efficacy of therapy is that of acute herpes zoster. Notwithstanding authoritative opinions to the contrary, personal experience in treating nearly 200 patients between 1943 and 1982 and the reports of many others have firmly convinced me that regional sympathetic block, alone or combined with somatic nerve block, achieved with a long-lasting local anesthetic and done within the first 4 to 6 days of the onset of symptoms [tingling in the distribution of the nerve(s) or on the first day of vesicular eruptions] produces prompt relief of pain, decreases severity and duration of the eruption, seems to prevent the spread of the disease, and decreases the incidence of postherpetic neuralgia by at least 30%. Although antiviral drugs are said to produce beneficial effects, they do not provide prompt relief of pain. In view of this, it is recommended that antiviral therapy be combined with sympathetic interruption for synergistic action and a greater decrease in the incidence of postherpetic neuralgia. On the other hand, delaying therapy beyond 15 to 20 days of the eruption results in a progressive decrease in beneficial effects and an increase in the incidence of post-herpetic neuralgia.

Relation Between Distribution of Secondary Hyperalgesia and Referred Pain

Another important characteristic in the relation between secondary hyperalgesia and referred pain is their distribution. Initially, abdominal visceral disease produces referred pain in the midline and frequently without evidence of secondary hyperalgesia in the referred area. This is what Ross (83), Lewis (52), and Cohen (16,16a) called "true visceral pain." Within hours hyperalgesia begins to appear and at the peak of the pathophysiology, the hyperalgesia is distributed in nearly all of the dermatomes supplied by the neural segments that supply the viscera with afferent fibers. However, the referred pain may remain in the midline or shift to one side, but its distribution is more limited than that of hyperalgesia to large patches or areas. Figures 3.3 and 3.4 illustrate this phenomenon. It is to be noted in Fig. 3.4 that diseases of the gallbladder produce hyperalgesia bilaterally in all of the dermatomes supplied by the spinal cord segments that supply this viscus, but the pain is usually located in a large, limited area often on the right side, and this may be due to extension of the inflammation to the parietal structures producing parietal referred pain.

Effects on Referred Pain and Hyperalgesia of Anesthetizing the Area of Reference

One of the most controversial and confusing problems of referred pain and the associated hyperalgesia and hyperesthesia is the effect produced by infiltrating the

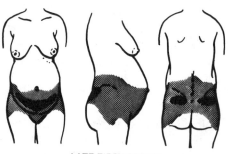

LATE FIRST STAGE

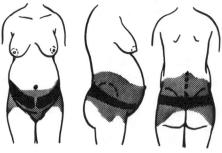

LATE FIRST STAGE

FIG. 3.3. Distribution of hyperalgesia and pain during the late first stage of labor.

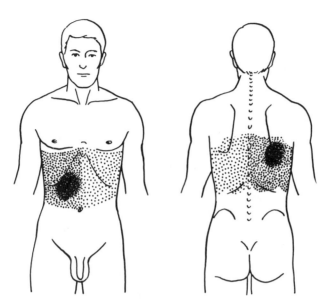

FIG. 3.4. The distribution of referred pain and hyperalgesia due to disease of the gallbladder. [From ref. 11(c).]

area of reference with a local anesthetic. In 1926 Lemaire (49) reported that anesthesia of the abdominal wall produced by the injection of 0.5% procaine solution in four patients with intra-abdominal visceral disease resulted in pain relief and the associated hyperalgesia and muscular rigidity disappeared. Subsequently, similar results were reported by Weiss and Davis (93) on 25 patients and by Morley (71) on 13 patients with referred pain due to visceral disease. Morley also reported that the pain and hyperalgesia referred to the shoulder as a consequence of diaphragmatic irritation could be eliminated or diminished by infiltration of local anesthetic in that region.

Theobald (90) reported the relief of pain of the early first stage of labor by anesthetization of the skin of the lower abdomen, an observation reported by Rose (82) 12 years before and subsequently substantiated by Abrams (1) and many others. Theobald (90) also reported the relief of pain in the reference zone resulting from dysmenorrhea or from faradic stimulation of the uterus. In his classic experimental studies of pain from the gastrointestinal tract using an inflatable balloon, Jones (41) reported that "it was possible to inflate with novocaine the skin area at which pain was experienced, for example, in the midepigastrium following distension of the first portion of the duodenum with resulting abolition of the local reference of pain." Cohen (16,16a) described the cases of two patients who had had previous amputation of the left arm near the shoulder and who subsequently developed anginal pain in the chest and the phantom limb with physical effort, and this was relieved with rest. In one patient block of the brachial plexus relieved the pain that occurred with effort in the phantom limb but not in the chest. In the other patient who, before brachial plexus block, developed pain in the phantom limb after he had walked 120 to 150 yards with no incline at a rate of 96 paces per minute, and after a further 50 yards the pain spread to the chest and neck. After the brachial plexus block was achieved, no discomfort appeared on walking until a distance of 200 yards had been covered, at which point he felt pain and constriction in the neck, but not in the phantom limb, and at 600 yards he developed severe chest pain and a mild burning sensation in the phantom limb.

Notwithstanding these and other reports on the efficacy of superficial analgesia in partially or wholly relieving referred pain and hyperalgesia caused by deep somatic or visceral disease, others reported negative results. Woollard et al. (99) attempted to confirm Morley's findings by stimulating the phrenic nerve, which was exposed prior to avulsion. They noted that although stimulation produced pain in the distribution of the fourth cervical segment, it was not reduced by anesthetization of the skin of this area. Similar negative reports were made by Lewis (52), McLelland and Goodell (63), and others [see ref. 7(a) for references].

The obvious discrepancies reported above have prompted several explanations. Theobald (89) suggested that the divergence of the results obtained by Morley (71) and those by Woollard et al. (99) could be attributed to the difference in the intensity of the stimulus they applied: with a mild stimulus, the referred pain was eliminated, but with severe referred pain, it was not. In support of this hypothesis, he submitted experimental data that demonstrated that mild referred pain in the lower abdominal wall consequent to weak faradic stimulation of the cervix could be relieved by just needling the affected cutaneous area. A further increase in the current caused pain that could not be relieved by needling but frequently could be relieved by injecting 5 ml of saline solution intradermally. A still further increase in the current caused pain that could not be relieved by saline but could be eliminated by injection of 1% procaine. In nearly every patient studied, by raising the current, a point was ultimately reached at which the pain persisted in spite of the injection of large amounts of local anesthetic and was usually referred to the same cutaneous area that was anesthetized. I [8(a)] have observed in a significant number of parturients that mild labor pain of the early first stage can be virtually eliminated by infiltrating the skin of the lower abdominal wall with a local anesthetic, whereas the severe pain of the late first stage was not affected appreciably. However, paracervical block, which interrupts nociceptive pathways from the uterus including the cervix, completely relieved the pain and hyperalgesia. These results provide additional evidence that the referred pain and the secondary hyperalgesia are due to spinal cord mechanisms and will persist as long as the site of noxious stimulation remains.

The results of these and other studies provide additional evidence that referred pain and secondary hyperalgesia are due to the convergence of cutaneous and visceral afferents in the spinal cord. When the nociceptive input from visceral afferents is not strong, elimination of the cutaneous afferent input is sufficient to eliminate the referred pain. However, with intense visceral input the central barrage from the viscera or deep somatic structures is sufficient to break through and produce referred pain even when the cutaneous input is eliminated.

CLINICAL IMPLICATIONS OF HYPERALGESIA AND PAIN

Because therapy of hyperalgesia is discussed elsewhere in this volume (see chapter by Bullitt) I will briefly comment on the function of pain. It is well-known that transient acute pain, as occurs when an individual touches a hot stove or steps on a sharp object, promptly alerts the individual and causes him to withdraw the limb immediately and thus avoid further damage. In addition, acute pain associated with severe injuries involving deep somatic structures, such as fractures or sprains, imposes limitation of action and therefore tends to prevent further damage or aggravation of pathophysiology. Similarly, acute pain of visceral disease has the biologic function of warning the individual that something is wrong; it prompts him to consult a physician and is used by a physician as an aid in making the diagnosis.

Although this biologic function of acute pain has been appreciated, what is not generally realized, even by many physicians, is that in many instances the warning signal (pain) comes too late to avoid injury and if persistent may prove deleterious to the organism. This includes the pain that is experienced after most pathologic processes have been initiated as is the case with certain visceral diseases, nerve injury, and neoplasms. Severe postoperative and posttraumatic pain not only have no biologic function, but if not adequately relieved produce abnormal physiologic and psychologic reactions that often cause complications, as emphasized below. Similar deleterious effects result if the severe pain of acute myocardial infarction and acute pancreatitis, for example, are not effectively relieved after they have served their biologic function. Indeed, even severe pain associated with such a physiologic process as parturition, if allowed to persist, will produce deleterious effects on the mother, the force of labor, and the fetus and newborn. I will first discuss briefly the responses to tissue injury and then consider the pathophysiologic effects of pain and associated hyperalgesia and allodynia and their prevention and therapy in regard to moderate to severe postoperative and posttraumatic pain and the pain of childbirth. In the United States these three conditions afflict some 30 million persons annually, and unfortunately in the majority of patients the pain and associated responses are not properly managed and the patient incurs increased morbidity and, at times, mortality [11(a)].

Human Responses to Tissue Injury

To provide a background for the understanding of why severe postoperative and posttraumatic pain and the pain of childbirth are deleterious to the organism, it is necessary to consider briefly the local, segmental, suprasegmental, and cortical responses to injury.

Tissue destruction, whether from crush injury, fracture, operation, or internal disease, results in biochemical changes and autonomic reflex responses, which in the past were considered important in maintaining homeostasis but more recently have been viewed as maladaptive responses. The local biochemical changes, which include liberation of intracellular algogenic substances into the extracellular fluid surrounding nerve endings and alteration of their microenvironment, stimulate and sensitize nociceptors to induce local pain, tenderness, and primary hyperalgesia. The nociceptors thus activated, also transduce the noxious stimuli into impulses that are transmitted to the neuraxis, wherein, after being subjected to modulating influences, they stimulate and sensitize cells in the spinal cord and brain stem to produce segmental and suprasegmental responses and eventually reach the cerebrum to produce pain sensation and perception and psychologic and physiologic responses.

Segmental Responses

Intense nociceptive barrage produces stimulation and sensitization of neurons in the dorsal horn, as well as interneurons and neurons located in the anterior and anterolateral cord. Stimulation and sensitization of somatomotor neurons result in skeletal muscle spasm, which decreases excursion of the abdominal and chest muscles and thus decreases chest wall compliance and impairs ventilation. Moreover, reflex muscle spasms through positive feedback loops generate and sustain nociceptive impulses from the muscles and thus aggravate the pain and discomfort. Although some recent writers have suggested that this is a new concept, it was duly emphasized a century ago by MacKenzie (58–60) and subsequently by many others [7(b),16,28,46,52,53,56]. It is also important to note that reflex muscle spasm very often is associated with muscular hyperalgesia and allodynia that persist for a considerable period of time after the spasm and pain disappear.

Stimulation of sympathetic preganglionic neurons in the anterolateral horn of the spinal cord causes an increase in cardiac work and myocardial oxygen consumption and if severe enough causes cardiac arrhythmia [see ref. 7(a) for references]. Sympathetic hyperactivity also decreases gastrointestinal tone, which may progress to ileus, and decreases the tone of the urinary tract and reduces urinary output. Sympathetic hyperactivity often causes intense segmental cutaneous vasoconstriction, which in somatic structures produces algogenic substances that may be responsible for secondary hyperalgesia (46). Severe intense vasoconstriction in the splanchnic bed may cause intestinal ischemia, which results in hypoxic tissue damage and release of toxic substances that enhance shock in a traumatized patient (55). Injury in the abdomen or chest may also provoke a variety of segmental reflexes including viscerocutaneous, cutaneovisceral, viscerovisceral, and reflexes between deep somatic structures and viscera (46).

Sensitization of dorsal horn neurons, interneurons, and anterior horn neurons caused by afferent barrage from stimulation of C fibers from muscles, joints, and the periosteum produce a long latency, long duration facilitation that affects cells in lamina I and deeper laminae and thus triggers a very prolonged increased excitability of these cells (94–98). Since the characteristics of these phenomena will be discussed in detail by other authors, only a brief summary is given here. Based on both experimental and clinical evidence, the sensitization spreads not only in those segments that receive input from the affected nociceptive fibers, but with time it causes changes of neurons in adjacent spinal segments that become involved in the expansion of the area of hyperalgesia, allodynia, reflex muscle spasm, and other segmental responses. Although the facilitation is triggered by the arrival of impulses in C fibers from deep tissue, it is sustained by an intrinsic spinal cord process. C fibers innervating muscles cause a more prolonged sensitization than those that supply the skin (92). This prolonged increase of excitability of the central cells in the neuraxis is probably the basis for the widespread prolonged cutaneous and deep tenderness, hyperalgesia, allodynia, and frequent bouts of intense skeletal muscle spasm that produce excruciating pain. The sensitization may persist for days or even weeks after an operation or injury in deep somatic structures of the back or joints. Consequently, bouts of excruciating pain can be provoked by non-nociceptive stimulation such as body movement.

Suprasegmental Responses

Suprasegmental reflex responses result from nociceptive-induced stimulation of medullary centers of ventilation and circulation, hypothalamic (predominantly sympathetic) centers of neuroendocrine function, and some limbic structures. These responses consist of hyperventilation, increased hypothalamic neural sympathetic tone, and increased secretion of catecholamines and other catabolic hormones. The increased neural sympathetic tone and catecholamine secretion add to the effects of spinal reflexes and further increase cardiac output, peripheral resistance, blood pressure, cardiac workload, and myocardial oxygen consumption (94). In addition to catecholamine release there is an increased secretion of cortisol, adrenocorticotropic hormone (ACTH), glucagon, cAMP, antidiuretic hormone, growth hormone, renin, and other catabolically acting hormones, with a concomitant decrease in the anabolically acting hormones insulin and testosterone (5,42,94). This type of endocrine secretion, characteristic of the stress response, produces widespread metabolic effects, including increased blood glucose, free fatty acids, blood lactate, and ketones, as well as a generalized increased metabolism and oxygen consumption. The endocrine and metabolic changes result in substrate utilization from storage to central organs and injured tissue and lead to a catabolic state with a negative nitrogen balance. The degree and duration of these endocrine and metabolic changes are related to the degree and duration of tissue damage, and many of these biochemical changes last for days (5).

Cortical responses, in addition to and including the perception of pain as an unpleasant sensation and negative emotion, initiate the psychodynamic mechanisms of anxiety, apprehension, and fear. These in turn produce cortically mediated increases in blood viscosity, clotting time, fibrinolysis, and platelet aggregation. Indeed, cortisol and catecholamine responses to anxiety usually exceed the hypothalamic response that is provoked directly by nociceptive impulses reaching the hypothalamus.

Postoperative and Posttraumatic Pain

The local, segmental, and neuroendocrine stress responses that produce pain and hyperalgesia and cause widespread biochemical and metabolic disturbances were long considered the "obligatory" phase of postoperative and posttraumatic injury that were intended to act as homeostatic responses that accelerated healing. However, recent advances in nutrition, anesthesia, and surgery suggest that these responses are not necessarily essential for survival and restitution of the patient to a normal status. Consequently, the emphasis has been shifted to the importance of increased demand on various organs, pulmonary complications, thromboembolism, myocardial infarction, impaired muscle metabolism, fatigue, and weakness that prolong hospitalization and convalescence and, consequently, delay return to work. These deleterious effects, which were previously considered (justly or unjustly) to be caused by surgical imperfections or less than optimal anesthesia, or both, are the consequences of the persistent pain and the persistent and enhanced associated reflex responses. These considerations have led to studies of the effective methods of modulating the responses to surgical and accidental trauma. Kehlet (42) has suggested that, with the availability of blood, current nutritional and other therapies, and modern anesthesia and surgery, the stress response is not needed and indeed may have become maladaptive. The morbidity in high-risk surgical and trauma patients might therefore be reduced by preventing or eliminating the pain and the associated hyperalgesia and the aforementioned responses with local or regional analgesia or other therapeutic modalities. Presented below are data that show that local and regional analgesia, during and after the operation, not only obviates or minimizes pain and suffering for the patient but decreases or eliminates the stress response, decreases complications, enhances healing, and thus reduces the period of hospitalization and convalescence.

Local Anesthesia

Recent studies have shown that the neuroendocrine response to surgery and other trauma can be blunted or eliminated by neural blockade with a local anesthetic that can be given by local infiltration or epidural or subarachnoid block. This confirms the hypothesis of anociassociation proposed some 80 years ago by Crile (17), who suggested that nociceptive impulses provoked by an operation could be blocked by prior infiltration of a local anesthetic in the operative site, thus preventing the impulses from reaching the neuraxis and avoiding some of the harmful effects of surgery. Crile suggested that, if the patient required general anesthesia, infiltration of the operative site with a local anesthetic after the patient was unconscious, but prior to the operation, would prevent shock. In the first edition of my book [7(a)], published in 1953, I cited over 50 reports on the use of various forms of regional anesthesia to prevent nociceptive input during and after surgical operation to avoid or minimize complications. More recently, comprehensive reviews on this subject have been written by Kehlet (43) and in the second edition of *The Management of Pain* [11(b)].

The efficacy of local anesthetic infiltration or field block of the operative site in obviating the afferent barrage to the spinal cord and the aforementioned responses have been demonstrated by a number of workers. McQuay and associates (64) studied the effects of different types of anesthesia and premedication administered to 929 patients for orthopedic surgery and found that the median time to the first request for postoperative analgesia was as follows. Among 514 patients who received general anesthesia, the median time to the first request for opioids was less than 2 hr; among the 216 who had opioid premedication and general anesthesia, it was about 5 hr; among 117 patients managed with local anesthesia alone, it was 8 hr after the operation; and among the 82 patients who received both opioid premedication and local anesthesia, the median time was more than 9 hr. The percentages of patients who required intraoperative opioids were 44, 39, 11, and 7, respectively. These data emphasize the efficacy of local infiltration in eliminating the afferent barrage from deep somatic structures that have been shown in animals to produce sensitization of spinal cord neurons.

Similar results were reported by Teasdale and associates (87) who carried out a randomized controlled trial to compare local anesthesia with general anesthesia for short-stay inguinal hernia repair. They noted that, postoperatively, patients in the local anesthesia group did not require systemic analgesics for 8 to 10 hr, compared with 2 to 3 hr in patients managed with general anesthesia. Moreover, patients in the local anesthesia group could walk, eat, and pass urine much earlier than those in the general anesthesia group. Other reports of local infiltration analgesia suggest that this technique produces effective pain relief for 12 to 16 hr and a consequent decrease in the total amounts of opioids required during the postoperative period (29,72). Moreover, the local analgesia can be extended for several days by placing a catheter with multiple openings in the wound at the end of the operation and then injecting the local anesthetic for several days (72). This not only reduces the incisional pain but probably eliminates the secondary hyperalgesia as a source of nociceptive input.

An impressive example of the efficacy of local anesthetic infiltration in obviating spinal cord sensitization was reported in 1948 by Reynolds and Hutchins (78), who had noted that hyperalgesia in the area of referred pain did not develop if dental treatment was carried out with local anesthesia. This prompted them to carry out a controlled study in which symmetrical cavities on both sides of the mouth were filled using equal technical skill. The only difference was that on one side they produced block of the nerves that supplied the teeth, while on the other side regional analgesia was avoided and the procedure was intentionally a bit rough. In all cases mechanical stimulation of the maxillary antrum resulted in severe referred pain in the teeth and hyperalgesia in the overlying skin, whereas the referred pain and hyperalgesia never occurred on the side in which infiltration anesthesia of the nerves that supplied to the teeth had been used. In commenting on this report in 1953, I stated that this constituted "strong evidence that an initial excessive bombardment of nociceptive impulses had set up a modified functional state (a central excitatory state) in the central nervous system which was continuously reinforced by a steady but not particularly excessive train of impulses from the periphery." This speculation has been confirmed during the 1980s by contributors to this volume and others.

Regional Anesthesia

In the 1970s and 1980s studies on the effects of regional anesthesia and general anesthesia on the function of the cardiovascular, respiratory, hepatic, and other organ systems and on the neuroendocrine response in patients undergoing surgery provided convincing evidence that properly executed regional anesthesia, which blocks all afferent input from the site of surgical operation used before, during, and after the operation for 2 to 3 days not only obviates postoperative pain but also the sensitization of spinal cord and brain stem neurons and the consequent reflex and neuroendocrine responses that otherwise would result from the nociceptive input. This can be easily achieved with placement of a catheter into the epidural or subarachnoid space or with a catheter with its tip near major nerves and injecting the local anesthetic intermittently or by continuous infusion. I cite only a few examples on the efficacy of major regional anesthesia.

Pflug and associates (75), while in my department, compared the efficacy of continuous epidural analgesia during and following the operation and the efficacy of intraoperative general anesthesia and postoperative opioid analgesia on 17 patients who had major hip surgery. They noted that, postoperatively, those in the regional analgesia group had good pain relief, which permitted better ventilation, and had a much more benign postoperative course manifested by early ambulation and early return of appetite than the group that was managed with general anesthesia for the operation and with opioids postoperatively. The mean hospital stay was 4.7 days with regional analgesia as compared with 8.9 days for those managed with systemic analgesics.

A more recent study by Yeager and associates (100) entailed a randomized controlled clinical trial to compare the effects of continuous epidural anesthesia for surgery and analgesia for postoperative pain relief with those of general anesthesia during the surgery and systemic analgesics postoperatively. All 53 patients in the study were considered high risk because of severe preexistent disease and the magnitude of the anticipated surgical procedure. Table 3.1 summarizes the most pertinent results of the study. Similar results were reported by Cuschieri and co-workers (18) in 75 patients who underwent cholecystectomy. Modig et al. (69) compared continuous epidural anesthesia and analgesia, used during and after the operation, with general anesthesia on patients undergoing total hip replacement and noted a much lower incidence of thromboembolism with epidural anesthesia than with general anesthesia. They demonstrated that continuous epidural anesthesia for surgery and analgesia for 24 hr thereafter obviated the increase in fibrinolysis inhibition activity in serum for as long as 7 days. Moreover, patients with epidural anesthesia manifested high concentrations of plasminogen activators and decreased activation of factor VIII.

Another study by Brandt and associates (14) compared the influence of general anesthesia with halothane with that of continuous epidural anesthesia or analgesia on postoperative nitrogen balance in 12 women undergoing elective abdominal hys-

TABLE 3.1. *Epidural anesthesia and analgesia in high-risk surgical patients*

Group I	Group II
Anesthesia	Anesthesia
Epidural with local anesthesia	>50 μg/kg fentanyl
General anesthesia	>35 μg/kg fentanyl
	and nitrous oxide
Nitrous ox. & opioids	<35 μg/kg fentanyl
	and inhalation
	anesthesia
Postoperatively	Postoperatively
Epidural local anesthesia and opioids	Parenteral opioid (PRN)

	Group I	Group II
ASA classification	2.79/0.55	2.78/0.78
Age	71.2/10.0	71.5/7.7
Type of operation		
Intraabdominal	13	11
Intrathoracic	5	2
Major vascular	10	12
Total	28	25

Postoperative course

Parameter	Group I	Group II
Mortality	0	4
Morbidity		
Cardiovascular	4	13
Respiratory	1	8
Other complications	4	16
No. of patients with one or more complications	9(32%)	19(76%)
Economic impact		
Intensive care unit	2.5	5.7
Intubation (hr)	7.1	81.8
Hospital costs ($)	11,218	20,380
Physician costs ($)	3,801	5,134

Results obtained in high-risk surgical patients managed with continuous epidural anesthesia/analgesia and general anesthesia and systemic opioids.
From ref. 100.

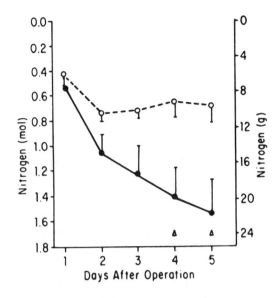

FIG. 3.5. Cumulative nitrogen balance in 12 patients. Patients who had epidural analgesia (○) were in nitrogen balance from the second day after the operation, whereas those who had general anesthesia (●) showed a negative balance throughout the study. This provided impressive evidence that blockade for 24 hr has a lasting effect on urinary nitrogen excretion. (From ref. 14.)

terectomy. As noted in Fig. 3.5, although the epidural anesthesia was continued for only 24 hr, the beneficial effects on cumulative nitrogen balance persisted for 5 to 7 days, thus emphasizing the importance of interrupting the afferent barrage during the operation and the first day, postoperatively, in producing longer lasting benefits.

Another example of the efficacy of the prophylactic use of regional anesthesia in preventing pain and hyperalgesia was a study by Bach and associates (2), carried out in 25 patients with severe persistent preoperative limb pain due to occlusive vascular disease who were scheduled to undergo amputation. One group of 11 patients received a continuous lumbar epidural blockade with bupivacaine to achieve complete pain relief for 72 hr prior to amputation, while a control group of 14 patients with similar history of pain were treated with nonopioid and opioid analgesia administered by standard methods. All 25 patients received epidural or spinal anesthesia for the amputation and opioids and nonopioid analgesics after the procedure. The incidence of phantom limb pain among the patients who had received preoperative regional analgesia was 27% at 6 days and 0% at 6 months and 1 year, whereas in the control group, the figures were 64%, 38%, and 27%, respectively (Fig. 3.6). These results suggest that eliminating the nociceptive input prior to the operation reduces or eliminates sensitization in the spinal cord.

Finally, I cite personal experiences with 11 hip operations for various iatrogenic complications and eventual hip replacement and four low back operations for spinal stenosis and herniated disks. Of these, eight were done with spinal anesthesia for the surgery and continuous epidural analgesia with dilute solution of local anesthetic for 3 to 4 days postoperatively, while the other seven were done with general anesthesia and postoperative opioid analgesics given parenterally or by patient-controlled analgesia. On each of the seven occasions in which the operation was done with general anesthesia, I experienced bouts of severe reflex spasm of my quadriceps muscle (after hip surgery) or in the low paraspinal and gluteal muscles after back surgery. The bouts of reflex spasm usually began in the second or third day postoperatively and were usually provoked by slight movement of my torso or an attempt to ambulate. Following none of the eight operations done with regional anesthesia

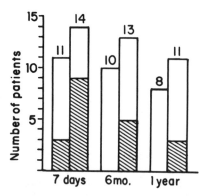

FIG. 3.6. The incidence of postamputation phantom limb pain (▨) in two groups of patients as discussed in text. (Modified from ref. 2.)

did I experience these painful phenomena. The studies by Woolf and Wall (92,95–98) probably explain the basis of this phenomenon. It is of interest to note that on two occasions continuous epidural opioid analgesia provided relief of the incisional pain but did not prevent the totally unexpected bouts of severe reflex muscle spasm and the attendant excruciating pain. The addition of a dilute solution of local anesthetics to the continuous epidural opioids terminated bouts of reflex spasm. This and the study by Ruthberg (84) make it obvious that epidural opioids are not as effective in blocking nociceptive afferent input as are local anesthetics or a combination of local anesthetics and opioids.

CLINICAL ASPECTS OF PAIN AND HYPERALGESIA DURING CHILDBIRTH

Although the proponents of natural childbirth, psychoprophylaxis, and Lamaze techniques continue to insist that human labor, being a physiologic process, should not be painful and support the claim by stating that childbirth among primitive people is painless, there is now overwhelming evidence that, even among those well prepared, human labor is a painful process. Indeed, Melzack and associates (65,66) used the McGill Pain Questionnaire to measure pain during labor and delivery and found that the Pain Rating Index score was higher in both primiparas and multiparas including those who had taken "educated" (natural) childbirth classes, than in cancer pain, chronic back pain, phantom limb pain, postherpetic neuralgia, toothache, and arthritis. This prompted Melzack to title one of his presentations "The Myth of Painless Childbirth" (66).

Labor and vaginal delivery produce tissue damage, particularly in the cervix and lower uterine segment and perineum, which, like other tissue damage from other causes, results in pain and hyperalgesia and the various responses already mentioned. These usually produce deleterious effects on the mother, on the forces of labor, and on the fetus and newborn.

Maternal Effects

The pain during human parturition produces several effects.

1. There are a three- to fivefold increase in ventilation, with a consequent increase in PaO_2 to about 100 mm Hg, a decrease in $PaCO_2$ from the pregnant level of 32 mm

Hg to values of 20 and even as low as 10 mm Hg, and a concomitant increase in pH to 7.5 to 7.6 (9) (Fig. 3.7). Such severe respiratory alkalosis causes constriction of cerebral vessels and possible changes in mentation and carpopedal spasms and may cause constriction of spinal arteries and thus impair placental blood perfusion. With the onset of the relaxation phase, pain no longer stimulates respiration so that hypocapnia causes a transient period of hypoventilation that decreases the maternal PaO_2 by 10% to 50% and even more if the mother has received an opioid that enhances the depressant effects of respiratory alkalosis. When maternal PaO_2 falls below 70 mm Hg, the fetus develops a low PaO_2 and late decelerations—signs of potential fetal distress (39) (Fig. 3.8). These are virtually eliminated with continuous epidural analgesia (Fig. 3.9).

2. Catabolic-acting hormones increase. Human studies have shown that severe pain and anxiety during active labor often cause increases in plasma levels of 300%

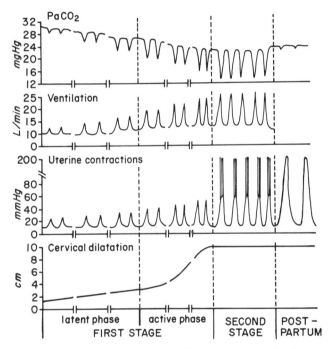

FIG. 3.7. Schematic representation of ventilatory changes during labor in an unpremedicated gravida. Note the correlation of the stages of labor as reflected by the Friedman's curve (bottom tracing), the frequency and intensity of uterine contractions, minute ventilation, and arterial carbon dioxide tension (top tracing). Early in labor uterine contractions are slight and are associated with mild pain, causing only small increases in minute ventilation and decreases in the $PaCO_2$. As labor progresses, however, the greater intensity of contractions causes greater changes in ventilation and $PaCO_2$. During the active phase, contractions with an increased intrauterine pressure of 40 to 60 mm Hg cause severe pain, which acts as an intense stimulus to ventilation with a consequent reduction of the $PaCO_2$ to 18 to 20 mm Hg. During the second stage the reflex bearing down efforts further increase intrauterine pressure and distend the perineum, producing consequent additional pain that prompts the parturient to ventilate at a rate almost twice that of early labor and causing a commensurate reduction in the $PaCO_2$. Pudendal block relieves the perineal pain, but the patient can still effectively bear down voluntarily. These efforts decrease the respiratory rate and consequently decrease minute volume ventilation, resulting in a smaller reduction in the $PaCO_2$ than was present before the block. (Modified from ref. 9.)

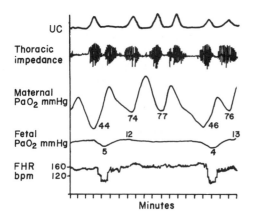

FIG. 3.8. Continuous recording of uterine contractions (UC), maternal thoracic impedance, maternal transcutaneous oxygen tension (PaO₂), fetal oxygen tension, and fetal heart rate (FHR) in a primipara 120 min before spontaneous delivery of an infant with an Apgar score of 7. Marked hyperventilation during uterine contractions was followed by hypoventilation or apnea between contractions. With the parturient breathing air during and after the first and fourth periods of hyperventilation, the maternal PaO₂ fell to 44 and 46 mm Hg, with a consequent decrease in fetal PaO₂ and variable decelerations, which reflected fetal hypoxia. (Modified from ref. 39.)

to 600% of epinephrine, 200% to 400% of norepinephrine, 200% to 300% of cortisol, and significant increases in corticosteroids and ACTH (48). These increases are greatly minimized by continuous epidural analgesia.

3. The pain and catecholamines added to the muscular work of labor cause marked increases in cardiovascular function including increases in cardiac output of

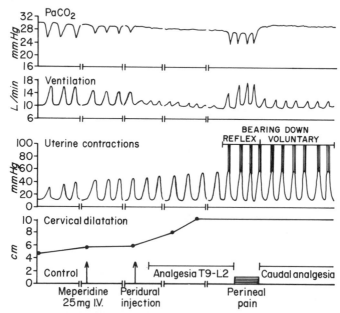

FIG. 3.9. Schematic representation of the effects of analgesia on ventilation based on measurements in a primipara. At 5-cm cervical dilatation, 25 mg of intravenous meperidine resulted in partial relief of pain and consequently produced smaller changes in ventilation and PaCO₂. Subsequent induction of segmental epidural analgesia produced complete pain relief, which eliminated maternal hyperventilation and PaCO₂ changes without affecting uterine contractions. During the second stage the onset of perineal pain and initiation of reflex bearing down efforts caused a concomitant increase in ventilation and a slight decrease in the PaCO₂, which were eliminated with the induction of low caudal (S1–S5) analgesia. (From ref. 9a.)

40% to 50% or higher, and some have an increase of 100% and a further increase of 20% to 30% during each painful contraction (36). These increases are also minimized by continuous epidural analgesia (Fig. 3.10).

4. There are marked metabolic changes including increases in free fatty acids and lactate levels leading to maternal acidosis that is transferred to the fetus, and these can be reduced by continuous epidural analgesia (Fig. 3.11).

5. The pain of labor also increases release of gastrin and decreases the gastrointestinal tone with a consequent delay in gastric emptying that causes retention of food and fluid for as long as 36 hr. Opioids and general anesthesia enhance these effects, whereas continuous epidural analgesia may decrease them. Induction of general anesthesia may cause regurgitation of stomach contents and their aspiration into the tracheobronchial tree, which in the past has been a major cause of maternal mortality [8(b)].

6. Severe labor pain can produce serious long-term emotional disturbances that might adversely affect the parturient's mental health, influence her relationship with her baby during the first few crucial days, and affect her sexual relations with her husband (22).

Effects on Labor

Through increased secretion of catecholamines and cortisol, pain and emotional stress can either increase or decrease uterine contractility and thus influence the duration of labor. Generally pain and anxiety in many parturients increase epinephrine and cortisol levels, thus decreasing uterine activity and prolonging the labor, or can even produce "incoordinate uterine contractions" that greatly prolong labor. All of these effects on the mother have an impact on the fetus, and consequently on the newborn. Continuous epidural analgesia has proven effective in the treatment of incoordinate uterine contractions (12).

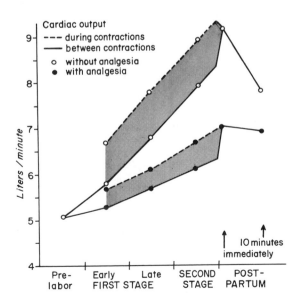

FIG. 3.10. Cardiac output during various phases of labor between contractions and during contractions. In a group of patients laboring without analgesia, the progressive increases between contractions and the further increases during each contraction were much greater than corresponding changes in a group of patients who received continuous epidural analgesia. [Developed from data of Ueland et al. in ref. 8(c).]

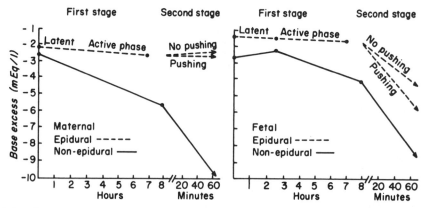

FIG. 3.11. Representation of mean changes in extent of maternal (*left*) and fetal (*right*) metabolic acidosis during the first and second stages of labor observed in a group of "clinically acceptable ideal" parturients managed without lumbar epidural analgesia and in two similar groups of parturients managed with epidural analgesia, of which those in one group retained a bearing down reflex and those in the other group did not and were delivered by outlet forceps. Note the significant metabolic acidosis among the nonepidural group of parturients, whereas those given an epidural analgesia experienced little or no change in their acid-base status. Fetuses born of mothers managed without epidural analgesia also developed impressive metabolic acidosis during the first stage and an even greater degree during the second stage. Fetuses of mothers given epidural analgesia had no change in acid base during the first stage, but there was a time-dependent increase in metabolic acidosis during the second stage, although the rate of increase was less than in the nonepidural analgesia group and least if the mother did not bear down during the second stage. (Modified from ref. 16b.)

Effects on the Fetus and Newborn

During labor the intermittent reduction of intervillous blood flow during the peak of a contraction leads to a temporary decrease in placental gas exchange. This impairment is often further increased by pain-induced severe hyperventilation with consequent alkalosis that diminishes uterine blood flow and impairs the transfer of oxygen from mother to fetus. Maternal hypoxemia during uterine relaxation and umbilical vasoconstriction with a consequent decrease in umbilical blood flow and a reduction in uterine blood flow provoked by an increase in norepinephrine and cortisol release can occur. As previously mentioned, these can be markedly reduced by eliminating the pain and the associated responses with continuous epidural analgesia (73,74).

Effects of Pain Relief

During recent years there has been a massive amount of evidence that complete pain relief achieved with continuous epidural analgesia prevents or diminishes many of these alterations in maternal function and obviates their deleterious impacts on the fetus and newborn. Some of these effects on maternal function of pain and anxiety, and their modification by epidural analgesia, are shown in Figs. 3.7–3.11.

REFERENCES

1. Abrams, A. A. (1950): Obliteration of pain at the site of reference by intradermal infiltration anesthesia in first-stage labor. *N. Engl. J. Med.*, 243:636.
2. Bach, S., Noreng, M. F., and Tjellden, N. U. (1988): Phantom limb pain in amputees during the first 12 months following limb amputation, after preoperative lumbar epidural blockade. *Pain*, 33:297.
3. Bauman, J. (1979): Treatment of acute herpes zoster neuralgia by epidural injection or stellate ganglion block. *Anesthesiology*, 51:523.
4. Behan, R. J. (1914): *Pain*. Appleton, New York.
5. Bessman, F. P., and Renner, V. J. (1982): The biphasic hormonal nature of stress. In: *Pathophysiology of shock, anoxia, and ischemia*, edited by R. A. Cowley and B. F. Trump, pp. 60–65. Williams & Wilkins, Baltimore.
6. Bessou, P., and Perl, E. R. (1969): Response of cutaneous sensory units with unmyelinated fibers to noxious stimuli. *J. Neurophysiol.*, 32:1025–1043.
7. Bonica, J. J. (1953): *The management of pain*. Lea & Febiger, Philadelphia (a. pp. 117–120; b. pp. 104–117).
8. Bonica, J. J. (1967): *Principles and practice of obstetric analgesia and anesthesia*. F. A. Davis, Philadelphia (a. p. 648; b. pp. 748–760; c. p. 80).
9. Bonica, J. J. (1973): Maternal respiratory changes during pregnancy and parturition. In: *Parturition and perinatology. Clinical anesthesia series*, vol. 10, no. 2, edited by G. F. Marx, pp. 9–21. F. A. Davis, Philadelphia.
9a. Bonica, J. J. (1980): *Obstetric analgesia and anesthesia*, 2nd ed. University of Washington Press, Seattle, p. 114.
10. Bonica, J. J. (1986): Pain of parturition. *Clin. Anesthesiol.*, 4:1.
11. Bonica, J. J. (1990): *The management of pain*, 2nd ed. Lea & Febiger, Philadelphia (a. pp. 159–179; b. pp. 177; c. p. 1219).
12. Bonica, J. J., and Hunter, C. A. (1969): Management in dysfunction of the forces of labor. In: *Principles and practice of obstetric analgesia and anesthesia*, edited by J. J. Bonica, pp. 1188–1208. F. A. Davis, Philadelphia.
13. Bonica, J. J., and McDonald, J. S. (1990): The pain of childbirth. In: *The management of pain*, 2nd ed, edited by J. J. Bonica, et al., pp. 1313–1343. Lea & Febiger, Philadelphia.
14. Brandt, M. R., et al. (1978): Epidural analgesia improves postoperative nitrogen balance. *Br. Med. J.*, 1:1106.
15. Campbell, J. N., et al. (1989): Peripheral neural mechanisms of nociception. In: *Textbook of pain*, edited by P. D. Wall and R. Melzack, pp. 22–45. Churchill Livingstone, Edinburgh.
16. Cohen, H. (1944): Mechanisms of visceral pain. *Trans. Med. Soc. Lond.* 64:65.
16a. Cohen, H. (1947): Visceral pain. *Lancet*, 2:933.
16b. Crawford, J. S. (1976): *Principles and practice of obstetric anesthesia*. Blackwell Scientific, Oxford (based on data of Pearson, J., and Davis, J. (1974): *Obstet. Gynaecol. Br. Cwlth.*, 81:971).
17. Crile, G. W. (1910): Phylogenetic association in relation to certain medical problems. *Boston Med. Surg. J.*, 163:893.
18. Cuschieri, R. J., et al. (1985): Postoperative pain and pulmonary complications: comparison of three analgesic regimens. *Br. J. Surg.*, 72:495.
19. Dan, K., Higa, K., and Noda, B. (1985): Nerve block for herpetic pain. In: *Advances in pain research and therapy*, vol. 9, edited by H. L. Fields, R. W. Dubner, and F. Cervero, pp. 831–838. Raven Press, New York.
20. Déjérine, J., and Roussy, G. (1906): Le syndrome thalamique. *Rev. Neurol. (Paris)*, 12:521–532.
21. Denmark, A. (1813): An example of symptoms resembling tic douloureux produced by a wound in the radial nerve. *Med. Clin. Times*, 4:48.
22. Deutsch, H. (1955): Psychology of pregnancy, labour and puerperium. In: *Obstetrics*, 11th ed. edited by J. P. Greenhill, pp. 349–360. W. B. Saunders, Philadelphia.
23. Dubner, R. (1991): Pain and hyperalgesia following tissue injury: new mechanisms and new treatments. *Pain*, 44:213.
24. Foerster, O. (1927): Die Leitungsbahnen des Schmerzgefühls und die chirurgische Behandlung der Schmerzzustände, Berlin. Urban and Schwarzenberg, Vienna.
25. Gellhorn, E., Gellhorn, H., and Trainor, J. (1931): Influences of spinal irradiations on cutaneous sensations. *Am. J. Physiol.*, 97:491.
26. Gowers, W. R. (1886): *A manual of diseases of the nervous system*. J. A. Churchill, London.
27. Hardy, J. D., Wolff, H. G., and Goodell, H. (1950): Experimental evidence on the nature of cutaneous hyperalgesia. *J. Clin. Invest.*, 29:115.
28. Hardy, J. D., Wolff, H. G., and Goodell, H. (1952): *Pain sensation and reactions*. Williams & Wilkins, Baltimore, pp. 173–238.
29. Hashimi, K., and Middleton, M. D. (1983): Subcutaneous bupivacaine for postoperative analgesia after herniorrhaphy. *Ann. R. Coll. Surg. Engl.*, 65:38.

30. Head, H. (1892): Thesis before the University of Cambridge. June 1892.
31. Head, H. (1893): On disturbances of sensation with especial reference to the pain of visceral disease. *Brain*, 16:1.
32. Head, H. (1920): *Studies in neurology.* Oxford University Press, London.
33. Head, H., and Campbell, A. W. (1900): The pathology of herpes zoster and its bearing on sensory localisation. *Brain*, 23:353.
34. Head, H., and Holmes, G. (1911): Sensory disturbances from cerebral lesions. *Brain*, 34:102–254.
35. Head, H., Rivers, W. H. R., and Sherren, J. (1905): The afferent nervous system from a new aspect. *Brain*, 28:99.
36. Hendricks, C. H., and Quilligan, E. J. (1956): Cardiac output during labour. *Am. J. Obstet. Gynecol.*, 71:953.
37. Hilton, J. (1863): *Rest and pain.* Bell & Daldy, London.
38. Holmes, G. (1919): *Contributions to medical and biological research.* Paul B. Hober, New York, pp. 239–246.
39. Huch, A., et al. (1977): Continuous transcutaneous monitoring of foetal oxygen tension during labour. *Br. J. Obstet. Gynecol.*, 84(suppl. 1):1.
40. Hunter, J., cited by MacKenzie, J. (1893): Some points bearing on the association of sensory disorders and visceral disease. *Brain*, 16:321–354.
41. Jones, C. M. (1943): Pain from the digestive tract. *Proc. Assoc. Res. Nerv. Ment. Dis.*, 23:274.
42. Kehlet, H. (1986): Pain relief and modification of the stress response. In: *Acute pain management,* edited by M. J. Cousins and G. D. Philips, pp. 49–75. Churchill Livingstone, New York.
43. Kehlet, H. (1988): Modification of responses to surgery by neural blockade: clinical implications. In: *Neural blockade,* 2nd ed., edited by M. J. Cousins and P. O. Bridenbaugh, pp. 145–190. J. B. Lippincott, Philadelphia.
44. Kellgren, J. H. (1937–38): Observations on referred pain arising from muscles. *Clin. Sci.* 3:176.
45. Kellgren, J. H. (1939): On the distribution of pain arising from deep somatic structures with charts of segmental pain areas. *Clin. Sci.*, 4:35.
46. Kuntz, A. (1953): *The autonomic nervous system,* 4th ed. Lea & Febiger, Philadelphia, pp. 402–432.
47. Lange, C. (1875): Nogle bemärkungen am neuralgie und deres behandlung. *Hosp. Tid.*, 2:641.
48. Lederman, R. P., et al. (1978): The relationships of maternal anxiety, plasma catecholamines, and plasma cortisol to progresses in labour. *Am. J. Obstet. Gynecol.*, 132:495.
49. Lemaire, A. (1926): La perception des douleurs viscerales. *Rev. Med. Louvain*, 6:81.
50. Letievant, E. (1873): *Traite des sections nerveuses.* J. B. Baillière, Paris.
51. Lewis, T. (1937): The nocifensive system of nerves and its reaction, I and II. *Br. Med. J.*, 1:431.
52. Lewis, T. (1942): *Pain.* Macmillan, New York.
53. Lewis, T., and Hess, W. (1933–34): Pain derived from the skin and the mechanism of its production. *Clin. Sci.*, 1:39.
54. Lewis, T., and Kellgren, J. H. (1939): Observations relating to referred pain, visceromotor reflexes and other associated phenomena. *Clin. Sci.*, 4:47.
55. Lillehei, R. C., and Dietzman, R. H. (1974): Circulatory collapse in shock. In: *Principles of surgery,* 2nd ed. edited by S. I. Schwartz, pp. 133–164. McGraw-Hill, New York.
56. Livingston, W. K. (1947). *Pain mechanisms.* Macmillan, New York.
57. Loh, L., Nathan, P. W., and Schott, G. (1981): Pain due to lesions of the central nervous system removed by sympathetic block. *Br. Med. J.*, 282:1026.
58. MacKenzie, J. (1892): Association of sensory disorders and visceral disease. *Med. Chron.*, August.
59. MacKenzie, J. (1893): Some points bearing on the association of sensory disorders and visceral disease. *Brain*, 16:321.
60. MacKenzie, J. (1908): *Symptoms and their interpretation.* Shaw and Sons, London.
61. Martyn, S. (1864): On the physiological meaning of inframammary pain. *Br. Med. J.*, 10:296.
62. McAuliffe, G. W., Goodell, H., and Wolff, H. G. (1943): Experimental studies on headache: pain from the nasal and paranasal structures. *Assoc. Res. Nervous Ment. Dis.*, 23:185.
63. McLelland, A. M., and Goodell, H. (1943): Pain from the bladder, ureter and kidney pelvis. *Proc. Assoc. Res. Nerv. Ment. Dis.*, 23:252.
64. McQuay, H. J., Carroll, D., and Moore, R. A. (1988): Postoperative paediatric pain—the effects of opiate premedication and local anaesthetic blocks. *Pain,* 33:291.
65. Melzack, R., et al. (1981): Labour is still painful after prepared childbirth training. *Can. Med. Assoc. J.*, 125:357.
66. Melzack, R. (1984): The myth of painless childbirth (the John J. Bonica Lecture). *Pain,* 19:321.
67. Mitchell, S. W. (1872): *Injuries of nerves and their consequences.* Smith Elder, London.
68. Mitchell, S. W., Moorehouse, G. R., and Keen, W. W. (1864): *Gunshot wounds and other injuries of nerves.* J. B. Lippincott, Philadelphia.

69. Modig, J., et al. (1983): Role of extradural and of general anesthesia in fibrinolysis and coagulation after total hip replacement. *Br. J. Anaesth.*, 55:625.
70. Morgagni, H. (1761): De sedibus et causis morborum, book ii., letter xx., article 30.
71. Morley, J. A. (1931): *Abdominal pain*. William Wood, New York.
72. Owen, M., Galloway, D. J., and Mitchell, K. G. (1985): Analgesia by wound infiltration after surgical excision of benign breast lumps. *Ann. R. Coll. Surg. Engl.*, 67:130.
73. Pearson, J. F., and Davies, P. (1973): The effect of continuous lumbar epidural analgesia on maternal acid-base balance and arterial lactate concentration during the first stage of labour. *J. Obstet. Gynaecol. [Br.]*, 80:218.
74. Pearson, J. F., and Davies, P. (1973): The effect of continuous lumbar epidural analgesia upon fetal acid-base status during the first and second stage of labour. *J. Obstet. Gynaecol. [Br.]*, 81:971.
75. Pflug, A. E., et al. (1974): The effects of postoperative peridural analgesia on pulmonary therapy and pulmonary complications. *Anesthesiology*, 41:8.
76. Pollock, L. J., and Davis, L. (1935): Visceral and referred pain. *Proc. Assoc. Res. Nerv. Ment. Dis.*, 15:210; *Arch. Neurol. Psychiatr.*, 34:1041; *Arch. Neurol. Psychiatr.*, 57:277, 1947.
77. Porter, K. M., and Davies, J. (1985): The control of pain after Keller's procedure—a controlled, double-blind prospective trial with local anesthetic and placebo. *Ann. R. Coll. Surg. Engl.*, 67:293.
78. Reynolds, O. E., and Hutchins, H. C. (1948): Reduction of central hyperirritability following block anesthesia of peripheral nerve. *Am. J. Physiol.*, 152:658.
79. Riddoch, G. (1938): The clinical features of central pain. *Lancet*, 234:1093–1098, 1150–1156, 1205–1209.
80. Riopelle, J. M., Naraghi, M., and Grush, K. P. (1984): Chronic neuralgia incidence following local anesthetic therapy for herpes zoster. *Arch. Dermatol.*, 120:747.
81. Robertson, S., Goodell, H., and Wolff, H. G. (1947): Studies on headache: the teeth as a source of headache and other pain. *Arch. Neurol. Psychiatry*, 57:277.
82. Rose, D. (1929): Local anesthesia in first and second stage labor. *N. Engl. J. Med.*, 201:117.
83. Ross, J. (1887): Segmental distribution of sensory disorders. *Brain*, 10:333.
84. Ruthberg, H. (1985): Endocrine-metabolic response to upper abdominal surgery: influence of extradural analgesia. Thesis, Linköping University, Linköping, Sweden.
85. Schmidt, R. (1908): *Pain*. J. B. Lippincott, Philadelphia, pp. 350–362.
86. Sturge, W. A. (1883): Phenomena of angina pectoris, and their bearing upon the theory of counterirritation. *Brain*, 5:492.
87. Teasdale, C., et al., (1982): A randomized controlled trial to compare local with general anaesthesia for short-stay inguinal hernia repair. *Ann. R. Coll. Surg. Engl.*, 64:238.
88. Tenicela, R., Lovasik, D., and Eaglstein, W. (1985): Treatment of herpes zoster with sympathetic blocks. *Clin. J. Pain*, 1:64.
89. Theobald, G. W. (1941): *Referred pain. A new hypothesis*. Colombo.
90. Theobald, G. W. (1946): Some gynaecological aspects of referred pain. *J. Obstet. Gynaecol. Br. Emp.*, 53:309.
91. Thomas, D. F. M., Lambert, W. S., and Lloyd, W. K. (1983): The direct perfusion of surgical wounds with local anesthetic solution: an approach to postoperative pain. *Ann. R. Coll. Surg. Engl.*, 65:226.
92. Wall, P.D., and Woolf, C. J. (1984): Muscle but not cutaneous C-afferent input produces prolonged increases in excitability of the flexion reflex in the rat. *J. Physiol. (Lond.)*, 356:443–458.
93. Weiss, S., and Davis, O. (1928): Significance of afferent impulses from the skin in the mechanism of visceral pain. *Am. J. Med. Sci.*, 176:517.
94. Wilmore, D. W., et al. (1976): Stress in surgical patients as a neurophysiologic reflex response. *Surg. Gynecol. Obstet.*, 142:257.
95. Woolf, C. J. (1983): Evidence for a central component of postinjury pain hypersensitivity. *Nature*, 308:686–688.
96. Woolf, C. J., and Wall, P. D. (1986): The brief and the prolonged facilitatory effects of unmyelinated afferent input on the rat spinal cord are independently influenced by peripheral nerve injury. *Neuroscience*, 17:1199.
97. Woolf, C. J., and Wall, P. D. (1986): A dissociation between the analgesic and antinociceptive effects of morphine. *Neurosci. Lett.*, 64:238.
98. Woolf, C. J., and Wall, P. D. (1986): The relative effectiveness of C primary afferent fibres of different origins in evoking a prolonged facilitation of the flexor reflex in the rat. *J. Neurosci*, 6:1433–1443.
99. Woollard, H. H., Roberts, J. E. H., and Carmichael, E. A. (1932): Inquiry into referred pain. *Lancet*, 1:337.
100. Yeager, M. P., et al. (1987): Epidural anesthesia and analgesia in high-risk surgical patients. *Anesthesiology*, 66:729.

Hyperalgesia and Allodynia,
edited by W. D. Willis, Jr.
Raven Press, Ltd., New York © 1992.

4

Possible Clues About the Evolution of Hyperalgesia from Mechanisms of Nociceptive Sensitization in *Aplysia*

Edgar T. Walters

Department of Physiology and Cell Biology, University of Texas Medical School at Houston, Houston, Texas 77225

Hyperalgesia is defined as an increased response to a stimulus that is normally painful, whereas the closely related term allodynia is defined as pain due to a stimulus that does not normally evoke pain (31). Because pain is defined in terms of subjective emotional experience, one cannot apply these definitions directly to the behavior of species unable to report their feelings. Nonetheless, *Homo sapiens* is a product of biological evolution, so one can assume that many of the physiological mechanisms underlying hyperalgesia and allodynia were inherited by humans from ancestral species. Some of these mechanisms may be relatively primitive and widely available for study in other species. The proportion of living species that could have inherited a given mechanism from a common ancestor will depend on the time elapsed since the appearance of the mechanism during evolution. An example of a primitive set of mechanisms is that underlying the action potential, which are remarkably similar in nearly all animals (23). An example of a mechanism that evolved relatively recently is immunoglobulin-mediated humoral immunity, which is found only in tetrapod vertebrates and is most highly developed in mammals (38). Although the comparative study of cellular mechanisms related to hyperalgesia and allodynia is just beginning, I will review recent studies suggesting the involvement of both primitive and recently evolved mechanisms in these phenomena.

BIOLOGICAL FUNCTIONS OF HYPERALGESIA AND ALLODYNIA

It is important to consider selection pressures that may have driven the evolution of the mechanisms of hyperalgesia and allodynia. These phenomena are usually produced by noxious stimulation and are most pronounced after serious injury. Some of the more obvious benefits of hyperalgesia and allodynia include (a) a decrease in the likelihood that a person will exacerbate an injury by moving an injured body part, (b) an increase in the sensitivity of the body part to potentially threatening contact, and (c) an increase in the speed and vigor of defensive responses to threatening contact. Such threats may be quite serious following injury because a weakened organism is more vulnerable to attack, and chemical and visual signals generated by wounds can attract predators and parasites (e.g., refs. 11,29). Because

45

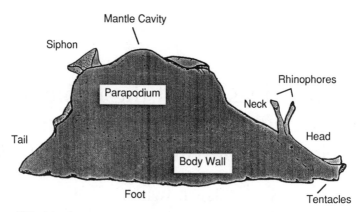

FIG. 4.1. Side view of the gastropod mollusc *Aplysia californica.*

virtually all animals are subject to injury from predators, parasites, competitors, or random physical assaults of the environment, injury-induced hypersensitivity should benefit many species. The ubiquity of such threats is indicated by the presence of well-developed defensive responses to noxious stimulation in nearly all animals that have been examined and in protozoans (e.g., ref. 25).

Although the adaptiveness of cutaneous hypersensitivity in protecting a wound from further attack would suggest that injury-induced hypersensitivity is widespread in the animal kingdom, until recently nociceptive sensitization had only been examined systematically in a handful of mammalian species. Sensitization following noxious stimulation has been reported in lower vertebrates (37) and a few invertebrates, including crayfish (28), leech (7), and octopus (54), but little is known about the function or mechanisms of these alterations. The most extensive analysis of nociceptive sensitization in a nonmammalian species has been in the large marine mollusc *Aplysia californica* (Fig. 4.1). A consideration of similarities and differences in mechanisms of nociceptive sensitization in groups as highly divergent as gastropod molluscs and mammals may offer clues about the evolution of mechanisms of hyperalgesia and allodynia.

NOCICEPTIVE PLASTICITY IN *APLYSIA*

Aplysia displays profound changes in behavior after noxious stimulation, perhaps because its soft body, unprotected by a hard exoskeleton or shell, makes it particularly vulnerable to the dangers that follow sublethal injury in a hostile environment. Behavioral and neurophysiological alterations produced by noxious stimulation of *Aplysia* can be divided functionally into three phases: injury detection, escape, and recuperation (Fig. 4.2) (51). These overlapping phases correspond to periods of immediate facilitation, short-term inhibition, and long-term facilitation of defensive responses and are somewhat similar to postinjury behavioral phases proposed for mammals by Bolles and Fanselow (6) and Wall (48). Mechanisms contributing to each phase occur in various types of neurons (20), but analysis has focused on two populations of nociceptive mechanosensory neurons: the LE neurons, which innervate the siphon, and the VC neurons, which innervate most of the rest of the body

Phase 1. Injury Detection	Phase 2. Escape	Phase 3. Recuperation
Period: 0.1 sec-10 min	1 sec-30 min	10min-1 month

Functions: • Severity appraisal
• Localization
• Compensation for destruction of nociceptive channels
• Defensive response triggering
• Anticipation
	• Flight
	• Inhibition of competing responses
		• General inactivity (healing)
		• Defensive readiness (sensitization)
		  a. General
		  b. Wound specific
		  c. Cue specific

Mechanisms: • Nociceptor activation
  a. Frequency code
  b. Wide dynamic range
• Activation of defensive circuits (Somatotopic organization)
• Nociceptor facilitation
  a. Afterdischarge
  b. PTP
  c. HSF
  d. Hyperexcitability
  e. ADEM
• Motor facilitation
	• Activity in circuits generating escape behavior
	• Nociceptor inhibition
	  a. Presynaptic inhibition (neuromodulation)
	  b. Activity-dependent inhibition
	• Inhibition of motor and interneurons controlling other behaviors
		• Inhibition of circuits controlling feeding, reproduction, etc.
		• Nociceptor facilitation
		  a. ADEM
		  b. Axon injury signals
		  c. Lower threshold
		  d. Less accommodation
		  e. Afterdischarge
		  f. Synaptic facilitation
		  g. Sprouting
		• Motor facilitation

FIG. 4.2. Three-phase model of the functions and general mechanisms of nociceptive plasticity in *Aplysia*. The times for each phase indicate the approximate beginning and end of the phase relative to the noxious stimulus. ADEM, activity-dependent extrinsic modulation; HSF, heterosynaptic facilitation; PTP, posttetanic potentiation. (From ref. 51.)

(reviewed in ref. 51). Each sensory population has peripheral terminals in the skin connected by long axons to somata and presynaptic terminals within central ganglia. Cells in both clusters have a wide dynamic range, responding with one or a few action potentials to stimuli of moderate intensity and with longer and higher frequency bursts as stimulus intensity is increased. These sensory neurons are classified as nociceptors (44) because they respond maximally to stimuli that injure the body.

Phase 1: Injury Detection

A brief facilitatory phase of plasticity, which might be functionally similar to short-term hyperalgesia, immediately follows noxious stimulation of *Aplysia*. Immediate facilitatory effects contribute to injury detection in at least two ways. First, a strong, injurious stimulus is likely to destroy nociceptor axons at the site of injury. Combined recordings from sensory, motor, and interneurons and from effector organs indicate that the intensity of reflexive responses to noxious stimulation depends on the number of nociceptors activated, the number and frequency of spikes generated in each nociceptor, and the amount of transmitter released per spike, as well as properties of other cells in the circuit (51). An injurious stimulus immediately activates both the damaged and undamaged nociceptors innervating the stimulated area. In addition, within a fraction of a second a facilitatory effect occurs, which compensates for the destruction of nociceptor axons. This effect begins when active nociceptors excite modulatory interneurons that release facilitatory neuromodulators such as serotonin (5-HT) (21) on the sensory cell body, the presynaptic terminals, and probably the peripheral terminals. The combination of spike activity and modulatory input produces a large depolarizing afterpotential in the soma (53) and perhaps other parts of the nociceptor, which generates an afterdischarge, prolonging the afferent signal from the damaged region for up to several seconds after the initial discharge (10). Because much of the afterdischarge is generated in the centrally located soma of the sensory neuron, it occurs even in cells that are disconnected from their peripheral terminals during injury. The result is that interneurons and motor neurons receive massive synaptic input from nociceptors innervating the traumatized region, which thus inform the CNS about the occurrence, location, and severity of injury, even when many of these nociceptors are disconnected from the periphery by the injury.

A second contribution of short-term facilitatory processes to injury detection occurs with noxious stimuli that do not immediately produce injury but would be damaging if the stimulus were prolonged or repeated. Nociceptors show brief (seconds to minutes) heterosynaptic facilitation, posttetanic potentiation (PTP), and enhancement of peripheral excitability (9,24,51). The enhancement of nociceptor sensitivity and synaptic output is amplified in active nociceptors, so continued or repeated noxious stimulation to the same region progressively increases the effectiveness of signals from the activated nociceptors. Summation of excitatory inputs and facilitation of excitability occur in at least some of the defensive interneurons and motor neurons, enhancing the responsiveness of the motor control circuit. Spontaneous firing rates of defensive motor neurons increase, leading to neuromuscular facilitation (20). All of these mechanisms act synergistically to produce rapid "windup" of defensive responses to threatening cutaneous stimulation. Windup insures that a decision to withdraw is made quickly when the animal is confronted with persistent, insidious stimuli, and it prepares the animal to respond maximally if more severe stimulation follows.

Phase 2: Escape

The second phase of nociceptive plasticity occurs during escape locomotion and may be functionally similar to some forms of analgesia in humans. Nociceptive reflexes are inhibited, and in *Aplysia,* as in mammals (6,48), this inhibition probably prevents less urgent behavior patterns (e.g., local withdrawal responses) from interfering with the organism's attempts to escape from a potentially mortal threat. The transient inhibition of defensive reflexes involves neuromodulation of sensory neurons, interneurons, and perhaps motor neurons (reviewed in ref. 51). Much less is known about these mechanisms than about facilitatory mechanisms in *Aplysia.*

Phase 3: Recuperation

This phase involves functions similar to those of long-term hyperalgesia. It begins about 10 min after injury, when the animal stops locomoting (often after taking shelter in a crevice). *Aplysia* can remain motionless for days after severe injury and may show exaggerated withdrawal responses and a low threshold for escape locomotion for weeks, especially if contact is made near the wound. This is illustrated in Fig. 4.3, which shows site-specific (wound-specific) sensitization produced by a brief,

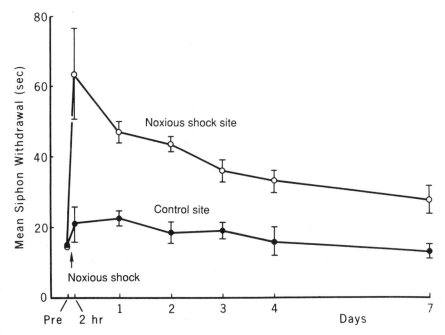

FIG. 4.3. Long-term, site-specific sensitization induced by noxious tail shock in *Aplysia*. Weak electrical test stimuli were delivered to marked sites on either side of the tail in the freely moving animal. Strong noxious shock (10 0.5-sec trains, 60 Hz AC, at 5-sec intervals) was then delivered close to one test site. The duration of siphon withdrawal responses to the test stimuli delivered close to the site of noxious stimulation was significantly enhanced compared to the distant test site for at least 1 week afterward. (From ref. 49.)

45-sec sequence of noxious shock to one side of the tail. Sensitization was revealed by an enhancement of siphon withdrawal responses to weak test stimuli delivered near the traumatized site, but was not observed when weak test stimuli were delivered at a distance from the traumatized site (49). However, if noxious stimuli are repeated several times over a period of hours or days, the sensitization can generalize to test sites distant from the site of trauma (19,36).

Both site-specific and general sensitization are associated with alterations in the nociceptors. A 45-sec sequence of noxious shock to the tail causes general facilitation of the synapses of inactive nociceptors, which lasts about 30 min (50). Specific synaptic facilitation (five times the magnitude of general facilitation and lasting at least a day) occurs in nociceptors that are activated by the noxious stimulus (50). These cells also show long-lasting enhancement of the excitability of the soma, expressed as an increased probability that afferent spikes will generate an afterdischarge in the soma (Fig. 4.4) (see also ref. 42). Peripheral terminals and/or axons of the nociceptors also change; a week after one side of the tail is injured or shocked, mechanosensory thresholds of nearby nociceptors are lowered and receptive fields are enlarged in the vicinity of the injury (5). If strong shock is repeated over hours or days, long-lasting physiological changes also occur in nociceptors that have unstimulated receptive fields (19). These changes have been correlated with morphological alterations in the central region of the neuron; the number of presynaptic varicosities and synaptic active zones doubles (3,4).

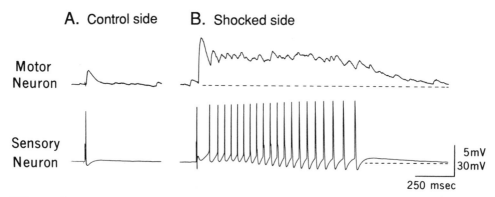

FIG. 4.4. Correlates of long-term, site-specific sensitization in nociceptive sensory neurons of *Aplysia*. One day after noxious shock was delivered to one side of the body the CNS was removed, and sensory and motor neurons innervating the shocked and unshocked sides were examined. **A:** Typical synaptic connection between a tail sensory neuron and tail motor neuron innervating the unshocked, control side of the tail. The connection was tested by activating the sensory neuron with a 10-msec depolarizing pulse injected into the soma. **B:** The same test procedure on the side that had experienced noxious shock revealed a larger synaptic potential in the motor neuron and an afterdischarge of 20 spikes in the sensory neuron. (From ref. 50.)

EVIDENCE FOR PRIMITIVE ORIGINS OF SOME HYPERALGESIA MECHANISMS

At a functional level, nociceptive sensitization in *Aplysia* and mammals displays a number of similarities. In both groups, facilitatory alterations occur in the first stages of nociceptive processing, within wide dynamic range nociceptors in *Aplysia* (Fig. 4.5) and in primary nociceptors and secondary wide dynamic range spinal interneurons in mammals (Fig. 4.6). Both nociceptive systems (57) show intensity-dependent enhancement of central and peripheral excitability, enlargement of receptive fields, activity-dependent plasticity, and maximal expression following nerve injury (see below). Moreover, some of the same mediators are used by each system (Figs. 4.5 and 4.6). Such similarities could be (a) accidental, (b) due to convergent evolution of independent mechanisms in response to common selection pressures (analogy), or (c) due to conservation of primitive mechanisms that had evolved in ancestors common to both molluscs and mammals (homology). Homologous features in molluscs and mammals would be very primitive, since the last common ancestor of these groups lived 600 to 700 million years ago during the Precambrian era, before most of today's animal phyla had become established (Fig. 4.7) (30,55).

Many studies have shown that sensitizing effects in *Aplysia* nociceptors can be induced by neuromodulators, such as 5-HT, released from facilitatory interneurons and by activity-dependent enhancement of the effects of these extrinsic modulators (ADEM) (reviewed in refs. 1,9,51). Sensitizing effects are expressed in the soma and synapses within seconds or minutes. Recently we found that many of the same effects in the soma and synapses can be induced by crushing the cells' axons under conditions in which spike activity and neuromodulator release are severely reduced (52). The crush-induced effects occur after a latency of 2 or more days, depending

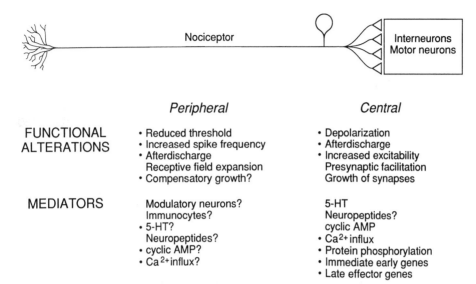

FIG. 4.5. Functional alterations and mediators implicated in nociceptive sensitization in *Aplysia. Question marks* indicate properties for which evidence is indirect. *Dots* indicate features that have also been observed in mammals (compare Fig. 4.6). (Modified from ref. 57.)

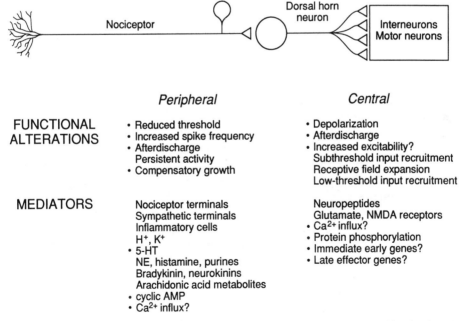

FIG. 4.6. Functional alterations and mediators implicated in nociceptive sensitization in mammals. *Dots* indicate features that have also been observed in *Aplysia* (compare Fig. 4.5). (Modified from ref. 57.)

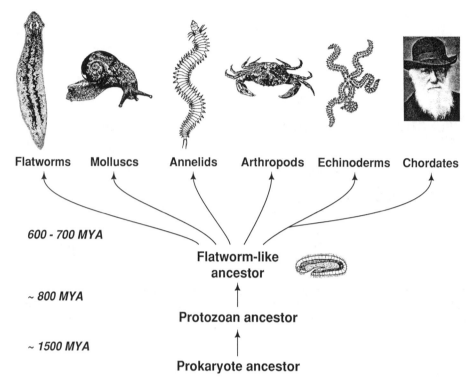

FIG. 4.7. Simplified phylogenetic tree showing primitive relationship between molluscs and chordates. The last common ancestor of the animal groups depicted was probably a flatworm-like organism that lived 600 to 700 million years ago (MYA). Only a few major groups, of special interest to neurobiologists, are shown. The arthropods are now considered by some systematists to comprise several different phyla. (Based on information in refs. 30 and 55.)

on the distance of the crush from the soma, and persist for weeks. These sensitizing effects include decreases in action potential threshold, accommodation, and after-hyperpolarization and increases in action potential duration, afterdischarge, and synaptic transmission. The long latency, axonal specificity, and large magnitude of the plasticity observed after crushing axons under conditions minimizing neuromodulator release and ADEM all suggest that induction signals are generated at a site of axonal injury and conveyed centrally by retrograde axonal transport. The injury signals might originate within the axon itself, by either the production of chemical messengers or an interruption of the retrograde transport of trophic factors. Injury signals might also originate in interactions of the damaged axon with extracellular messengers released from damaged cells or hemocytes attracted to the site of injury (2). This finding indicates a close relationship between mechanisms of nociceptive sensitization and adaptive reactions to cellular injury in *Aplysia* nociceptors. Under normal conditions, peripheral injury would produce all three sets of signals: release of neuromodulators, generation of action potentials in the nociceptors, and slow transport of intracellular signals within damaged axons.

In mammals peripheral sensitization and hyperalgesia are most intense and prolonged when nerves are injured. Marked hyperexcitability occurs in outgrowing sprouts at sites of axonal injury and also in sensory somata in dorsal root ganglia

(14). This suggests that axonal injury may directly produce intracellular signals contributing to hypersensitivity and sprouting in the damaged mechanosensory neurons. Intrinsic axonal signals may complement extrinsic chemical signals, such as prostaglandins, received from other cells. Hyperexcitability of the soma has been reported following axotomy in many other neurons in various phyla (47). Thus, data from diverse species indicate that sensitizing changes can be produced by cellular injury or by signals closely associated with cellular injury. If true, some of these mechanisms might be very primitive.

It seems likely that the earliest animals were subject to injury by various biological and physical assaults (51). Adaptive responses to cellular injury may have been particularly useful in primary mechanosensory neurons (among the earliest neurons) (8), because their peripheral branches are exposed to surface trauma. Injury-induced adaptive responses to the destruction of peripheral sensory branches could include regenerative sprouting from axon stumps, collateral sprouting from undamaged branches of injured sensory neurons, and an increase in the sensitivity and signaling effectiveness of damaged and undamaged peripheral branches (as well as central soma and synapses) of the sensory neuron. All of these responses would help to maintain sensation in body surface partially deprived of sensory innervation. Furthermore, these responses might have evolved from primitive cellular repair and signal compensation mechanisms that were originally triggered directly by cellular injury (51).

One can begin to assess the relative contributions of homologous and analogous mechanisms to nociceptive sensitization in *Aplysia* and mammals by searching for the involvement of common molecular mediators. Too little is known about the underlying molecular mechanisms in either group to draw firm conclusions about the sources of functional similarities, but some interesting comparisons are beginning to emerge at these levels. One molecular difference is already apparent. In *Aplysia* and mammals repeated noxious stimulation causes a long-lasting, cumulative depolarization in various nociceptive neurons. Much of this depolarization in mammalian dorsal horn neurons is due to voltage-dependent unblocking of N-methyl-D-aspartate (NMDA) receptor-regulated ion channels (reviewed in ref. 57). However, NMDA receptors and voltage-dependent relief of Mg^{2+} block have not been described in invertebrates. This suggests that the NMDA receptor–ion channel complex may be a relatively recent evolutionary development.

On the other hand, there are some indications of common molecular mechanisms contributing to plasticity in these divergent groups. Perhaps the most interesting current candidates for conserved mechanisms involve two ubiquitous intracellular signaling systems, the Ca^{2+} and cAMP pathways.

cAMP, Ca^{2+}, AND NOCICEPTIVE PLASTICITY

Many of the short- and long-term effects of noxious stimulation in *Aplysia* nociceptors appear to be mediated by cAMP. Synthesis of this second messenger in nociceptors is stimulated by extrinsic neuromodulators such as 5-HT released after noxious stimulation (35). In activated cells undergoing ADEM, Ca^{2+} coming into the cell during each spike enhances adenylate cyclase activity (1,9), causing cAMP synthesis to be amplified. Via a protein kinase (A-kinase), cAMP rapidly reduces K^+ conductances (closing "S" K^+ channels and Ca^{2+}-dependent K^+ channels), thus enhancing excitability (reviewed in refs. 9,24,51). By delaying action potential re-polarization at presynaptic terminals, the reduction in K^+ conductance increases Ca^{2+} influx and transmitter release. Some effects of cAMP in *Aplysia* nociceptors have been shown to last for hours, days, or longer; these include enhanced soma excitability (43), synaptic facilitation (41), altered protein synthesis (17), and growth of varicosities (33).

cAMP may produce similar effects in vertebrate mechanosensory neurons. For example, it appears to mediate the peripheral sensitizing effects on primary sensory neurons of directly acting hyperalgesic agents (adenosine and various eicosanoid products of arachidonic acid) (45,46). cAMP has been implicated in depression of K^+ conductances in mechanosensory neuron somata of mouse (22), chick (15), and lamprey (56). Indirect evidence suggests that cAMP may also be involved in injury-related growth of axonal processes in vertebrate sensory neurons. Membrane-permeant cAMP analogs promote neurite extension in cultured embryonic rat sensory neurons (e.g., ref. 39). Moreover, regeneration of peripheral sensory nerves is as-sociated with increased adenylate cyclase activity, and this regeneration is enhanced by forskolin in frog and hamster nerves (26,27). It is not known if cAMP synthesis in vertebrate sensory neurons is activity dependent. However, adenylate cyclase in rat and bovine brain, as in *Aplysia* neurons, is regulated by Ca^{2+}-calmodulin (16), which suggests a capacity for activity dependence. An interesting observation in this regard is that collateral sprouting of rat nociceptors into denervated skin is enhanced by spike activity in central portions of the neurons (34). This suggests that ADEM in the dorsal root ganglia might be involved in the induction of peripheral growth (see discussion in ref. 5).

The limited data available from *Aplysia* and vertebrate sensory neurons suggest an overly simplistic, but testable model in which short- and long-term nociceptive plasticity are triggered by increases in intracellular levels of Ca^{2+} and cAMP (Fig. 4.8). The model is based on the idea that Ca^{2+} and cAMP are major signals for two complementary aspects of injury: (a) Ca^{2+} influx during spike activity provides in-jury information at the cellular level, informing an injured sensory neuron that it has been damaged and (b) cAMP synthesized in response to the binding of extracellular modulators provides information to each sensory neuron about the severity of injury at the tissue or organismic level.

The Ca^{2+} signal occurs at the site of peripheral damage, at the synapses, and within the soma of the damaged neuron. Locally, Ca^{2+} enters through ruptured mem-brane and (with Mg^{2+}) directly stimulates repair mechanisms (axon constriction and vesiculation), sealing ruptured membrane (18). Peripheral depolarization occurs, generating action potentials, which propagate to synapses, causing Ca^{2+} influx, syn-aptic transmission, and short-term synaptic plasticity (PTP). Ca^{2+} influx during ac-tion potentials also occurs in the soma, where it may regulate various Ca^{2+}-sensitive proteins, including transcription factors involved in long-term plasticity (32). The size of the Ca^{2+} signal in the soma and synapses will depend on the frequency and duration of injury-induced firing. Similar degrees of firing might, however, be pro-duced by either restricted or extensive damage to the peripheral arbor. Thus, the rapid Ca^{2+} signal in the soma may be an excellent signal for the occurrence of injury to peripheral branches of the cell, but it may be an unreliable indicator of the extent of peripheral injury.

The soma can estimate the extent of peripheral injury on the basis of two addi-tional sources of information. First, slow, cell-specific intra-axonal signals (the levels

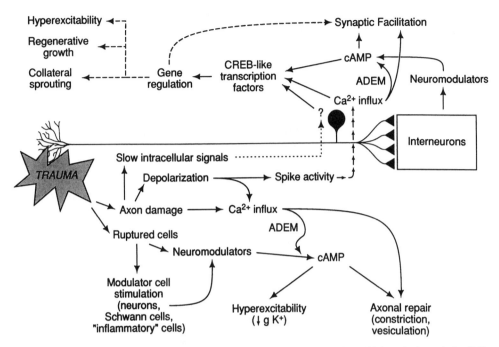

FIG. 4.8. A simple cAMP/Ca^{2+} convergence model for the induction of injury-induced plasticity in nociceptive sensory neurons. It is expected that other second and third messengers will also play important roles (see text). CREB-like transcription factors, nuclear proteins similar to the cAMP response element-binding proteins; ADEM, activity-dependent extrinsic modulation.

of which may directly reflect the extent of cellular injury) will eventually arrive from injured branches by retrograde axonal transport. Second, much more rapid signals are available from neuromodulators released onto mechanosensory neurons from modulatory neurons (including neuroendocrine cells) activated by input from nociceptors. These signals may be mediated intracellularly by various second messengers but, as discussed above, cAMP may be particularly important, at least in *Aplysia* nociceptors. The level of cAMP should indicate the extent of injury to the organism since the larger and more severe the injury to the animal, the greater the release of neuromodulators. A sensory neuron can use the Ca^{2+} signal to decide whether an injury involves its own peripheral arbor. It can then use the cAMP signal to estimate the severity of the injury at the organismic level. If there has been a severe injury and its own branches are involved, the cell can assume that the damage to its branches is likely to be extensive and rapidly alter protein synthesis (which occurs in the soma) to meet the anticipated cellular repair and signal compensation needs (5). Within a day or so, depending on the distance of the soma from the site of injury, the slow axonal injury signals will arrive to take over at least some of the regulation of adaptive changes in protein synthesis (52).

Neuromodulators are also released peripherally from ruptured cells, modulatory neurons (e.g., via axon reflexes or sympathetic terminals), Schwann cells, and inflammatory cells (hemocytes or immunocytes in invertebrates, see ref. 2). As in the soma, these neuromodulators probably stimulate the production of many different second messengers, but cAMP may play a particularly important role. cAMP synthesis is enhanced in active sensory neurons because of the Ca^{2+} sensitivity of adenylate cyclase (providing a mechanism for ADEM). As described above, cAMP rapidly causes a number of sensitizing effects in various parts of the sensory neuron, in addition to triggering long-term alterations.

Recent results suggest that long-term sensitization in *Aplysia* involves changes in gene expression induced by cAMP and that these effects of cAMP involve activation of a cAMP response element-binding (CREB) protein. CREB binds to the CRE DNA sequence, leading to an increase in transcription (12). The CRE sequence and at least one CREB protein appear to be very similar in molluscs and chordates. An interesting feature of the CREB protein is that it can be activated by either A-kinase or Ca^{2+}-calmodulin-dependent protein kinase II, and CREB activity is stimulated in an additive manner when the CREB protein is phosphorylated by both kinases (13). Therefore, this transcription activator is a convergence point for cAMP and Ca^{2+}. Because serious injury involving damage to the neuron's peripheral arbor should result in high levels of both Ca^{2+} and cAMP, the CREB protein is in an ideal position to sum these messages and initiate long-term, adaptive responses by gene regulation. Given that noxious stimulation may lead to the activation of other signals inside *Aplysia* sensory neurons, such as C-kinase (40), it is interesting that the CREB protein is also phosphorylated by C-kinase and casein kinase II. It should be kept in mind, however, that the CRE sequence is probably just one of many sites that can regulate gene expression in response to second and third messengers activated by noxious stimulation.

The $cAMP/Ca^{2+}$ convergence hypothesis is highly speculative, and many of the supporting data are indirect. For example, many of the biophysical and biochemical studies were performed in isolated, cultured neurons. Nonetheless, this hypothesis shows that novel molecular predictions can emerge from considering the possibility that some mechanisms of hyperalgesia are primitive and widely distributed in the animal kingdom. Given the analytic advantages of simpler nervous systems and the power of comparative approaches, examination of such hypotheses in a variety of species may prove useful for efforts to decipher cellular and molecular mechanisms underlying hyperalgesia and allodynia.

ACKNOWLEDGMENTS

I am grateful to Drs. Pramod Dash and Andrea Clatworthy for comments on the ideas presented in this chapter. Supported by National Institute of Mental Health grant MH38726 and National Science Foundation grant BNS9011907.

REFERENCES

1. Abrams, T. W., and Kandel, E. R. (1988): Is contiguity detection in classical conditioning a system or a cellular property? Learning in *Aplysia* suggests a possible molecular site. *Trends Neurosci.*, 11:128–135.
2. Alizadeh, H., Clatworthy, A. L., Castro, G. A., and Walters, E. T. (1990): Induction of an immune reaction in *Aplysia* is accompanied by long-term enhancement of sensory neuron excitability. *Soc. Neurosci. Abstr.*, 15:597.
3. Bailey, C. H., and Chen, M. (1983): Morphological basis of long-term habituation and sensitization in *Aplysia*. *Science*, 220:91–93.
4. Bailey, C. H., and Chen, M. (1988): Long-term memory in *Aplysia* modulates the total number of varicosities of single identified sensory neurons. *Proc. Natl. Acad. Sci. USA*, 85:2373–2377.

5. Billy, A. J., and Walters, E. T. (1989): Long-term expansion and sensitization of mechanosensory receptive fields in *Aplysia* support an activity-dependent model of whole-cell sensory plasticity. *J. Neurosci.*, 9:1254–1262.
6. Bolles, R. C., and Fanselow, M. S. (1980): A perceptual-defensive-recuperative model of fear and pain. *Behav. Brain Sci.*, 3:291–323.
7. Boulis, N. M., and Sahley, C. L. (1988): A behavioral analysis of habituation and sensitization of shortening in the semi-intact leech. *J. Neurosci.*, 8:4621–4627.
8. Bullock, T. H., and Horridge, G. A. (1965): *Structure and function in the nervous systems of invertebrates*. W. H. Freeman, San Francisco.
9. Byrne, J. H. (1987): Cellular analysis of associative learning. *Physiol. Rev.*, 67:329–439.
10. Clatworthy, A. L., and Walters, E. T. (1988): Sensitization and sensory signals in *Aplysia*. II. Modulation of central bursting and spike conduction. *Soc. Neurosci. Abstr.*, 14:609.
11. Curio, E. (1976): *The ethology of predation*. Springer-Verlag, Berlin.
12. Dash, P. K., Hochner, B., and Kandel, E. R. (1990): Injection of the cAMP-responsive element into the nucleus of *Aplysia* sensory neurons blocks long-term facilitation. *Nature*, 345:718–721.
13. Dash, P. K., Karl, K. A., Colicos, M. A., Prywes, R., and Kandel, E. R. (1991): cAMP response element-binding protein is activated by Ca^{2+}/calmodulin- as well as cAMP-dependent protein kinase. *Proc. Natl. Acad. Sci. USA*, 88:5061–5065.
14. Devor, M. (1989): The pathophysiology of damaged peripheral nerves. In: *Textbook of pain*, edited by P. D. Wall and R. Melzack, pp. 63–435. Churchill Livingstone, London.
15. Dunlap, K. (1985): Forskolin prolongs action potential duration and blocks potassium current in embryonic chick sensory neurons. *Pflugers Arch.*, 403:170–174.
16. Eliot, L. S., Dudai, Y., Kandel, E. R., and Abrams, T. W. (1989): Ca^{2+}/calmodulin sensitivity may be common to all forms of neural adenylate cyclase. *Proc. Natl. Acad. Sci. USA*, 86:9564–9568.
17. Eskin, A., Garcia, K. S., and Byrne, J. H. (1989): Information storage in the nervous system of *Aplysia*: specific proteins affected by serotonin and cAMP. *Proc. Natl. Acad. Sci. USA*, 86:2458–2462.
18. Fishman, H. M., Tewari, K. P., and Stein, P. G. (1990): Injury-induced vesiculation and membrane redistribution in squid giant axon. *Biochim. Biophys. Acta*, 1023:421–435.
19. Frost, W. N., Castellucci, V. F., Hawkins, R. D., and Kandel, E. R. (1985): Monosynaptic connections made by the sensory neurons of the gill- and siphon-withdrawal reflex in *Aplysia* participate in the storage of long-term memory for sensitization. *Proc. Natl. Acad. Sci. USA*, 82:8266–8269.
20. Frost, W. N., Clark, G. A., and Kandel, E. R. (1988): Parallel processing of short-term memory for sensitization in *Aplysia*. *J. Neurobiol.*, 19:297–334.
21. Glanzman, D. L., Mackey, S. L., Hawkins, R. D., Dyke, A. M., Lloyd, P. E., and Kandel, E. R. (1989): Depletion of serotonin in the nervous system of *Aplysia* reduces the behavioral enhancement of gill withdrawal as well as the heterosynaptic facilitation produced by tail shock. *J. Neurosci.*, 9:4200–4213.
22. Grega, D. S., and Macdonald, R. L. (1987): Activators of adenylate cyclase and cyclic AMP prolong calcium-dependent action potentials of mouse sensory neurons in culture by reducing a voltage-dependent potassium conductance. *J. Neurosci.*, 7:700–707.
23. Hille, B. (1987): Evolutionary origins of voltage-gated channels and synaptic transmission. In: *Synaptic function*, edited by G. M. Edelman, W. E. Gall, and W. M. Cowan, pp. 163–176. John Wiley, New York.
24. Kandel, E. R., and Schwartz, J. H. (1982): Molecular biology of learning: modulation of transmitter release. *Science*, 218:433–444.
25. Kavaliers, M. (1988): Evolutionary and comparative aspects of nociception. *Brain Res. Bull.*, 21:923–931.
26. Kilmer, S. L., and Carlsen, R. C. (1984): Forskolin activation of adenylate cyclase *in vivo* stimulates nerve regeneration. *Nature*, 307:455–457.
27. Klein, H. W., Kilmer, S., and Carlsen, R. C. (1989): Enhancement of peripheral nerve regeneration by pharmacological activation of the cyclic AMP second messenger system. *Microsurgery*, 10:122–125.
28. Krasne, F. B., and Glanzman, D. L. (1986): Sensitization of the crayfish lateral giant escape response. *J. Neurosci.*, 6:1013–1020.
29. Lapage, G. (1958): *Parasitic animals*. Cambridge University Press, Cambridge.
30. Meglitsch, P. A., and Schram, F. R. (1991): *Invertebrate zoology*. Oxford University Press, New York.
31. Merskey, H. (1986): Pain terms: a current list with definitions and notes on usage. *Pain*, suppl. 3:S216–S221.
32. Morgan, J. I., and Curran, T. (1989): Stimulus-transcription coupling in neurons: role of cellular immediate-early genes. *Trends Neurosci.*, 12:459–462.
33. Nazif, F., Byrne, J. H., and Cleary, L. J. (1991): cAMP induces long-term morphological changes in sensory neurons of *Aplysia*. *Brain Res.*, 539:324–327.

34. Nixon, B. J., Doucette, R., Jackson, P. C., and Diamond, J. (1984): Impulse activity evokes precocious sprouting of nociceptive nerves into denervated skin. *Somatosens. Res.*, 2:97–126.
35. Ocorr, K. A., Tabata, M., and Byrne, J. H. (1986): Stimuli that produce sensitization lead to elevation of cyclic AMP levels in tail sensory neurons of *Aplysia. Brain Res.*, 371:190–192.
36. Pinsker, H. M., Hening, W. A., Carew, T. J., and Kandel, E. R. (1973): Long-term sensitization of a defensive withdrawal reflex in *Aplysia. Science*, 182:1039–1042.
37. Razran, G. (1971): *An east-west synthesis of learned behavior and cognition.* Houghton Mifflin, Boston.
38. Roitt, I. M., Brostoff, J., and Male, D. K. (1989): *Immunology.* C. V. Mosby, St. Louis.
39. Rydel, R. E., and Greene, L. A. (1988): cAMP analogs promote survival and neurite outgrowth in cultures of rat sympathetic and sensory neurons independently of nerve growth factor. *Proc. Natl. Acad. Sci. USA*, 85:1257–1261.
40. Sacktor, T. C., and Schwartz, J. H. (1990): Sensitizing stimuli cause translocation of protein kinase C in *Aplysia* sensory neurons. *Proc. Natl. Acad. Sci. USA*, 87:2036–2039.
41. Schacher, S., Castellucci, V. F., and Kandel, E. R. (1988): cAMP evokes long-term facilitation in *Aplysia* sensory neurons that requires new protein synthesis. *Science*, 240:1667–1669.
42. Scholz, K. P., and Byrne, J. H. (1987): Long-term sensitization in *Aplysia*: biophysical correlates in tail sensory neurons. *Science*, 235:685–687.
43. Scholz, K. P., and Byrne, J. H. (1988): Intracellular injection of cAMP induces a long-term reduction of neuronal K+ currents. *Science*, 240:1664–1666.
44. Sherrington, C. S. (1947): *The integrative action of the nervous system.* Cambridge University Press, Cambridge.
45. Taiwo, Y. O., Bjerknes, L. K., Goetzl, E. J., and Levine, J. D. (1989): Mediation of primary afferent peripheral hyperalgesia by the cAMP second messenger system. *Neuroscience* 32:577–580.
46. Taiwo, Y. O., and Levine, J. D. (1990): Direct cutaneous hyperalgesia induced by adenosine. *Neuroscience*, 38:757–762.
47. Titmus, M. J., and Faber, D. S. (1990): Axotomy-induced alterations in the electrophysiological characteristics of neurons. *Prog. Neurobiol.*, 35:1–51.
48. Wall, P. D. (1979): On the relation of injury to pain. *Pain*, 6:253–264.
49. Walters, E. T. (1987): Site-specific sensitization of defensive reflexes in *Aplysia*: a simple model of long-term hyperalgesia. *J. Neurosci.*, 7:400–407.
50. Walters, E. T. (1987): Multiple sensory neuronal correlates of site-specific sensitization in *Aplysia. J. Neurosci.*, 7:408–417.
51. Walters, E. T. (1991): A functional, cellular, and evolutionary model of nociceptive plasticity in *Aplysia. Biol. Bull.*, 180:241–251.
52. Walters, E. T., Alizadeh, H., and Castro, G. A. (1991): Similar neuronal alterations induced by axonal injury and learning in *Aplysia. Science*, 253:797–799.
53. Walters, E. T., and Byrne, J. H. (1983): Slow depolarization produced by associative conditioning of *Aplysia* sensory neurons may enhance Ca^{2+} entry. *Brain Res.*, 280:165–168.
54. Wells, M. J. (1975): Evolution and associative learning. In: *"Simple" nervous systems*, edited by P. N. R. Usherwood and D. R. Newth, pp. 445–473. Crane-Russak, New York.
55. Willmer, P. (1990): *Invertebrate relationships: patterns in animal evolution.* Cambridge University Press, Cambridge.
56. Womble, M. D., and Wickelgren, W. O. (1989): Activation of adenylate cyclase by forskolin prolongs calcium action potential duration in lamprey sensory neurons. *Brain Res.*, 485:89–94.
57. Woolf, C. J., and Walters, E. T. (1991): Common patterns of plasticity contributing to nociceptive sensitization in mammals and *Aplysia. Trends Neurosci.*, 14:74–78.

Hyperalgesia and Allodynia,
edited by W. D. Willis, Jr.
Raven Press, Ltd., New York © 1992.

5

Alterations in the Responsiveness of Cutaneous Nociceptors

Sensitization by Noxious Stimuli and the Induction of Adrenergic Responsiveness by Nerve Injury

*Department of Physiology, University of North Carolina at Chapel Hill,
Chapel Hill, North Carolina 27599*

Primary afferent neurons ("receptors") strongly activated by innocuous events typically give a lessened response (habituate) on repeated stimulation, a feature noted in early electrophysiological recordings from single afferent fibers. The cycle of recovery to maximal ("rested") responsiveness for repeated identical stimuli varies substantially with the type of sensory unit (3). An example of marked habituation on stimulus repetition for a myelinated fiber "touch receptor," of the type associated with Haarscheibe, appears in Fig. 5.1. Habituation is not characteristic only of mechanoreceptors. The responses of a cutaneous C-fiber warming unit with an unmyelinated afferent fiber in Fig. 5.2 are substantially lessened to repetition of a warming sequence than appeared initially. Thus, habituation to repeated stimuli is neither a function of the general class of cutaneous sensory unit nor a feature directly determined by the size of the afferent fiber in a peripheral nerve.

SENSITIZATION OF CUTANEOUS NOCICEPTORS

Early work in defining cutaneous nociceptors that were promptly excited by noxious heating uncovered a sharp contrast to habituation (2,43). The cutaneous C-fiber units called polymodal nociceptors (CPMs) have thresholds for heating and mechanical stimuli substantially higher than those of a number of other types of afferent units innervating the same skin areas and give graded responses to overtly tissue-damaging intensities of mechanical, heat, and irritant chemical stimuli. Ordinarily, CPMs have no ongoing or background discharge in the absence of prior activation, one of several features setting them apart from "specific" thermoreceptors that usually exhibit considerable ongoing discharge at physiological skin temperatures. On the other hand, many CPMs develop ongoing discharge after a single vigorous activation; a striking example is shown in Fig. 5.3A for the initial activation of a cat

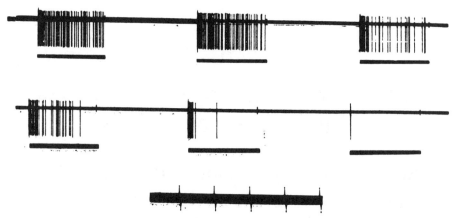

FIG. 5.1. Responses elicited from a cutaneous type I receptor with a myelinated afferent fiber by identical successive stimuli to a receptive spot illustrating habituation. The duration of the mechanical stimuli is shown by the horizontal bars. Time marker shows 1-sec pulses. (From ref. 23.)

CPM from hairy skin. Notably, the majority of CPM units, on repeated heating, give more vigorous responses at particular cutaneous temperatures than on first stimulation. Figure 5.3B and C illustrates this in plots of discharge frequency as a function of temperature for a first and second heating of a cat CPM. These phenomena are not species specific. A similar type of C-fiber nociceptor in monkey hairy skin also typically shows enhanced responses with repeated heat activation (28,29). The difference in response for the initial exposure of the CPM unit to noxious heat in Fig.

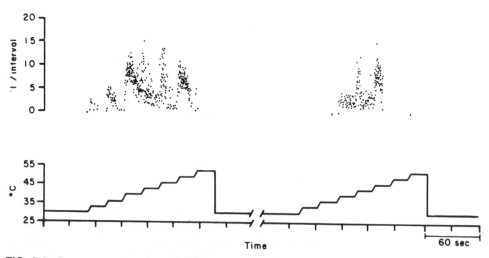

FIG. 5.2. Responses of a warming receptor to the increases in thermode temperature from 30° to 51°C as shown in the *lower trace*. Each *dot* represents an impulse plotted as 1/interval from the previous impulse. A second heating sequence was repeated 5 min after the first. (From ref. 51.)

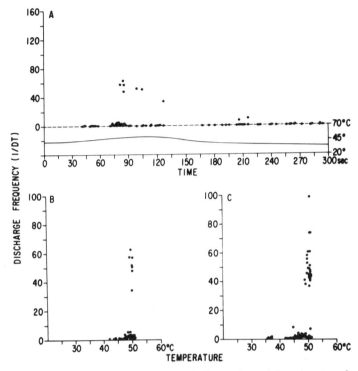

FIG. 5.3. Responses to heating of a cutaneous C-fiber polymodal nociceptor of cat hairy skin. **A:** Instantaneous frequency indicated by *dots* above the *broken line* (as in the convention of Fig. 5.2) and thermode temperature by the *solid line* below it. **B:** Replot of the initial 150 sec of A as 1/interval as a function of thermode temperature. **C:** The first 150 sec of a second initial heating test plotted as in B. (From ref. 43.)

5.4A and those to the third (Fig. 5.4B) and fifth (Fig. 5.4C) cycle of stimulation documents a dramatic increase in the number of impulses and discharge frequency with stimulus repetition.

Increases in responsiveness of cutaneous nociceptors on repeated activation is not a feature unique to cutaneous CPMs. Fitzgerald and Lynn (15) showed that myelinated fiber mechanical nociceptors of the skin, which do not respond promptly to heat initially, become responsive to heat upon prolonged or repeated stimuli. Activity generated by these mechanical nociceptors is also enhanced after further repetition of cutaneous heating (Fig. 5.5).

Decreases of nociceptor threshold often occur as a result of repeated heat stimuli. Figure 5.6A graphs the discharge frequency of a cat CPM as a function of time in parallel with a stepped heating stimulus. Figure 5.6B redisplays these data in a plot of discharge frequency as a function of temperature; all discharges except one occurring during the cooling phase were evoked in the last step heat increase to about 52°C. Application of the same heating sequence a second time (Fig. 5.6C) evoked discharges at lower temperatures. A third repetition of the temperature stimulus (Fig. 5.6D) produced essentially the same discharge pattern as that which appeared at a 5° lower temperature than during the first trial. The initiation of background discharge after heat stimuli complicates estimation of threshold CPM alterations in

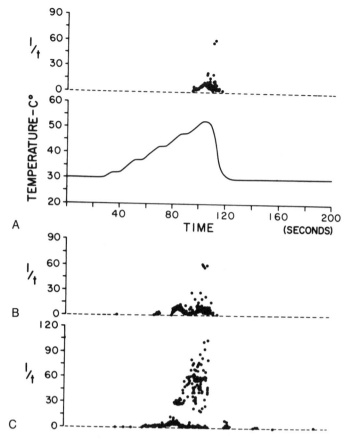

FIG. 5.4. Responses of a primate CPM to repeated noxious heating of the receptive field with a small contact thermode. Plots constructed as in Fig. 5.2. The illustrated sequence of temperature increase and sudden cooling was repeated at 200-sec intervals. **A,** first heating cycle; **B,** third heating cycle; **C,** fifth heating cycle. Plots were aligned by superimposing the analogue records of the heating cycle. (From ref. 28.)

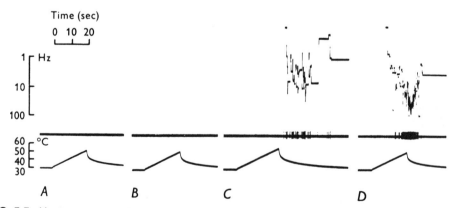

FIG. 5.5. Heat responses of rabbit high-threshold mechanoreceptor with a myelinated afferent fiber. **A,B:** Two heat stimuli to 50°C fail to produce any firing. **C:** Heat stimulus terminating at 55°C evokes discharges immediately after the heating ceased. **D:** Fourth stimulus to 50°C evokes a vigorous discharge both during heating and for some seconds afterward. *Bottom traces,* Thermode-skin temperature; *middle traces,* action potentials recorded from the sural nerve; *top traces,* (C and D), instantaneous frequency of the discharges. (From ref. 15.)

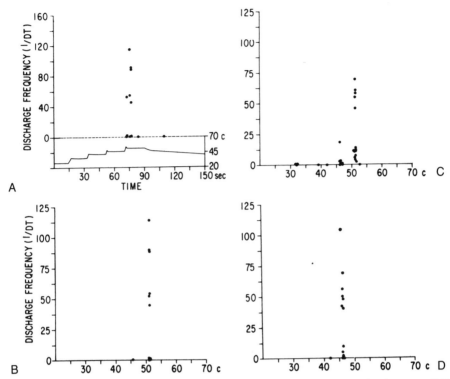

FIG. 5.6. Discharges of a cat CPM during successive cycles of skin heating by a small ther- mode. Nerve discharges plotted as in Fig. 5.2. **B:** "Instantaneous" discharge frequency (ver- tical axis) as a function of thermode temperature for the test shown in **A** (see Fig. 5.2); **C:** Plot of second heat test identical to A 150 sec after A. **D:** Plot of third heat test (150 sec) during which the highest temperature was 5°C lower than for A–C. (From ref. 2.)

many cases. To provide insight into the range of modification of both overall re- sponse and threshold, observations on five primate CPM units from hairy skin with low background discharge even after repeated cycles of exposure to noxious heat are shown in Fig. 5.7. A progressively larger number of impulses were generated in all five units for three repetitions of a stereotyped thermal cycle, although when a fourth and fifth cycle were used, the increase was either less notable or replaced by a decrease relative to the third stimulation (Fig. 5.7A). Threshold (Fig. 5.7B) for these same five units judged by the first impulse after the beginning of the increasing temperature sequence (as in Fig. 5.4) also showed progressive decreases with re- peated heating, although the magnitude and progression of the threshold changes varied considerably from one unit to another. These changes are noteworthy from the viewpoint of possible relationships between afferent messages from a class of sensory units and sensory experience.

Enhanced responsiveness and a lowering of threshold of cutaneous nociceptors certainly are consonant with a link to primary cutaneous hyperalgesia of the type associated with inflammation-producing injury and inflammatory responses. The ap- pearance of background activity must also be considered as a factor in pain in the absence of external stimulation from injured tissue or inflamed tissues. Sensitization

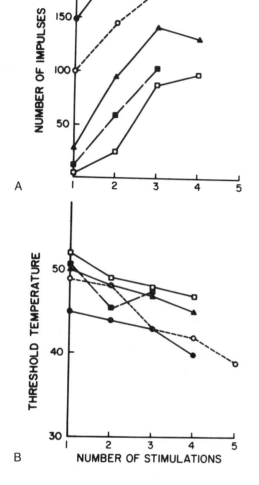

FIG. 5.7. Effects on primate CPMs of repeated exposure to noxious heat. Heating of the receptive field as Fig. 5.4A was repeated every 200 sec using a small contact probe covering the receptive field for mechanical stimuli. As in Fig. 5.4, the maximal temperature was about 53°C. Each symbol refers to a different unit; a given symbol identifies the same unit in both parts. **A:** Total number of impulses recorded during the heating cycle are plotted as a function of the cycle sequence. **B:** Threshold temperature for evoked discharge (one impulse during a temperature step). The five units had low background discharge rates throughout (>1/10 sec). (From ref. 28.)

as a phenomenon appears to set nociceptors apart from low-threshold sense organs of the same tissues.

Do sensitization and the changes it reflects indicate that nociceptors are not subject to habituation and fatigue? Not at all, and this has been a consideration associated with misunderstanding. Some time ago it was pointed out that, although at times obscured by the processes of sensitization, CPMs and other cutaneous nociceptors exhibit distinct habituation or fatigue (2,28). An indication of this appears in Fig. 5.7A for two units (filled circles and filled triangles) by the lesser responses they exhibit in the last test(s) of the responses to heating than in the previous. An example of the interplay between the enhanced responsiveness in sensitization and habituation/fatigue appears in the evoked activity of the monkey CPM unit of Fig. 5.8; the total number of impulses generated during stereotyped heating cycles repeated at various intervals is plotted. The progressively increased numbers of impulses generated in the first three of a sequence of rapidly (ca. 3 min) repeated heating cycles

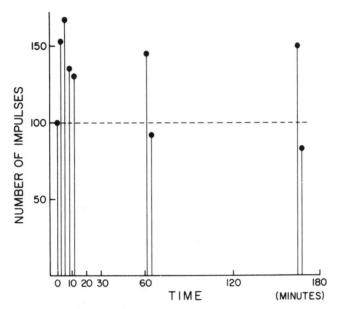

FIG. 5.8. A primate CPM response to repeated, identical noxious heat stimulation cycles. A small contact thermode was rigidly fixed on the receptive field (see Fig. 5.4). The minimal interval between cycles was 200 sec. Each *filled circle* indicates the total number of impulses for the 180 sec beginning with the start of the stepwise heating as a function of time relative to the time of the first stimulation. *Dotted horizontal line* indicates the response to the first cycle. (From ref. 28.)

were followed by return toward initial levels in the fourth and fifth cycles, presumably due to fatigue. A rest (no stimulation) of approximately 50 min resulted in an apparent return of the enhanced responsiveness seen in the second and third trials; however, retesting about 3 min later reduced the response to the control level. This sequence of regained enhanced responsiveness and its disappearance on quick retrial repeated after another protracted period without stimulation. Thus, nociceptors may sensitize but they also exhibit habituation and/or fatigue. Moreover, similar to other sense organs, their receptive characteristics can be deactivated by stimuli strong enough to destroy the receptive terminals (not shown), which also may mask sensitization.

Deactivation of the receptive apparatus is sometimes not given proper attention when stimuli to different cutaneous tissues and subcutaneous tissues are compared arbitrarily on the basis of physical measures of intensity. The various tissues of intact mammals in ordinary life are not subject to identical external circumstances and the afferent units terminating in each tissue appear adapted to respond to levels of stimuli common for the host tissue. In other words, what is noxious for one region of skin or tissue may not be tissue threatening for another.

MECHANISMS OF NOCICEPTOR SENSITIZATION

Given that nociceptors are by definition most effectively excited by near-damaging or frankly damaging stimuli, a possible relationship to another process regularly associated with such events, inflammation, has provided clues to the underlying mechanisms. The inflammatory process is complex. The changes involved include dilation of blood vessels with an associated increased local blood flow, the extravasation of plasma into the extracellular space, and a substantial aggregation and enhanced activity of certain white blood cells. The extensively documented importance of diffusible agents in mediating the vascular and cellular aspects of inflammation (17,20) inspired us to examine the possible contributions of some of these same substances to the sensitization of cutaneous nociceptors. Our attention was directed to exploration of mechanisms by which a noxious stimulus at one point of the skin could modify the responsiveness of receptor whose peripheral receptive field was located nearby because of a common appearance of background discharge in nociceptive units with receptive fields bordering areas of frank tissue damage (44). Such lateral spread of a sensitizing influence may be related to skin type (6,15).

Our early descriptions of sensitization lumped enhanced response, lowering of threshold, and initiation of ongoing discharge (2). On the other hand, subsequent observations suggested that dissociation of the evoked response from ongoing activity could occur. For instance, repeated, exceptionally strong stimulation of the receptive field sometimes resulted in cessation of responses to previously adequate stimuli for protected periods while the ongoing activity persisted. On occasion, the converse also was observed, that is, enhancement of responsiveness without a concomitant or parallel increase in background discharge. The five primate CPM units of Fig. 5.7 are examples (background for each after several trials of noxious heat stimulation was under 1 impulse/10 sec). Such dissociation may reflect different processes in the generation of evoked and background impulses or different loci for initiation of ongoing and stimulus-initiated impulses.

The putative involvement of cellular and chemical constituents of blood in the initiation and maintenance of changes associated with inflammation (17) raises the issue of blood as a source of agents leading to sensitization of nociceptors. For this reason, we turned to an *in vitro* preparation of the rabbit ear, perfused through the great auricular artery with an oxygenated substitute for serum, to further study nociceptor sensitization, a preparation permitting minimal trauma in immediate vicinity of receptive field region. CPMs of the *in vitro* rabbit ear are remarkably similar to those found *in vivo* (8,44,51). *In vitro* determined thresholds, mechanical and heat-evoked responses and heat-evoked sensitization appear essentially the same as those *in vivo* in the hairy skin of the hindlimb of other mammals (8,44,51). Figure 5.9 shows the discharge pattern of a CPM recorded *in vitro* to repeated heat stimulation cycles. The enhanced response for the second cycle of stimulation compared to the first is evident as is the notable increase in ongoing discharge during the periods when the cutaneous temperature was unchanging. Thus, circulating blood was not essential for either the enhanced response or the ongoing activity. However, the possibility that blood-borne agents were somehow involved could not be completely eliminated because even after several hours of perfusion with an artificial, acellular solution, some blood constituents probably remain in the tissue.

Figure 5.10 provides a quantitative description of the range of CPM sensitization *in vitro* using the thermal test of Fig. 5.9; the total number of impulses generated during each of a succession of heating trials repeated at 10-min intervals is pictured for a series of units relative to those generated in the first trial. In Fig. 5.10 the results from each unit are arranged arbitrarily from the smallest difference between the first and subsequent tests to the largest. This manipulation shows that enhancement of the number of impulses generated by a stereotyped noxious heat sequence is regular

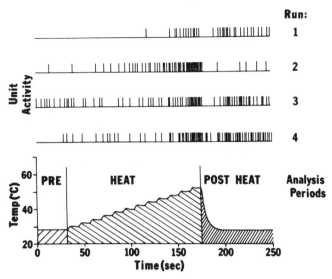

FIG. 5.9. Example of responses of a rabbit CPM from the great auricular nerve recorded *in vitro* to repeated heating–cooling cycles. Lines labeled 1–4 show discharges recorded as a function of time in successive trials at 10-min intervals. The lowest graph illustrates the stimulus temperature sequence for each trial. Periods PRE, HEAT, and POST HEAT mark phases used for analyses (see Table 5.1, Figs. 5.10–5.13; ref. 16). (From ref. 8.)

but quite variable from one unit to another under conditions in which care is taken not to destroy the terminal tissue by suprathreshold temperatures.

One approach to the question of a chemical mediator in sensitization is to apply substances locally or through the vasculature and examine their effect on responsiveness. Although the method can establish the capacity of an individual agent to produce a change in the target, it does not prove that the substance in question is actually involved in a biological process. This caveat particularly applies when the quantities of an agent required for effective action appear to be many times greater than could be expected in life. An alternative is to use more or less selective antagonists or blocking substances to dissect out the contribution of particular mediators. The combination of both agonist and antagonist manipulations can provide convincing evidence that particular substances and their cellular receptors are involved in a process.

A variety of substances have been shown to be produced or released when tissue is injured; these include but are not limited to increased concentrations of K^+, kinins such as bradykinin, histamine, serotonin, and various breakdown products of arachidonic acid including prostaglandins and leukotrienes. All of these have the potential directly or indirectly to influence the excitability of nerve terminals. Bradykinin in particular has been the subject of considerable interest, both because it is algogenic and, as shown by a number of investigations, can directly excite discharges from nociceptors. Interestingly, Szolcsányi (55) reported that of the various sensory units in the rabbit ear, only CPM units were excited by bradykinin in concentrations as low as one might expect to find in injured tissues. Other chapters in this volume will deal explicitly with bradykinin effects. The following concentrates on the parts played by other possible chemical mediators in sensitization.

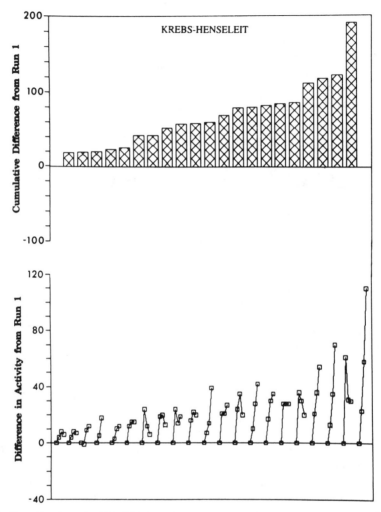

FIG. 5.10. Sensitization of rabbit CPMs recorded *in vitro* under control conditions. **Upper:** Net (algebraic sum) difference (±) between impulses evoked during the first stepwise heating sequence and impulses evoked during subsequent (2, 3, and 4) repetitions for each unit (*vertical bars*). **Bottom:** For each unit the difference between the number of impulses evoked during the heat period in every trial relative to the first trial. The value for the first of four trials (*interconnected squares*) for each unit was taken as the base (0 difference). To illustrate the range of variation, data from individual CPMs are arranged left to right according to the magnitude of net difference. (From ref. 8.)

ARACHIDONIC ACID METABOLITES

A considerable body of medical and common experience has shown that aspirin, indomethacin, and a number of other nonsteroidal agents suppress inflammation and the pain associated with it. It is broadly accepted that the mechanism of such nonsteroidal anti-inflammatory action is through the suppression of prostaglandin formation in the metabolism of arachidonic acid (4,17), although some argue that the evidence is not sufficient to preclude other mechanisms (17). Prostaglandins of the

E category (PGEs) appear in tissue fluids after burn and other injuries (12,13,25,26) but do not necessarily directly initiate pain (9,12,21) or excite sensory neurons (31). On the other hand, PGEs are reported to sensitize some CPMs (18,37) and to induce hyperalgesia in experimental situations (12,14,40). We recently showed that nonsteroidal anti-inflammatory agents (NSAIDs) established to inhibit prostaglandin formation by the cyclooxygenase pathway suppressed heat-induced sensitization of cutaneous CPMs *in vitro* (8). Figure 5.11 summarizes the suppression of sensitization by indomethacin and dipyrone in some but not all CPM units (cf. Figs. 5.10 and 5.11). Indomethacin at two concentrations (3 and 28 μm) and dipyrone (1 mm) blocked sensitization in about one-half of the tested units, whereas the other part of the test group continued to show a pattern and magnitude of sensitization similar to those exhibited by controls. Close examination of the results from individual units in Fig. 5.11 (lower) shows that in the presence of either NSAID, sensitization was blocked for some units, whereas others, after an enhanced response to a second test, gave lesser responses in further trials. In addition to prostaglandins, another major

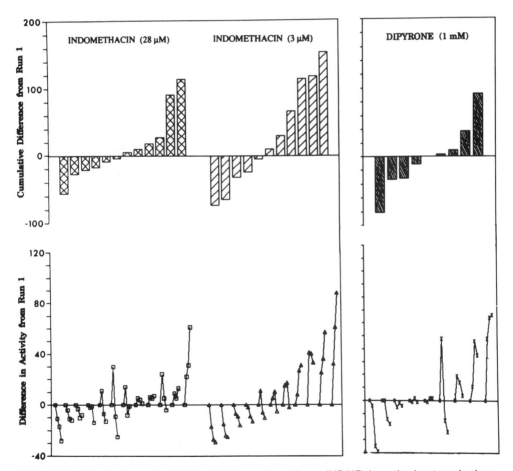

FIG. 5.11. Effects of nonsteroidal anti-inflammatory drugs (NSAIDs) on the heat-evoked activity of CPMs. See fig. 5.10 for conventions. Agents and doses given above each set of observations (bar graphs above and interconnected symbols below). (From ref. 8.)

group of eicosanoids, the leukotrienes, stem from arachidonic acid by way of the lipoxygenase metabolic path. Both reduction (50) and enhancement of nociceptive activity (37) by leukotrienes have been reported. In the absence of access to a selective lipoxygenase inhibitor, we used an agent (BW755C) reported to have significant suppressive actions on both cyclooxygenase and lipoxygenase pathways to challenge sensitization. The results obtained with BW755C (Fig. 5.12) were comparable to those seen for presumed selective cyclooxygenase suppressors. To the extent that BW755C blocks leukotriene production, these observations suggest that the latter's contribution to the sensitization process of CPMs is small. In contrast, prostaglandins appear to participate directly or indirectly to sensitization for some, but not all, cutaneous sensory units classified as CPMs.

The results shown in Figs. 5.11 and 5.12 offer a possible explanation for previous failures to demonstrate effects of indomethacin alone on sensitization (27,44), since in those earlier analyses only averages of the response of a population of units were compared. Given the apparent separation of CPM units into two groups in recent work (8), one set in which several NSAIDs blocked sensitization and another in

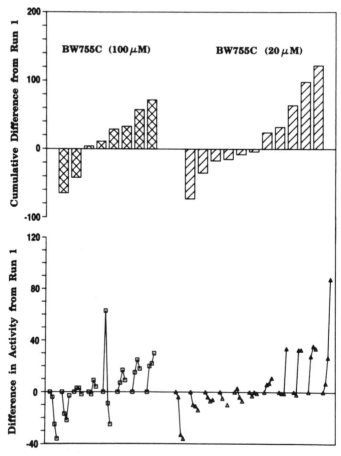

FIG. 5.12. Effects of a dual cyclooxygenase/lipoxygenase inhibitor, BW755C, on the heat-evoked activity of rabbit CPMs *in vitro*. See Figs. 5.10 and 5.11 for conventions. (From ref. 8.)

which sensitization was not notably affected, conclusions similar to those reached earlier would have again been drawn had the data been pooled. These results imply the existence of more than one process or mechanism leading to sensitization of CPMs and possibly other cutaneous nociceptors. The observations also with NSAIDs appear consistent with the finding that injection of PGEs sensitizes or enhances the response of only some C-fiber nociceptors (18,37).

The split in the actions of prostaglandins and prostaglandin inhibitors in terms of the C-fiber nociceptor population has implications for hyperalgesia and the treatment of inflammatory pain. Clinical experience amply documents the inability of NSAIDs to alleviate some types of pain of peripheral tissue origin. There is also good evidence for the existence of several types of nociceptors with substantially different signaling characteristics and responsiveness to specific stimuli (5,45,55). Therefore, only part of the population of afferent units with probable importance in cutaneous

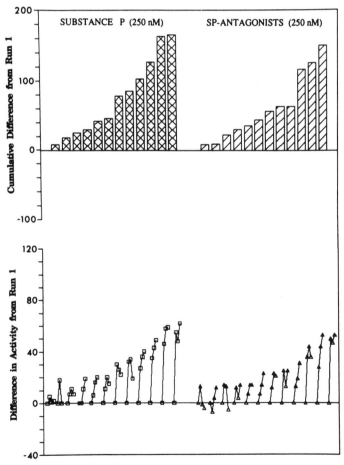

FIG. 5.13. Effects of substance P (SP) and SP-antagonists (dPdT)-SP or (dPPdT)-SP, on the heat-evoked activity of rabbit CPMs recorded *in vitro*. See Figs. 5.10 and 5.11 for conventions. Observations for the two SP-antagonists (see text) were combined since no difference between them was found. (From ref. 8.)

pain would have enhanced responsiveness suppressed by NSAIDs. Looked upon in another way, these data suggest the presence of two in some way similar but not identical C-fiber cutaneous nociceptors that exhibit prompt responses to both mechanical and heat stimuli.

Substance P

Vasodilation and fluid extravasation are prominent features of acute inflammation. Both changes have been known for years to follow antidromic stimulation of unmyelinated afferent fibers. These antidromic nerve effects are argued to be produced through the intermediary of the release of substance P (SP) from the peripheral terminals of the unmyelinated fibers (19,32–34,36,42,56). While SP itself is not pain producing (54), it has been reported to have a weak excitatory effect on nociceptors (16,30,39). The vasodilation and plasma extravasation evoked by antidromic C-fiber activation can be blocked by inactive SP analogues (34). For these reasons, we tested the possible contribution of SP to CPM sensitization (8). Using the experimental arrangement employed for testing the NSAIDs, concentrations of SP shown to produce vasodilation and loss of fluid from the vasculature, given intra-arterially during the heat stimulation testing of a series of CPMs, did not notably affect sensitization (Fig. 5.13). Similarly, inactive SP analogues that effectively antagonize the vascular changes induced by antidromic impulses in C-fibers produced no evident change in sensitization evoked by repeated noxious heat stimulation (Fig. 5.13, right panel). In the *in vitro* preparation, the weak excitatory effects reported for SP itself were not evident, although some units had an ongoing discharge after several exposures to heat that appeared greater than for the control population. Thus, SP directly or indirectly does not appear to be a major factor in cutaneous sensitization, at least in the absence of blood-borne elements.

INJURY OF PERIPHERAL NERVES

Injury of peripheral nerves, particularly relatively large mixed nerves of the limbs or bodily injuries that involve a substantial distribution of peripheral nerves, are sometimes followed by aberrant pain syndromes. The pain is usually described as having a burning quality, initially referred to the region innervated by damaged nerves and was given the name causalgia in the descriptions by Weir Mitchell et al. (38) from the American Civil War. Although classically the pain is described as appearing some days or weeks after the injury, recent literature often mentions that burning pain may appear shortly after the injury; however, it is not clear whether such reports include special care to separate the pain of the acute trauma from the persisting discomfort. In association with the prominent burning pain, most cases of causalgic syndromes have a distinct hypoesthesia and hypoalgesia to pin prick and suffer intense pain from normally nonpainful stimuli (allodynia). Many subjects also have alterations in perspiration and changes in the local circulation of the region involved. It has been recognized that sympathetic innervation has an important part in this syndrome since the work of Leriche (35), and chemical or surgical interruption of the sympathetic supply to the affected region often offers temporary or even permanent relief. Many present-day authors place the syndrome as described originally by Mitchell et al. into a larger class often called reflex sympathetic dystrophies, which may lack one or more of these features.

There have been a number of theories about the possible etiology and mechanisms underlying causalgia and the reflex sympathetic dystrophies. Given the central themes of partial denervation, spontaneous or inappropriate burning pain, and involvement of the sympathetic supply, mechanisms such as ephaptic connections between efferent sympathetic postganglionic fibers and afferent neurons in the injured nerves or sympathetic excitation of nerve fibers in neuromas have been suggested (11,41). Although sympathetic stimulation (SS) excites some cutaneous sensory units in the absence of acute inflammatory changes (57), SS does not excite nociceptors (1,22,46,51). For this reason, recent hypotheses have emphasized central neural factors in association with partial denervation as the predominant underlying mechanism (24,46). The missing link in this history has been the lack of tests of the effects of partial nerve injury on sympathetic effects on nociceptors.

Over the past several years, we (47–49) have specifically addressed this question using the innervation of the rabbit ear *in vivo*. In our model, the great auricular nerve was partially damaged under sterile conditions in several ways: by a cut, a pair of ligatures tied tightly enough to impede venous flow, or stretching the perineurium sufficiently to embarrass its circulation for several minutes. The lesions were chosen to replicate types of nerve injury clinically associated with causalgia or reflex sympathetic dystrophies. In a terminal experiment under anesthesia, recordings from teased nerve filaments were made from single unmyelinated afferent fibers *central* to the lesion site. A branch of the artery supplying most of the ear was cannulated for close arterial injection of norepinephrine and other agents. The sympathetic trunk was isolated and made available for electrical stimulation just distal to the superior cervical ganglion. Single units were selected for study by stimulation of the nerve *distal* to the lesion site; this meant that all fibers conducted across the lesion site. Units conducting at C velocity with an elevated threshold for mechanical stimulation of the receptive field, typical of CPM units, were tested for the direct effects of SS, intravascular adrenergic agents, or such manipulations on heat-evoked responses. Only those sensory units with a C afferent fiber and an elevated threshold for mechanical stimulation and at some stage in the analysis shown to have responses to heat typical of a polymodal nociceptor were included in the analyses. Therefore, all of the elements studied had an afferent fiber conducting across the injury site and the characteristic response to skin stimulation for CPMs. The recovery of receptive characteristics by sensory units with peripheral C afferent fibers after transection of the great auricular nerve at a point equivalent to our injuries has been shown to require more than 30 days (52).

Originally, we looked for subtle effects, possibly manifest upon sensitization. As a consequence, we went through an elaborate process of testing the units for sensitization in the absence and presence of sympathetic stimulation in control and injured nerve populations, as appears in the data shown in Table 5.1. In the course of these studies, some CPM units from injured nerve were found to be directly excited by SS (Fig. 5.14, Table 5.2). This was in sharp distinction to the effects of SS on units recorded from normal nerves (1,53) (Table 5.2). The direct response to sympathetic stimulation appeared as a series of impulses beginning some seconds after sympathetic stimulation was initiated and usually outlasting the period of stimulation. In those units in which SS evoked responses directly, the effect was consis-

TABLE 5.1. *Responses to a thermal stimulus (mean number of impulses ± SEM) of rabbit CPMs from normal (control) and injured nerves*

Nerve injury (n)	Phase	Stimulus 1 (no. of impulses)	Stimulus 2 (no. of impulses)
Control (28)	Pre	0.43 ± 0.17	0.71 ± 0.23
	Stim	16.79 ± 1.35	32.79 ± 4.88[a]
	Total	34.54 ± 3.54	53.86 ± 8.62
Control + SS (12)	Pre	0.25 ± 0.18	0.33 ± 0.19
	Stim	14.67 ± 1.33	15.58 ± 2.38
	Total	27.25 ± 4.52	30.00 ± 6.60
Partial cut + SS (24)	Pre	0.71 ± 0.35	1.21 ± 0.40
	Stim	14.83 ± 1.21	29.79 ± 4.45[a]
	Total	35.83 ± 5.26	57.33 ± 8.69[a]
Stretch + SS (14)	Pre	0.50 ± 0.36	1.14 ± 0.54
	Stim	12.14 ± 0.79	23.36 ± 4.67
	Total	36.57 ± 7.38	57.29 ± 10.25[a]
Ligature + SS (12)	Pre	1.17 ± 0.44	0.83 ± 0.30
	Stim	18.25 ± 2.29	33.25 ± 3.70[a]
	Total	46.08 ± 5.52[a]	67.25 ± 8.58[a]

[a]$P<0.05$ versus control + SS.
Total indicates impulses recorded during the preliminary (Pre), stimulatory (Stim), and recovery phase (Pre and Stim and recovery) during a 250-sec stimulus cycle (see Fig. 5.9). *P* values obtained by one-way ANOVA and Fisher's test.
From ref. 49.

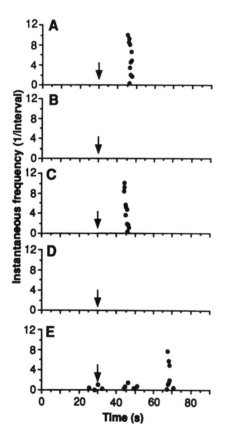

FIG. 5.14. Responses by rabbit CPMs recorded in the great auricular nerve *in vivo* to close arterial injection of norepinephrine 17 days after partial cut injury of that nerve. *Arrows* indicate time of injection of norepinephrine (200 ng/0.2 ml). **A**, initial injection; **B**, 15 min after intravenous yohimbine 1.0 mg/kg; **C**, 51 min after B; **D**, after infiltration of receptive field with lidocaine (0.25%); **E**, 91 min after receptive field infiltration with lidocaine. The unit was not excited by vasopressin (0.6 units) injected intra-arterially, a dose that produced a temperature drop at the receptive field identical to that produced by norepinephrine injection. (From ref. 49.)

TABLE 5.2. *Direct excitation of CPM units by SS or close arterial injection of norepinephrine and the effects of α-adrenergic receptor antagonists*

Type	Sympathetic stimulation			Norepinephrine		
	n	Excited		*n*	Excited	
Control	27	0		15	0	
Lesion	101	20		71	31	
Agent	Ab.	Decr. >50%	Un.	Ab.	Decr. >50%	Un.
Yohimbine	4	1	0	14	0	0
Rauwolsine				4	0	0
Prazosin				0	2	1

n, number of units tested (before heat stimulation); Excited, number of units exhibiting discharges within 180 sec after SS or norepinephrine (2 × SEM greater than background). Control, units from unoperated animals; Lesion, units from nerves with lesions, mostly partial cut, 15 to 40 days after nerve damage. The lower section shows the number of excited units for which a reversible complete (Ab.) or partial (Decr. >50%) block of discharge evoked by SS or norepinephrine was produced. Un, unchanged. Agents were given intravenously and produced 20 to 30 mm Hg decreases in systemic arterial pressure [yohimbine (0.3–1 mg/kg), rauwolsine (1 mg/kg), and prazosin (0.1 mg/kg)]. Most units directly excited by SS were also tested with and responded to norepinephrine injections.
From ref. 49.

tently repeatable and could be mimicked by intra-arterial injection of small quantities (200 ng) of norepinephrine. Approximately one of five CPM units from injured nerve was directly excited by SS; a somewhat higher percentage responded to intra-arterial injections of norepinephrine (Table 5.2). All but a few observations of direct excitation of CPM units were from nerves injured less than 30 days previously, and, therefore, the afferent fibers had not degenerated and regenerated.

The direct responses to both SS and norepinephrine were consistently blocked or reduced substantially in a reversible fashion by competitive antagonists of α_2-adrenergic receptors, such as yohimbine and rauwolsine. An example is shown in Fig. 5.14A–C). Prazosin, a competitive adrenergic receptor blocker acting preferentially at α_1 sites, was less effective in blocking the norepinephrine excitation than the α_2 blockers. A β-adrenergic receptor blocker (propranolol) did not interfere with direct excitation. Figure 5.14 also shows that injection of a local anesthetic (lidocaine) into the receptive field reversibly blocked the effects of norepinephrine injection and SS (not shown). Block of the direct excitation by a local anesthetic in the peripheral receptive field was consistent. It seemed unlikely that the direct excitatory effects of SS and norepinephrine were the product of vasoconstriction because an equivalent drop of temperature at the receptive field produced by intra-arterial injection of vasopressin did not excite units responding to norepinephrine (Fig. 5.14).

SS 5 min prior to a thermal test (e.g., Fig. 5.9) produced no detectable effect on the average response to the initial sequence of stimulation, but *suppressed* the expected degree of sensitization for CPM units from control nerves [Table 5.1 and Fig. 5.15 (control and SS)]. The suppression of sensitization was less evident or absent in CPMs from injured nerve and seemed related to the time after nerve injury (Fig. 5.15). In fact, sensitization on the average seemed to have been enhanced in units recorded from 10 to 20 days after nerve injury. Figure 5.16 shows that some units recorded from injured nerves showed sensitization in the presence of SS that was substantially greater than that seen in a control group. Figure 5.16 also indicates that in injured nerve, absence of sensitization in the presence of SS for individual units

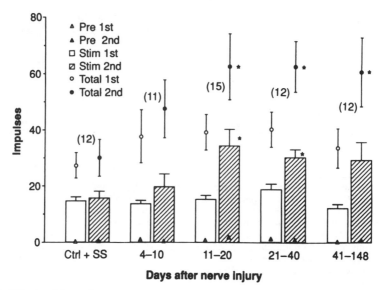

FIG. 5.15. Effects of time after nerve lesion on average response of CPMs to repeated thermal stimulation. Stimulation pattern was similar to that illustrated in Fig. 5.9. *Open bars* and *open symbols*, first heating cycle; *shaded bars* and *filled symbols*, second heating cycle. The ipsilateral sympathetic trunk was stimulated for 30 sec, 5 min before beginning of the heating cycle (Pre). *Total* indicates the impulses recorded during the *pre*liminary heating. (Stim) and recovery (post-heat) phase (see Fig. 5.9 for conventions). Numbers of units for each category are in parentheses. Control + sympathetic stimulation (Ctrl + SS), units from uninjured nerves. Days 4–10, 11–20, 21–40, and 41–148, units recorded during the time frame indicated after the nerve lesion. Data from animals with different kinds of nerve lesions were pooled because the number of units at different survival times from each type of lesion was too small for valid comparison. Shown as mean ± SEM. *$P<0.05$ versus control + SS (Fisher's test). (From ref. 49.)

was less frequent than in normal nerve. Some units showing marked sensitization in the presence of SS were also directly excited by SS.

In summary, nerve injury induces sympathetic and adrenergic excitation of a proportion of CPMs in the damaged nerve. The direct excitatory adrenergic effects can be demonstrated at times after nerve injury too short to have allowed regeneration. Thus, CPM units showing such adrenergic excitation were either uninjured or too slightly injured to cause their peripheral fibers to degenerate. The adrenergic excitation is mediated by an α_2-like adrenergic receptor based on its susceptibility to pharmacological agents established to competitively block specific adrenergic receptors. The nerve injury also appears to induce sympathetic enhancement of sensitization in a proportion of CPM units from injured nerves with a peak effect 2 to 3 weeks after the nerve injury. The latter time course is similar to that described for supersensitivity to adrenergic agents after sympathetic denervation of effector organs (7,10). The adrenergic effect and excitatory action of SS occur at the receptive field of the CPM units because they can be blocked reversibly at that point. The mechanisms leading to denervation supersensitivity may be explained by the induction or upregulation of α_2-like adrenergic receptors in elements associated with the excitatory terminals of CPM units. These results on the induction of adrenergic responsiveness of a cutaneous nociceptor after partial nerve injury suggest that this

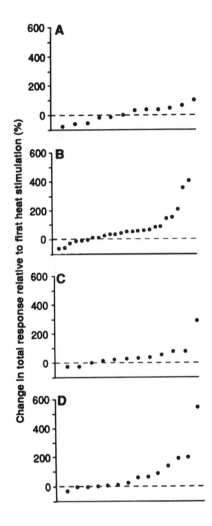

FIG. 5.16. Effects of SS on response of individual CPMs to a repeated thermal (heat) stimulation. For each unit the total response (see Table 5.1) to the first stimulation cycle was taken as 0; the plotted point represented the response to the second stimulation cycle relative to that of the first. Units arbitrarily arranged within each group from least to greatest difference. **A**, control + SS; **B**, partial cut + SS; **C**, ligature + SS; **D**, stretch + SS. (From ref. 49.)

process must be considered an etiological factor contributing to the development of causalgia and reflex sympathetic dystrophies and offers an explanation for the prominence of burning pain as a symptom in these syndromes.

ACKNOWLEDGMENTS

The substantial assistance of Ms. S. Derr in the preparation of this manuscript is gratefully acknowledged. Preparation of the report and most of the work described from the author's laboratory were supported by research grants NS10321 and NS14899 from the NINDS of the National Institutes of Health.

REFERENCES

1. Barassi, S., and Lynn, B. (1986): Effects of sympathetic stimulation on mechanoreceptive and nociceptive afferent units from the rabbit pinna. *Brain Res.*, 378:21–27.

2. Bessou, P., and Perl, E. R. (1969): Response of cutaneous sensory units with unmyelinated fibers to noxious stimuli. *J. Neurophysiol.*, 3:1025–1043.

3. Bessou, P., Burgess, P. R., Perl, E. R., and Taylor, C. B. (1971): Dynamic properties of mechanoreceptors with unmyelinated (C) fibers. *J. Neurophysiol.*, 34:116–131.

4. Bonta, I. L., Bray, M. A., and Parnham, M. J. ed. (1985): *The pharmacology of inflammation.* Elsevier, Amsterdam.

5. Burgess, P. R., and Perl, E. R. (1973): Cutaneous mechanoreceptors and nociceptors. In: *Handbook of sensory physiology, Vol. 2, Somatosensory system*, edited by A. Iggo, pp. 29–78. Springer, Berlin.

6. Campbell, J. N., and Meyer, R. A. (1983): Sensitization of unmyelinated nociceptive afferents in monkey varies with skin type. *J. Neurophysiol.*, 49:98–110.

7. Cannon, W. B., and Rosenblueth, A. (1949): *The supersensitivity of denervated structures.* Macmillan, New York.

8. Cohen, R. H., and Perl, E. R. (1990): Contributions of arachidonic acid derivatives and substance P to the sensitization of cutaneous nociceptors. *J. Neurophysiol.*, 64:457–464.

9. Crunkhorn, P., and Willis, A. L. (1971): Cutaneous reactions to intradermal prostaglandins. *Br. J. Pharmacol.*, 41:57–64.

10. Davies, B., Sudera, D., Sagnella, G., Marchesi-Saviotti, E., Mathias, C., Bannister, R., and Sever, P. (1982): Increased numbers of alpha receptors in sympathetic denervation supersensitivity in man. *Clin. Invest.*, 69:779–784.

11. Devor, M. (1983): Nerve pathophysiology and mechanisms of pain in causalgia. *J. Auton. Nerv. Syst.*, 7:371–384.

12. Ferreira, S. H. (1972): Prostaglandins, aspirin-like drugs and analgesia. *Nature New Biol.*, 240:200–203.

13. Ferreira, S. H. (1985): Prostaglandin hyperalgesia and the control of inflammatory pain. In: *Handbook of inflammation. The pharmacology of inflammation, vol. 5*, edited by I. Bonta, M. A. Bray, and M. J. Parnham, pp. 107–116. Elsevier, Amsterdam.

14. Ferreira, S. H., and Nakamura, M. I. (1979): Prostaglandin hyperalgesia, a cAMP/Ca^{2+} dependent process. *Prostaglandins*, 18:179–190.

15. Fitzgerald, M., and Lynn, B. (1977): The sensitization of high threshold mechanoreceptors with myelinated axons by repeated heating. *J. Physiol. (Lond.)*, 265:549–563.

16. Fitzgerald, M., and Lynn, B. (1979): The weak excitation of some cutaneous receptors in cats and rabbits by synthetic substance P (abstract). *J. Physiol. (Lond.)*, 293:66P–67P.

17. Gallin, J. I., Goldstein, I. M., and Snyderman, R. (1988): *Inflammation basic principles and clinical correlates.* Raven Press, New York.

18. Handwerker, H. O. (1976): Influences of algogenic substances and prostaglandins on the discharges of unmyelinated cutaneous nerve fibers identified as nociceptors. In: *Advances in pain research and therapy*, vol. 1, edited by J. Bonica and D. Albe-Fessard, pp. 41–45. Raven Press, New York.

19. Helme, R. D., Koschorke, G. M., and Zimmerman, M. (1985): Immunoreactive substance P release from skin nerves in the rat by noxious thermal stimulation. *Neurosci. Lett.*, 63:295–299.

20. Henson, P. M., and Murphy, R. C. (1989): *Mediators of the inflammatory process.* Elsevier, Amsterdam.

21. Horton, E. W. (1963): Action of prostaglandin E$_1$ on tissues which respond to bradykinin. *Nature*, 200:892.

22. Hu, S., and Zhu, J. (1989): Sympathetic facilitation of sustained discharges of polymodal nociceptors. *Pain*, 38:85–90.

23. Hunt, C. C., and McIntyre, A. K. (1960): Properties of cutaneous touch receptors in cat. *J. Physiol. (Lond.)*, 153:88–98.

24. Jänig, W. (1985): Organization of the lumbar sympathetic outflow to skeletal muscle and skin of the cat hindlimb and tail. *Rev. Physiol. Biochem. Pharmacol.*, 102:119–213.

25. Jonsson, C-E., Shimizu, Y., Fredholm, B., Granström, E., and Oliw, E. (1979): Efflux of cyclic AMP, prostaglandin E$_2$ and F$_{2\alpha}$ and thromboxane B$_2$ in leg lymph of rabbits after scalding injury. *Acta Physiol. Scand.*, 107:377–384.

26. Juan, H., and Lembeck, F. (1976): Release of prostaglandins from the isolated perfused rabbit ear by bradykinin, prostaglandins and acetylcholine. *Agents Actions*, 6:642.

27. King, J. S., Gallant, P., Myerson, V., and Perl, E. R. (1976): The effects of anti-inflammatory agents on the responses and the sensitization of unmyelinated (C) fiber polymodal nociceptors. In: *Sensory functions of the skin in primates*, edited by Y. Zotterman, pp. 441–454. Pergamon, Oxford.

28. Kumazawa, T., and Perl, E. R. (1977): Primate cutaneous sensory units with unmyelinated (C) afferent fibers. *J. Neurophysiol.*, 40:1325–1338.

29. Kumazawa, T., and Perl, E. R. (1978): Excitation of marginal and substantia gelatinosa neurons in the primate spinal cord: indications of their place in dorsal horn functional organization. *J. Comp. Neurol.*, 177:417–434.

30. Kumazawa, T., and Mizumura, K. (1979): Effects of synthetic substance P on unit-discharges of testicular nociceptors of dogs. *Brain Res.*, 170:553–557.
31. Lembeck, F., and Gamse, R. (1977): Lack of algesic effect of substance P on paravascular pain receptors. *Naunyn Schmiedebergs Arch. Pharmacol.*, 299:295–303.
32. Lembeck, F., Gamse, R., and Juan, H. (1977): Substance P and sensory nerve endings. In: *Substance P*, edited by U. S. von Euler and B. Pernow, pp. 160–181. Raven Press, New York.
33. Lembeck, F., and Holzer, P. (1979): Substance P as neurogenic mediator of antidromic vasodilation and neurogenic plasma extravasation. *Naunyn Schmiedebergs Arch. Pharmacol.*, 310:175–183.
34. Lembeck, F., Donnerer, J., and Barthó, L. (1982): Inhibition of neurogenic vasodilation and plasma extravasation by substance P antagonists, somatostatin and [D-Met², Pro⁵] enkephalinamide. *Eur. J. Pharmacol.*, 85:171–176.
35. Leriche, R. (1916): De la causalgie envisagée comme un névrite du sympathétique et de son traitement. *Presse Med.*, 24:178–180.
36. Lundberg, J. M., Saria, A., Rosell, S., and Folkers, K. A. (1984): Substance P antagonist inhibits heat-induced oedema in the rat skin. *Acta Physiol. Scand.*, 120:145–146.
37. Martin, H. A., Basbaum, A. I., Kwiat, G. C., Goetzl, E. J., and Levine, J. D. (1987): Leukotriene and prostaglandin sensitization of cutaneous high-threshold C- and A-delta mechanonociceptors in the hairy skin of rat hindlimb. *Neuroscience*, 22:651–659.
38. Mitchell, S. W., Morehouse, G. R., and Keen, W. W. (1864): *Gunshot wounds and other injuries of nerves*. Lippincott, Philadelphia.
39. Mizumura, K., Sato, J., and Kumazawa, T. (1987): Effects of prostaglandins and other putative chemical intermediaries on the activity of canine testicular polymodal receptors studied *in vitro*. *Pflugers Arch.*, 408:565–572.
40. Nakamura-Craig, M., and Smith, T. W. (1989): Substance P and peripheral inflammatory hyperalgesia. *Pain*, 38:91–98.
41. Nathan, P. W. (1947): On the pathogenesis of causalgia in peripheral nerve injuries. *Brain*, 70:145–171.
42. Olgart, L., Gazelius, B., Brodin, E., and Nilsson, G. (1977): Localization of substance P-like immunoreactivity from dental pulp. *Acta Physiol. Scand.*, 101:510–512.
43. Perl, E. R. (1972): Mode of action of nociceptors. In: *Cervical pain*, edited by C. Hirsch and Y. Zotterman, pp. 157–164. Pergamon Press, Oxford and New York.
44. Perl, E. R., Kumazawa, T., Lynn, B., and Kenins, P. (1976): Sensitization of high threshold receptors with unmyelinated (C) afferent fibers. In: *Progress in brain research. Somatosensory and visceral receptor mechanisms*, vol. 43, edited by A. Iggo and D. B. Ilyinsky, pp. 263–276. Elsevier, Amsterdam.
45. Perl, E. R. (1984): Pain and nociception. In: *Handbook of physiology—the nervous system III*, edited by I. Darian-Smith, pp. 915–975. American Physiological Society, Bethesda, MD.
46. Roberts, W. J., and Elardo, S. M. (1985): Sympathetic activation of A-delta nociceptors. *Somatosens. Res.*, 3:33–44.
47. Sato, J., and Perl, E. R. (1989): Sympathetic activation increases nociceptor responsiveness after nerve injury. *Soc. Neurosci. Abstr.*, 15:440.
48. Sato, J., and Perl, E. R. (1990): Peripheral nerve injury causes cutaneous nociceptors to be excited by activation of catecholamine receptors. *Soc. Neurosci. Abstr.*, 16:1072.
49. Sato, J., and Perl, E. R. (1991): Adrenergic excitation of cutaneous pain receptors induced by peripheral nerve injury. *Science*, 251:1608–1610.
50. Schweizer, A., Brom, R., Glatt, M., and Bray, M. A. (1984): Leukotrienes reduce nociceptive responses to bradykinin. *Eur. J. Pharmacol.*, 105:105–112.
51. Shea, V. K., and Perl, E. R. (1985): Sensory receptors with unmyelinated (C) fibers innervating the skin of the rabbit's ear. *J. Neurophysiol.*, 54:491–501.
52. Shea, V. K., and Perl, E. R. (1985): Regeneration of cutaneous afferent unmyelinated (C) fibers after transection. *J. Neurophysiol.*, 54:502–512.
53. Shea, V. K., and Perl, E. R. (1985): Failure of sympathetic stimulation to affect responsiveness of rabbit polymodal nociceptors. *J. Neurophysiol.*, 54:513–519.
54. Stewart, J. M., Getto, C. J., Nelder, K., Reeve, E. B., Krivoy, W. A., and Zimmerman, E. (1976): Substance P and analgesia. *Nature*, 262:784–785.
55. Szolcsányi, J. (1987): Selective responsiveness of polymodal nociceptors of the rabbit ear to capsaicin, bradykinin and ultra-violet irradiation. *J. Physiol. (Lond.)*, 388:9–23.
56. Tissot, M., Pradelles, P., and Giroud, J. P. (1988): Substance-P-like levels in inflammatory exudates. *Inflammation*, 12:25–35.
57. Wiesenfeld-Hallin, Z., and Hallin, R. G. (1984): The influence of the sympathetic system on mechanoreception and nociception. A review. *Hum. Neurobiol.*, 3:41–46.

Hyperalgesia and Allodynia,
edited by W. D. Willis, Jr.
Raven Press, Ltd., New York © 1992.

6

Nociception in Normal and Arthritic Joints

Structural and Functional Aspects

U. Hanesch, B. Heppelmann, K. Messlinger, and R. F. Schmidt

Institute of Physiology, University of Würzburg, D-8700 Würzburg, Germany

Diseases in joints are a major source of pain in human pathology. Present-day hypotheses about the origin and modulation of joint pain and pain in other deep tissues are based on the theory that pain is an independent sensation with its own specialized apparatus of sensors, conduction pathways, and centers. In recent years our group has been engaged in analyzing both the peripheral and the more central aspects of the nociceptive structures and processes involved in joint pain. This chapter summarizes some of this work, particularly on the peripheral aspects of articular nociception in regard to both its histology and its function. Some spinal and supraspinal aspects of articular nociception are dealt with in Chapter 18 by Schaible.

Special emphasis will be given to the recent finding that healthy articular tissue contains nocisensors (nociceptors) with thresholds so high that they cannot be excited by acute noxious stimuli (silent or "sleeping" nocisensors) (52,53). However, sensitization of these nocisensors as a consequence of pathological tissue alterations (e.g., by inflammation) will "awaken" them. Sensitization is probably brought about by algesic substances (mediators of inflammation, e.g., prostaglandins, bradykinin). The increase in sensory inflow resulting from the sensitization of peripheral nocisensors leads subsequently to a central component in the sensitization, which in turn modifies the perception of pain under these circumstances. Various processes, such as expression of c-fos-like protein, modification of the spinal composition of endogenous opioids, and release of neuropeptides, may be involved in this newly detected phenomenon (see elsewhere in this volume). Peripheral as well as central sensitization most likely contribute to hyperalgesia.

SENSORY OUTFLOW FROM THE NORMAL AND INFLAMED KNEE JOINT: AN OVERVIEW

The knee joint of the cat is mainly innervated by two nerves: the medial (MAN) and the posterior articular nerves (PAN) (21). Both of them have been analyzed histologically to determine their afferent and efferent fiber content. As can be seen from Table 6.1, each nerve contains approximately 650 afferent fibers, mainly of groups III and IV, and another 500 unmyelinated sympathetic efferents (43). In the group IV fiber range the maximum of the diameter distribution is between 0.3 and

TABLE 6.1. *Composition of the cat's articular nerves*

Fibers (group)	MAN		PAN	
I	—		27	(4%)
II	59	(9%)	149	(22%)
III	131	(21%)	94	(14%)
IV	440	(70%)	410	(60%)
Afferents	630	(100%)	680	(100%)
Sympathetic	500		515	

MAN, medial articular nerve; PAN, posterior articular nerve.

0.4 μm for the afferent fibers, whereas the maximum is around 0.8 to 0.9 μm for the sympathetic efferent ones (Fig. 6.1A) (27). The latter study and that of Langford and Schmidt (43) also allowed the determination of the respective numbers of each of the group I–III fibers (Fig. 6.1B; see also Table 6.1). Obviously, the majority of fibers in both nerves belongs to the fine afferent ones consisting of groups III and IV (MAN, 91%; PAN, 74%). The small contribution of the group I fibers in the PAN is presumably due to stray fibers joining in from muscle spindles of the Musc. popliteus (51).

Using this background and the results of studying the discharge characteristics of individual fine afferents (to be discussed below), it has been possible for the first time to estimate the number of afferent impulses reaching the spinal cord in response to a single simple flexion movement from the mid-position of the joint under both normal and inflamed conditions (25). Since sufficient data were only available for

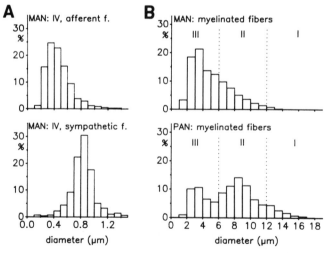

FIG. 6.1. Diameter distribution of unmyelinated and myelinated nerve fibers in articular nerves of the cat. **A:** Fiber size distribution of unmyelinated afferent (group IV) and sympathetic nerve fibers in the MAN. **B:** Comparison of the diameter distribution of myelinated nerve fibers in the MAN and PAN. The fibers were classified according to the classification of Boyd and Davey (7).

the MAN, the estimate has been restricted to that particular input (Table 6.2). In the normal joint 35% of the group III and 36% of the group IV afferents have a mean resting activity of 10 and 19 impulses per minute, respectively. Group II fibers are barely active at rest. Altogether this makes for some 1,800 impulses per 30 sec entering the spinal cord from a knee joint resting in mid-position (13,25,70). Actually, the functional significance of this resting discharge is not well understood. None of the discharges depends on the position of the joint. Thus, they do not seem to contribute to kinesthesia.

During inflammation both the percentage of fibers having resting activity and their mean discharge frequency increase. In the group III range 75% and in the group IV range 83% of the afferents are spontaneously active with a mean resting activity of 54 and 46 impulses per minute, respectively. Also, some of the group II afferents develop a slight resting activity. Both factors contribute to the increase of afferent activity from 1,800 to 11,100 impulses reaching the spinal cord within 30 sec with the joint in resting position (13,25,70). A similar increase in resting discharges has to be expected from the afferent units in the PAN. We propose that these combined impulses are the peripheral neurobiological correlate for pain at rest from an inflamed joint.

In the normal joint 89% of the group II, 45.5% of the group III, and 29.5% of the group IV afferents respond during a joint movement in its normal working range, i.e., they are of low threshold (26). In the MAN these percentages amount to 240 afferent fibers having low thresholds and 390 fibers having high ones. Again, it is not absolutely certain which type of information is signaled to the nervous system by these discharges. Most units respond to more than one type of joint movement (extension, flexion, inward and outward rotation). Thus, only in a very loose way can these discharges contribute to measuring joint movement and joint direction. The afferent volley during the simple flexion movement comprises approximately 4,400 impulses per 30 sec (including the resting discharges).

Inflammation of the joint reduces the mechanical thresholds of most of the afferent fibers regardless of their threshold under normal conditions. A movement in the normal working range of the joint, such as the test flexion used here, will now excite approximately 550 units in the MAN, and, in addition, the discharge rates of those low-threshold units having already been excited in the normal state are now much higher than previously. All in all in the MAN the afferent volley in response to the test movement now consists of some 30,900 impulses per 30 sec, i.e., about seven times more than under normal conditions (in individual afferents that have been studied consecutively under both normal and inflamed conditions, the afferent discharges sometimes increased more than 100-fold). This huge volley, together with

TABLE 6.2. *Influence of an acute inflammation*

Medial articular nerve	Joint		Change
	Normal	Inflamed	
Resting activity (impulses/30 sec)	1,800	11,100	×6.2
Low-threshold units	240 fibers	550 fibers	×2.3
Movement (impulses/30 sec)	4,400	30,900	×7.0

the corresponding one in the PAN, obviously transmits those messages responsible for the noxious reflexes and the pain perception when moving an inflamed joint (details on the response properties of fine articular afferents are discussed in a later section).

TERMINAL ARBORIZATION OF ARTICULAR AFFERENTS

Very little is known of the ultrastructure of the terminal areas of fine afferent nerve fibers in general and on the structure of nocisensors and their eventual specializations relative to other "free nerve endings" in particular. Therefore, we have carried out a number of studies devoted to these areas. We used serial sectioning of the terminal areas of group III and IV articular afferents of distances up to 300 μm, which were studied under the electron microscope and reconstructed three-dimensionally with computer assistance. All studies were on the medial aspect of the knee joint and done on tissue that had been sympathectomized earlier. Our methods are described in detail elsewhere (28).

As regards the course of the fine afferents in the articular tissue we found that the terminal twigs of the MAN filaments and, finally, of those fine afferents that were no longer surrounded by perineurium were running mainly in a thin superficial layer of the joint capsule and, in addition, on the inside and outside surfaces of the ligamentum patellae and ligamentum collaterale mediale. Barely any nerve fibers could be detected within the densely packed connective tissue of these areas.

The final portion of any group III afferent fiber can be conveniently separated into three major areas (30) (see also Fig. 6.6A): (a) The proximal portion of the afferent fiber is myelinated and runs within a perineural sheath. Most likely, action potentials are being conducted from Ranvier node to Ranvier node in this area. (b) More distally there is an intermediate portion that has lost its myelin at a last half Ranvier node but that is still running within the perineural sheath. However, its ultrastructure is already comparable to that of the distal portion described next. The length of the intermediate portion in our reconstructions was between 7 and 98 μm (3). The distal portion, free of myelin as the intermediate one, starts at the end of the perineural sheath. It runs into the tissue, splits up into several branches, and forms the sensory terminal tree. This terminal tree consists usually of two to four larger branches with a length of about 80 to 200 μm (Fig. 6.5). In addition, there are short side branches of lengths of 10 to 20 μm (Figs. 6.2 and 6.5). The branches innervate a predominantly two-dimensional area of tissue of about 150 × 200 μm (29).

The unmyelinated afferent group IV fibers have a proximal and a distal terminal portion. The proximal one is defined as that still running within the perineural sheath, the distal one as that outside (Fig. 6.5) (there is no intermediate portion since there is no myelin sheath). The major branches coming out of the distal portion are quite long, sometimes more than 300 μm. They have frequently short side branches of lengths of less than 10 μm (29). The fibers usually run parallel to vessels, but the distances to the vessel walls may vary considerably.

In the terminal areas of both fiber types mast cells can be found that are sometimes less than 2 μm from the nerve fibers. The distal portions are covered by Schwann cells, but this coverage is incomplete. Altogether about one-third of the membrane surface is not covered by these cells. These "bare areas" are particularly frequent at the so-called axonal beads (Figs. 6.2–6.5; see also

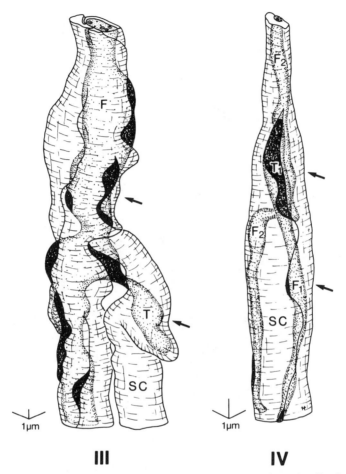

III   **IV**

FIG. 6.2. Three-dimensional reconstructions of 20-μm segments from the distal portion of one group III and two group IV nerve fibers. **Left:** Unmyelinated terminal portion of a group III fiber (F) with a short terminal branch (T). Bare areas of the axolemma, not covered by the Schwann cell (SC), appear densely dotted. **Right:** Sensory endings of two group IV nerve fibers (F₁, F₂) within the same Remak bundle. One fiber is passing the segment (F₂), whereas the other fiber (F₁) terminates (T₁). *Arrows* indicate the position of the microphotographs of cross-sections through axonal beads (III, upper arrow; IV, lower arrow) and end bulbs (III, lower arrow; IV, upper arrow) shown in Figs. 6.3 and 6.4.

below). The axonal beads near the bare areas show a fine filamentous axoplasma that is somewhat more electron dense than the neighboring cell plasma. These plasma modifications look similar to the receptor matrix described by Andres and von Düring (1).

As mentioned, the intermediate and final fiber sections display regular axonal thickenings that in three-dimensional reconstructions appear to be lined up like pearls on a string. These axonal beads contain an above average number of mito-chondria, glycogen granules, and vesicles (Figs. 6.3A and 6.4A) (29). Counting these beads showed that in group III fibers there are about seven beads per 100 μm of fiber length, whereas with the group IV fibers there are nine to 10 per 100 μm. In other

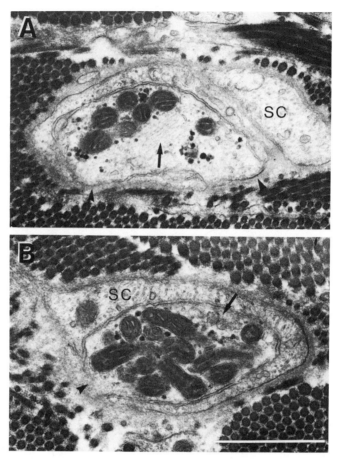

FIG. 6.3. Cross-sections through an axonal bead (**A**) and an end bulb (**B**) of a group III nerve fiber. **A:** Axonal bead with accumulations of mitochondria and glycogen granules. On two sides the bare axolemma bulges through gaps between Schwann cell processes (*arrowheads*). The neurofilament core of the sensory axon (*arrow*) consists mainly of parallel microfilaments and is marked by its lack of cell organelles. **B:** Axonal end bulb of a short side branch of the same nerve fiber. In addition to mitochondria and glycogen particles, this section contains larger dense core vesicles (*arrow*) but, in contrast to beads, no microtubules and no neurofilament core. Bar = 1μm.

words, the beads are smaller and more frequent in group IV than in group III fibers. Microtubules and microfilaments can be seen along the length of both terminal fiber types.

The group III fiber terminals have, in addition, in the center of their axoplasm a neurofilament core consisting of numerous microfilaments (Fig. 6.3A). In this area no organelles and barely any tubuli can be seen. This finding is absolutely for sensory endings of myelinated fibers, which can be identified by this feature (no neurofilament core has ever been seen in group IV terminals). It may be speculated that this neurofilament core serves as a "backbone" for the quite extended unmyelinated terminal areas of the group III afferents since, relative to the group IV fibers, they have a much lower ratio of surface area to volume. The group III afferents end in a

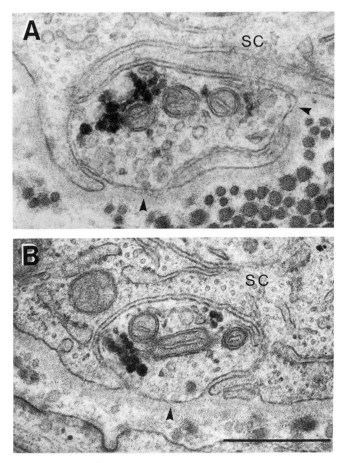

FIG. 6.4. Cross-sections through an axonal bead (**A**) and an end bulb (**B**) of a group IV nerve fiber. A: Axonal bead of the nerve fiber with mitochondria, glycogen particles, and various clear vesicles. A part of the axolemma lies bare from Schwann cell (SC) covering and is only separated by the basal lamina from the surrounding tissue (*arrowheads*). In contrast to group III fibers, a neurofilament core does not exist. B: Cross-section through the end bulb of the same nerve fiber. The axon shows the same organelle content as the axonal beads. On one side the bare axolemma bulges through a gap between Schwann cell processes (*arrowhead*). Bar = 0.5 μm.

terminal end bulb, which is comparable in size and contents to the axonal beads (Figs. 6.3 and 6.4). The difference is that the organelles (mitochondria, vesicles, glycogen granules) are irregularly distributed within the ending. Also, the neurofilament core is no longer visible. The group IV fibers do not have a terminal bulb but just taper off as a very thin ending.

Based on these results, we are now able to decide, with electron microscopy of a single section or after a very brief reconstruction (maximum 10 μm), whether a nerve fiber under investigation belongs to group III or IV, i.e., if it is myelinated or not in its more proximal portions. Also, with the group III fibers, it is now possible to decide whether the section is across an axonal bead or a terminal end bulb. This differentiation, however, is only possible in sympathectomized tissue, as, up to now,

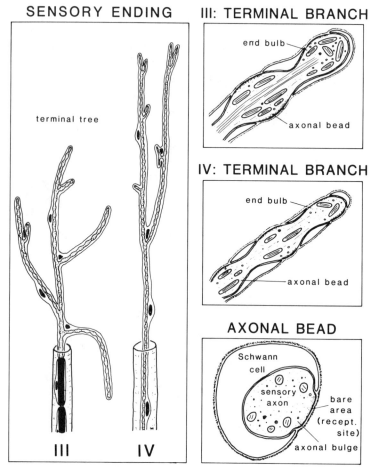

FIG. 6.5. Schematic drawings of group III and IV sensory endings in the knee joint capsule of the cat. A terminal tree is formed by several long and short branches of various orientations. The sensory axons consist of periodically arranged thick and thin segments forming spindle-shaped beads. The axolemma is not completely ensheathed by its accompanying Schwann cells; the bare areas presumably are the receptive sites.

no morphological criteria are known to distinguish between fine afferent and post-ganglionic sympathetic nerve fibers. In addition, these results do not give any clue to the function of the fiber under investigation.

THE CYTOPLASMIC CONTENT OF FINE AFFERENTS AND THEIR TERMINALS

As mentioned, neither the shape nor the area of innervation by the terminal portions of the fine afferent nerve fibers gives any clue to their function. Therefore, we studied the cytoplasmic content of the afferents to find out whether its appearance may offer any special clues regarding the sensory properties of these fibers. The first finding was that the mitochondria are not regularly distributed in the terminal regions: They accumulate in the axonal beads of both fiber types and in the end bulbs of the group III afferents. High concentrations of mitochondria are found in these areas, whereas in the thin fiber portions between the axonal beads barely any mitochondria can be seen. Another aspect is that the number of mitochondria, i.e., their density, increases considerably in the intermediate and, particularly, the distal portions of group III fibers relative to the proximal ones. This is illustrated in Fig. 6.6A, which shows the measurement of the mitochondria cross-section area relative to the

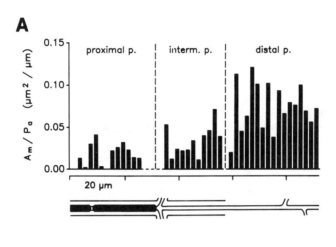

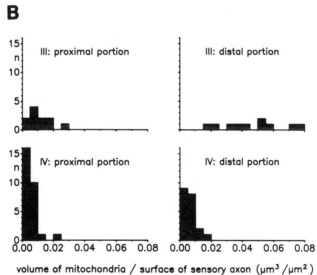

FIG. 6.6. Density of mitochondria in distal segments of fine afferent nerve fibers of the knee joint capsule. **A:** Variation of the cross-sectional area of mitochondria per perimeter of the sensory axon (A_m/P_a) in cross-sections of a group III nerve fiber at a distance of 2 μm. The nerve fiber was examined over a length of 92 μm from the last two myelinated segments of the proximal portion to a part of the unmyelinated distal portion showing a marked increase of the mitochondrial density in the distal portion. **B:** Mean surface density (volume of mitochondria per surface of the sensory axon) of the proximal and distal portion of group III (proximal, n = 11; distal, n = 10) and IV (proximal, n = 28; distal, n = 20) nerve fibers. In the proximal portion, the fibers of both groups show a low density of mitochondria, whereas in the distal portion of group III fibers the mean density is increased and varies over a wide range. In group IV fibers, the mean density is similar to that of the proximal portion.

fiber circumference over a total length of 92 μm, including the proximal, intermediate, and distal portions of that fiber.

Measurements of this type in many units revealed that the density of mitochondria may vary considerably from fiber to fiber. Therefore, in a population of 21 group III and 41 group IV afferents the average volume of mitochondria per surface area of the fiber has been determined over a length of 15 to 108 μm in steps of 1 μm. Calculating the "volume per surface area" relationship is somewhat unusual, but it is used here to highlight eventual differences in the relationship between the adenosine triphosphate- (ATP) producing organelles, namely, the mitochondria, and the energy-using structures, namely, the membranes of the afferent units. The results are illustrated in Fig. 6.6B: In the proximal areas of group III afferents we found an average surface density of 0.004 to 0.030 $μm^3/μm^2$. In contrast in the distal areas, we found both a considerable increase of these values and a much wider fluctuation of the measured surface densities (0.016–0.080 $μm^3/μm^2$).

Altogether the group IV terminals contain fewer mitochondria than the group III ones. Within any individual fiber profile we never saw more than four to seven cross-cut mitochondria at once. But since the fiber surface is also so much smaller, the surface density in the proximal part is comparable with that of the group III units (0.001–0.025 $μm^3/μm^2$). In contrast to the group III units, however, we did not see a significant increase in the density of mitochondria in the distal portion. Also no increase in the fluctuation of the values could be seen (0.003–0.019 $μm^3/μm^2$) (Fig. 6.6B).

If it is agreed that the total volume of mitochondria is proportional to the production and storage of ATP as a readily available pool of energy, then the results presented here point to considerable differences in the energy requirements between individual units of group III and IV fibers, particularly in the group III range. Actually, for skeletal muscle a linear relationship has been shown to exist between the oxidative capacity of this tissue and the total volume of mitochondria contained in it (75). Similar studies are not available for peripheral nervous tissue, with one exception: In the lobster muscle receptor organs a positive correlation has been found between the concentration of mitochondria and the electrophysiologic responses of these cells (50): Neurons with a low mechanical threshold and a long adaptation time showed a high density of mitochondria, whereas neurons with high mechanical thresholds and a short adaptation time contained significantly fewer mitochondria. As both cell types contain nearly the same amount of electrogenic pumps in their membranes (18), the functional character of these cells seems to be determined by their oxidative capacity (50).

Based on these findings, the following suggestions for the fine articular afferent fibers may be proposed: (a) Since the saltatory conduction of action potentials in the proximal portions of group III afferents requires only a small amount of energy, the density of mitochondria is low in these portions, whereas in the distal portions a much higher energy consumption requires the presence of larger numbers of mitochondria. (b) In the group IV fibers the differences in mitochondrial content between the proximal and distal portions are small because both areas use approximately the same amount of energy (mainly because of the lack of a myelin sheath). (c) The large variations in mitochondrial content, relative to energy consumption, of the terminal portions of various individual units most likely are related to differences in their sensory function.

As will be reported in a later section, large differences exist in the level of the mechanical threshold of fine articular afferent units (68). If we succeed in correlating these different findings, then the outcome may most likely be that high-threshold (nociceptive) fine afferents contain fewer mitochondria per surface area than low-threshold mechanosensitive units, because the high-threshold units are being activated much more rarely than the low-threshold ones. But it has to be appreciated that other sensory functions of these polymodal units (e.g., chemosensitivity) and perhaps efferent functions may complicate the issue.

In addition to mitochondria, glycogen granules, and vesicles, a large variety of neuroactive substances could be localized in the cytoplasma of articular primary afferent fibers. We focused our interest on the neuropeptides as they are found in all sensory ganglia of all species, especially in small-diameter neurons (for review, see ref. 32). There is some agreement that they seem to play a dual role: (a) modulating the transmission of (nociceptive?) information and (b) local effector functions (for reviews, see refs. 34,36,42). Of particular interest are the tachykinins substance P (SP) and neurokinin A (NKA), calcitonin gene-related peptide (CGRP), and somato-statin (SOM), which have been demonstrated in various dorsal root ganglia. There is good evidence that these neuropeptides play a key role in nociception. For example, it has been shown using the antibody microprobe technique that various types of noxious stimulation lead to the release of these peptides in the spinal cord (15–17,35,60,73).

In our experiments with retrograde labeling of MAN afferents with the fluorescent dye Fast Blue and with subsequent immunocytochemical staining (PAP method) of the dorsal root ganglia cells for the neuropeptides SP, NKA, SOM, and CGRP (for methods, see refs. 12,24), the major results were:

—SP and CGRP could be visualized without a colchicine treatment of the ganglia, i.e., without enhancing the concentration of peptides in the perikarya by inhibiting the axonal transport; in contrast, for quantitative analysis of the percentage of NKA- and SOM-containing cells, a colchicine treatment was necessary.

—SP-, NKA-, and SOM-like immunoreactivity (SP-, NKA-, SOM-li) was evenly distributed throughout the cytoplasm; CGRP-like immunoreactivity (CGRP-li) occurred as a bright and even staining across the cytoplasm, a punctate granule-like stain evenly distributed in the cytoplasm, or a combination of both.

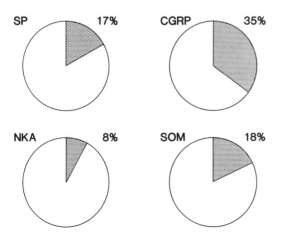

FIG. 6.7. Percentage of the articular afferents with a positive SP-, CGRP-, NKA-, and SOM-like immunoreactivity examined in the dorsal root ganglion cells of the MAN after a retrograde labeling with Fast Blue.

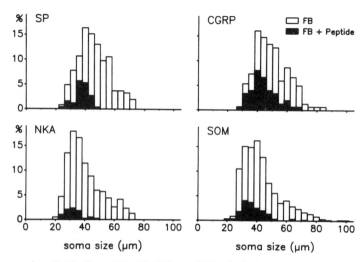

FIG. 6.8. Soma size distribution of the Fast Blue- (FB) labeled dorsal root ganglion cells of the MAN and the perikarya showing an additional SP-, CGRP-, NKA-, and SOM-like immunoreactivity. SP, NKA, and SOM are only found in small- or intermediate-sized perikarya ($<50\mu$m), whereas CGRP is also present in some large-sized dorsal root ganglion cells ($>50\mu$m).

—CGRP-li was found within 35% of the MAN neurons, SP-li and SOM-li in 17% and 18%, respectively, of the MAN afferents, NKA-li in only a small population of afferents; 8% were NKA positive (Fig. 6.7).

—The examined neuropeptides are nearly exclusively localized in small- to intermediate-sized cell bodies (<50 μm) (Fig. 6.8), which are known to give rise predominantly to group IV and some group III fibers.

—CGRP was found additionally in some large perikarya (>50 μm) (Fig. 6.8), which give probably rise to myelinated nerve fibers of groups I and II and to some group III fibers (three-fourths of CGRP-li is localized in small- and intermediate-sized, one-fourth is found in large perikarya).

As will be shown in the next section, our data suggest that roughly 60% of the MAN afferents have high mechanical thresholds, which make them candidates for nociceptors. Obviously not all of them contain the peptides just discussed. Even if it is assumed that only nociceptive afferents contain such peptides, only about 30% of them could contain SP or SOM, and no more than 10% of the nociceptors could contain NKA, and these percentages would have to be further reduced in view of the fact that low-threshold mechanosensitive neurons also contain one or the other type of these peptides (46). Thus, it is one of the major conclusions of this investigation that no simple correlation between the existence of a peptide in an afferent fiber and the sensory function of that fiber, e.g., nociception, seems to exist.

RESPONSE PROPERTIES OF ARTICULAR AFFERENTS

Group II articular afferent units (conduction velocity 21–65 m/sec) have no resting discharges and mostly low mechanical thresholds to movement. Actually, their vast majority is excited by gentle local stimuli and by movements in the working range of the knee joint. Although they encode pressure and particularly movement stimuli up to the noxious range, their responses were more closely related to the particular type of stimulus (e.g., movement in a specific direction) than to intensity (innoxious vs noxious). These results suggest that they are probably not involved in joint nociception and pain. Rather, they presumably subserve proprioceptive functions such as deep pressure sensation and kinesthesia (13).

In articular group III (conduction velocity 2.5–20 m/sec) and IV (<2.5 m/sec) afferent units, resting discharges occur in no more than one-third of all fibers. The frequency of these irregular discharges is low, usually below 0.5 Hz (68). In their response behavior to passive movements of the knee joint, the fine afferent units (groups III and IV) can be grouped together according to their movement sensitivity, ranging from units that are readily or only marginally activated by non-noxious events, through units that are only activated by noxious movements, to units that, despite being undoubtedly afferent, are not activated by any movements, even extremely noxious ones (silent or "sleeping" units). According to our measurements, approximately 55% of the group III and 70% of the group IV units either respond only to (potentially) noxious movements or fail to respond to movements completely (26,69). Units in the PAN can also be grouped into different categories. But, surprisingly, the vast majority of the group IV fibers do not respond to mechanical stimulation at all (23).

The units that are excited while the joint is being moved through its normal working range cannot be considered nociceptive. Fibers that are only activated by noxious stimuli (movements outside the normal working range against tissue resistance) can be referred to as nocisensors, as defined by the specificity theory. The function of those afferent units, which in the normal joint are not excited by any movements, remains open. In the normal joint it may be more an efferent than an afferent one (40).

INFLAMMATION-INDUCED CHANGES OF THE MECHANOSENSITIVITY OF ARTICULAR AFFERENTS

In our experimental model of acute arthritis the inflammation is induced in two steps. First, a 4% solution of kaolin suspended in distilled water is injected into the knee joint cavity using a lateral approach. Thereafter, the knee joint is rhythmically flexed and extended for 15 min. Finally, 0.15 to 0.3 ml of a 2% solution of carrageenan is injected into the joint cavity, and the joint is again flexed and extended for another 5 min. This procedure leads to a long-lasting inflammation with behavioral changes of the awake cat and histological signs of acute severe inflammation with cellular infiltration (11,23,71).

As a consequence of the inflammation there are profound changes in the resting and evoked discharge characteristics of fine articular afferents, as seen both in single units, which were observed under normal or inflamed conditions, and in individual primary articular afferents, which were continuously observed under normal conditions and while the joint became inflamed (11,23,70,72). During inflammation resting activity is observed in 75% of group III and 83% of group IV units of the MAN. The discharges are irregular and sometimes of high frequency. Both the percentages of units with resting activity and the frequencies of their discharges are more than twice as high as in the control sample. Their resting activity might represent the neural correlate of spontaneous pain, and the large number of fibers exhibiting resting activity under inflammatory conditions also implies (and has been confirmed by direct observations) that in any case there are numerous nociceptors (usually silent in the normal joint) that exhibit resting activity under these conditions (see earlier for an estimate of the size of the afferent inflow at rest and during a flexion movement of the normal and the inflamed joint).

Studying the movement sensitivity it was seen that nearly all fine afferent units from inflamed joints have low thresholds to movement, and most of them respond well to flexion and extension. The increase in the number of easily excitable afferents corresponds to the clear decrease in the number of units belonging to the other classes. In experiments using continuous observation of single units, our population studies were confirmed, namely, that the fibers, which in the normal joint mainly or exclusively respond to noxious movements, become very sensitive to movement when the joint is inflamed. The message "noxious" is now sent to the central nervous system, even if movement takes place in the normally innocuous range (71,72).

Also, it is striking that the remaining fraction of fibers that do not respond to movement is only very small in the inflamed joint. It follows from this that most of the units must have become sensitive to movement, as again confirmed in continuous observations. This makes it clear that units that do not respond to movement in the normal joint must also be regarded as nociceptors. Thus, they respond to movement only in the case of true tissue damage. This recruitment of a large population of fibers during the inflammatory process leads to a massive amplification of the afferent signals reaching the central nervous system (Table 6.2).

There are interesting differences in the time course of sensitization of the various types of articular afferents that were revealed by the continuous observation of single units (71). Low-threshold units, mainly in the group II and III fiber range, developed increased reactions foremost in the first hour after the injection of the inflammatory compounds, sometimes starting immediately after the injection (usually low-threshold group II units). In high-threshold afferents, including originally silent ones ("sleeping" nocisensors), the sensitization became evident within the second to third hour after induction of inflammation with a further increase later on.

FACTORS RESPONSIBLE FOR THE INFLAMMATORY SENSITIZATION

It is still an open question which of the many changes induced by the inflammation are responsible for the sensitization and excitation of the nocisensors. Mechanical factors (increase of the tissue turgor by cellular and interstitial edema) and thermal factors (increase in local temperature as a consequence of vasodilation, not the vasodilation itself) could in part be responsible for the sensitization, but we do not know of any clinical and experimental findings supporting such an assumption.

On the other hand, there are several good reasons to believe that chemical factors are the decisive component in the sensitization caused by inflammatory processes. In the inflamed tissue a large number of inflammatory mediators accumulate, for instance, bradykinin, prostaglandins, and leukotrienes (2,19,44,54). These are either locally released or synthesized. In several tissues such inflammatory mediators could either excite the nocisensors directly or could sensitize them for other stimuli (4,5,39,49,55,57,62,66,72). For instance, close arterial injection of prostaglandins into the joint tissue led to an increase of the afferent responses to joint movements as well as the subsequent injection of bradykinin (Figs. 6.9A and 6.10A) (5,72,74).

Interestingly, the probability of these sensitizing effects was different in populations of slowly conducting afferents with different mechanical sensitivity. Using prostaglandin I_2, a larger proportion of low-threshold fibers than of high-threshold fibers was sensitized to mechanical stimuli (Fig. 6.9B), whereas a smaller proportion of low-threshold fibers than of high-threshold fibers was sensitized to bradykinin (Fig. 6.10B). Many if not all knee joint afferents, however, differ in their responsiveness to distinct inflammatory mediators, leading to a pronounced diversity of their chemical sensitivity. As an example, most of the articular afferents tested are sensitive to prostaglandin I_2, whereas only a part of them is also sensitive to prostaglandin E_2 (Fig. 6.11).

Taking into account the mode of action of the various inflammatory mediators on fine afferents (e.g., percentage of fibers being excited and/or sensitized, time course

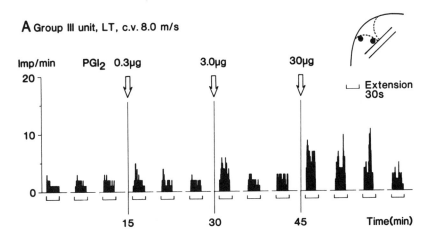

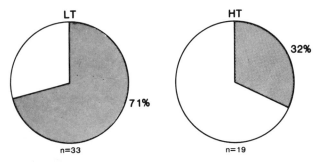

FIG. 6.9. Sensitization of afferents by prostaglandin I_2 (PGI$_2$) to passive movements of the knee joint. **A:** Responses to movements in a low-threshold group III unit with two receptive fields in the knee joint (displayed as impulses per second) showing increasing sensitization by injection of three different doses of PGI$_2$. **B:** Proportions of low-threshold (LT) and high-threshold (HT) group III and group IV units sensitized (*shaded area*) to movements by PGI$_2$.

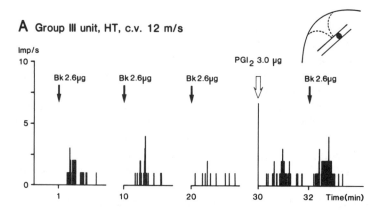

A Group III unit, HT, c.v. 12 m/s

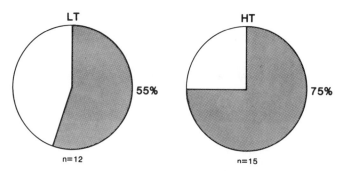

B Proportion of sensitized units

LT

55%

n=12

HT

75%

n=15

FIG. 6.10. Sensitization of afferents by prostaglandin I_2 (PGI_2) to an intra-arterial injection of bradykinin close to the knee joint. **A:** Responses to bradykinin (Bk) in a high-threshold group III unit with a receptive field in the region of the medial collateral ligament (responses displayed as impulses per second within 2 min after Bk injection). At min 30, PGI_2 was injected, causing an excitation and an increase of the following response to bradykinin. **B:** Proportions of low-threshold (LT) and high-threshold (HT) group III and IV units sensitized (*shaded area*) to bradykinin by PGI_2.

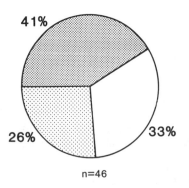

41%

26%   33%

n=46

FIG. 6.11. Proportions of group III and IV units that were sensitive (i.e., excited and/or sensitized) to both PGI_2 and PGE_2 (▒), PGI_2 alone (⬚), and insensitive to both (□). No unit was exclusively sensitive to PGE_2.

of the effect), it has to be assumed that several mediators act in concert ("inflammatory cocktail," see Handwerker and Reeh, Chapter 7) to produce the changes in the receptive properties observed during inflammation. This does not exclude that several other substances could participate in the sensitization processes. Such substances may include potassium ions, serotonin, histamine, and eventually also H^+ ions (pH) and catecholamines (31,58,61,62,76).

At present it appears that the neuropeptides do not play a major role in the sensitization process (34). Perhaps some of them induce the production of prostaglandin E_2 in synovial tissue (48), and these prostaglandins in turn act on joint afferents in an excitatory or sensitizing manner (72).

TRANSDUCTION MECHANISMS

In the preceding section prostaglandins and bradykinin have been mentioned as important inflammatory mediators. As a working hypothesis, they are supposed to evoke their effects by binding at receptors presumably on the membrane of sensory endings, thereby activating second messenger systems. So far, different second messenger systems have been proposed to be responsible for the effects of algogenic mediators at sensory endings. The hyperalgesia due to prostaglandins has been associated with the activation of the adenylate cyclase–cAMP-system (20,78). In different experimental approaches bradykinin seems to induce several intracellular events, such as the increase of intracellular cGMP (9,67,77), as well as the activation of phospholipase A_2 (3) and stimulation of prostaglandin synthesis (38,47,58,59).

Through the breakdown of phosphoinositides (22,37,56) bradykinin induces the production of second messenger molecules such as diacylglycerol (DAG), which activates protein kinase C (PKC) (64). PKC has been shown in cultured sensory neurons to be indeed involved in the mechanism of action of bradykinin (9), and recent *in vitro* observations suggested a critical role of PKC in the excitation of polymodal nociceptors (14,65).

Experimentally PKC can be activated by phorbol esters instead of the physiological second messenger DAG (10,45). Since phorbol esters are not metabolized and enter readily into the cell membrane, it is possible to bypass receptor-mediated cellular events and activate PKC directly. Therefore, in our knee joint model we used the phorbol ester phorbol 12,13-dibutyrate (PDBu) as an experimental stimulus to examine the role of PKC in the excitation of fine articular afferents, particularly with nociceptive properties.

As a result, in a large proportion of slowly conducting afferents PDBu caused excitation and/or sensitization to movements. For example, excitation occurred in 28% of group III and in 40% of group IV fibers of our population of 41 afferents (21 of group III and 20 of group IV). The excitation manifested itself as a beginning or an increase of ongoing (spontaneous) activity, which in most cases lasted more than 20 min (Fig. 6.12A). Furthermore, an enhancement of responses to passive movements of the joint, i.e., a sensitization, occurred in a large proportion of slowly conducting afferents. In summary, 37.5% of the low-threshold and 50% of the high-threshold fibers proved to be sensitive to PDBu. Thus, the sensitivity to PDBu was slightly more frequent in high-threshold than in low-threshold units.

This study provides the first data concerning the effects of activation of PKC by

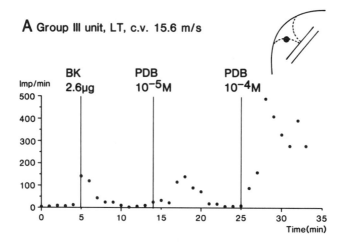

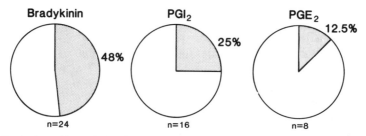

FIG. 6.12. Excitation of knee joint afferents to a close intra-arterial injection of different inflammatory mediators and phorbol ester. **A:** Responses of a group III unit to bradykinin (BK) and to two different doses of phorbol dibutyrate (PDB), displayed as impulses per minute. **B:** Proportions of group III and IV units excited by PDB (*shaded area*) in samples of units that are sensitive to bradykinin (excitation) or the prostaglandins PGI_2 and PGE_2 (excitation and/or sensitization).

phorbol esters on electrophysiologically characterized single sensory afferents. The current data show that PDBu can mimic the main actions of inflammatory mediators, first, the excitation and, second, the sensitization to mechanical stimuli of polymodal sensory afferents. The main difference between the effects of PDBu and those of inflammatory mediators is the relatively long duration of the PDBu effects. This is consistent with the idea that phorbol esters are poorly metabolized and therefore lead to a long-lasting activation of PKC (45).

In our experiments only about one-half of the bradykinin-positive afferents were also sensitive to PDBu (Fig. 6.12B). Since there is a proportion of units that did not react to PDBu in our study as well as in other investigations (9), PKC activation may not be the only mechanism by which sensory neurons can be activated by bradykinin. The proportion of units that were sensitive to both PDBu and prostaglandin I_2 or E_2 was rather small compared with the number of bradykinin-sensitive units (Fig. 6.12B). These data suggest that PKC activation may not be very important for the transduction of prostaglandin-mediated effects on sensory afferents. From these findings we conclude that the second messenger mechanisms triggered by bradykinin, on the one hand, and the prostaglandins, on the other, seem to be different.

STRUCTURE–FUNCTION RELATIONSHIPS: FIRST INSIGHTS

As outlined in the preceding sections and several other chapters in this volume, there are many new findings in the fields of electrophysiology, cytochemistry, and ultrastructure to characterize and identify slowly conducting fine afferent fibers, but there are some "missing links" between these various fields of research that prevent us from bringing together all our information to finally characterize a nociceptor and to distinguish it from other fine afferents. A particularly difficult gap to bridge concerns the relationship between structure and function. For instance, afferent fibers of groups II to IV, which are defined by their axon diameter and conduction velocity (6,7,21,63), are supposedly terminating in the knee joint either in corpuscular receptors (group II units) or in so-called "free nerve endings" (group III and IV units). But apart from some types of corpuscular receptors, this correlation is poorly confirmed and the borders between these groups are ill-defined. Furthermore, the primary processes of signal transduction and transformation of the generator potential to action potentials are probably independent and spatially separated, but we do not know where these processes take place. As described above we can discriminate three (group III) or two (group IV fibers) sections of peripheral nerve fibers, but what their relative role in the electrophysiological processes is remains open. Slowly conducting afferents show a variety of responses and response characteristics to mechanical, chemical, and thermal stimuli, and these properties are rather independent of their conduction velocity; on the other hand, the sensory endings of thinly myelinated and unmyelinated fibers can be found in different layers and associated with different histological structures of the knee joint capsule, which again may be a structural finding related to their functional properties. Finally, the ultrastructure of the terminal areas, as already outlined above, is also variable in respect to shape, free area (not covered by Schwann cells), and organelle content of the sensory axon, which may or may not be related to the physiological properties (see discussion above).

Regarding nociception and hyperalgesia, the following three questions are in the foreground of our interest: (a) Can we discriminate low- from high-threshold afferents by morphology? As outlined above, we are at present investigating the hypothesis that the content of mitochondria is different in these two functionally distinct types. (b) Is there a structural basis for polymodality? One possibility could be that the various terminal branches of a sensory ending have different histological structures (yet to be discovered) that subserve also different types of modality. (c) What happens in sensitization, i.e., what are the morphological, cytochemical, intracellular, or plasma membrane changes involved?

Our own attempt to make some progress in relating physiological, cytochemical, and morphological data in order to answer some of these questions is now concentrated on experiments at several morphological "levels."

At a rather "macroscopic level" we are trying to determine whether the various types of articular sensors show some differential in the location of their receptive fields on the joint capsule and the ligaments. For instance, we have looked at the distribution of receptive fields of polymodal sensors (those having mechano- and chemosensitivity) versus specific mechanosensitive units (no excitation to 2.6 μm bradykinin) but could not see any significant difference. On the other hand, there may be some differential in the distribution of low-threshold mechanosensitive versus very high threshold mechanosensitive receptive fields (those of movement category I vs movement category IV), the latter being almost entirely restricted to the triangle between the borders of the condyli of femur and tibia and the patellar ligament (i.e., "free" capsule on the articular cleft) (Fig. 6.13). This finding raises the question whether some silent nocisensors may be located in menisci, cruciate ligaments, or the infrapatellar fat body, all being close to the joint cavity where they are primarily exposed to an inflammation of the knee joint.

At the "histological level" we have started to mark receptive fields of functionally characterized group II to IV afferents for a subsequent histological study (both by light and electron microscopy). Such a morphological identification of sensory endings of physiologically pre-examined slowly conducting afferents was so far only tried by Kruger et al. (41) on testicular afferents. In our study first results of the examination of structure and function of identified sensory endings are as follow. (a) At the "preparative level" the microdissection of functionally mapped receptive fields showed that endings of high-threshold group III and IV afferents (nocisensor units) are more frequently related to ligaments (medial collateral and patellar ligaments) than low-threshold units. (b) At the "microscopic level" (histotopography of sensory endings) we have so far analyzed four group III units. Of these two were of high threshold (or nocisensors) and two were of low threshold. The high-threshold units were located in dense connective tissue (stratum fibrosum of capsule and ligament structure, respectively), the low-threshold units were located in soft connective tissue, related to delicate collagen fibers (Fig. 6.14) (reconstruction of low-threshold sensory ending). It will be interesting to see whether these findings can be confirmed and a general principle evolved from such measurements. (c) At the "ul-

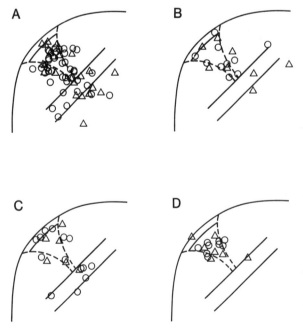

FIG. 6.13. Medial aspect of the cat's knee joint showing the distribution of the receptive fields of mainly slowly conducting afferents, categorized according to their mechanical sensitivity to movements. The contours of the patellar and collateral ligament are drawn with *solid lines,* the borders of the femoral and the tibial epicondylus *dotted.* **A,** movement category 1 (excited by innocuous passive movements of the knee); **B,** movement category 2 (poorly excited by innocuous movements); **C,** movement category 3 (only excited by noxious movements); and **D,** movement category 4 (not excited by movements). *Circles,* receptive fields of polymodal afferents, excited by mechanical stimuli and 2.6 μg bradykinin; *triangles,* receptive fields of mechanosensitive afferents, only excited by mechanical stimuli and not by bradykinin.

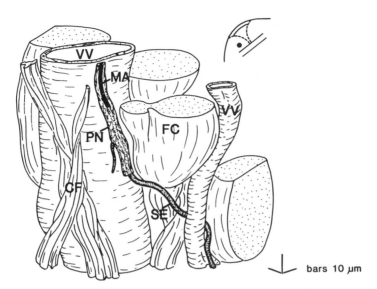

FIG. 6.14. Three-dimensional reconstruction of the sensory ending of a functionally characterized low-threshold (movement category 1) group III afferent nerve fiber with a conduction velocity of 9.6 m/sec and chemoreceptive properties, excited by bradykinin and PDB and weakly sensitized by prostaglandins. The sensory ending was located in soft connective tissue of the articular capsule on the femoral epicondyle. CF, collagen bundles; FC, fat cell; MA, myelinated axon; PN, perineurium; SE, sensory ending; VV, venous vessel.

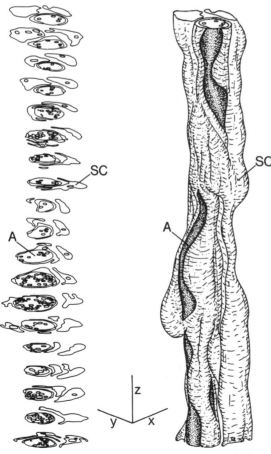

FIG. 6.15. Part of the sensory ending of a group III fiber with movement category 2 characteristics. **Left:** Contour plots of ultrathin cross-sections at 1-μm intervals, arranged by a computer program in a true-to-scale three-dimensional projection. x, y, z bars = 2μm. Morphometrical measurements of axon diameter and areal density of mitochondria were made on these sections. **Right:** Reconstruction showing surface details. Bare areas of the sensory axon, not covered by the Schwann cell processes, appear densely dotted. A, sensory axon, filled with mitochondria; SC, Schwann cell lamellae.

trastructural level" we have measured the axon diameter of two group III units with different conduction velocities. It was seen that the rapidly conducting group III unit (conduction velocity 12.8 m/sec) had indeed a thicker sensory axon within its terminal (mean diameter 1.6 μm) than the slowly conducting unit (conduction velocity, 6.4 m/sec; axon diameter, 1.1 μm) (Fig. 6.15). Morphometrical measurements of the content of the mitochondria (volume density) within the sensory axon of the latter unit (marginally activated by innocuous movements, i.e., category 2 unit, cf. Fig. 6.13) revealed a medium value compared to a random sample of other group III fibers (see discussion above).

It is immediately obvious from the brief sketch of our recent findings that many methodological difficulties make progress very slow in our attempt to relate structure, particularly ultrastructure, to function. Nevertheless, we consider these experiments a valuable tool in the study of structure-dependent characteristics of nociceptors and therefore will continue them.

SUMMARY AND CONCLUDING REMARKS

From the results summarized in this chapter it appears beyond reasonable doubt that the local tenderness (hyperalgesia) and the pain at rest and during movements of an inflamed joint have their peripheral origin in the increased sensitivity (decreased mechanical threshold plus enhanced responses to suprathreshold stimuli) of all types of articular afferent units. Most likely, the awakening of the silent or "sleeping" nociceptors is the most important single factor in producing the subjective sensations of tenderness and pain as well as the motor and autonomic reflexes observed in this and other inflammatory conditions (but not addressed in this review).

We are also convinced that chemical factors, namely, the so-called inflammatory mediators (e.g., bradykinin and other tachykinins, prostaglandins), are the decisive component in the sensitization caused by the inflammatory processes. But neither can a contribution of other factors (mechanical, thermal) be fully ruled out nor are we able to pinpoint exactly those substances having the most pronounced effects. The data currently available offer a bewildering scenario of individual patterns of chemosensitivity of single afferent units displaying tachyphylaxis to repeated applications of individual substances as well as potentiating effects when applying several such substances together or in close succession. Somewhat surprisingly, neuropeptides do not seem to play a major role in the sensitization process, at least not in the acute stage of an inflammation (almost nothing is known about the mechanisms of chronic sensitization, e.g., in a "tennis elbow").

There is a high degree of certainty regarding some of the histological findings on the innervation of the knee joint of the cat. These results include the composition of the two major joint nerves, MAN and PAN (number of afferent and efferent axons, percentages of the various fiber groups), their areas of innervation, the shape and dimensions of the terminal trees formed by the fine afferent axons, and the essential cytoplasmic contents of their axons. Unmyelinated afferent axons dominate the fiber spectrum, and together with the fine myelinated ones account for between 75% (PAN) and 90% (MAN) of the afferent fiber population.

The "hard core" functional and structural data mentioned above form a substantial background of knowledge formerly unavailable but now being used as a vantage point from which to tackle the most pressing questions in the unfolding story of the normal and pathophysiological mechanisms involved in articular nociception and pain. Some of these questions have been addressed here, particularly the transduction mechanisms in the afferent terminals and the structure–function relationships of the fine afferent units. The answers produced by these investigations will amplify our understanding of the peripheral nociceptive mechanisms in healthy and diseased tissue and thereby provide the ultimate basis from which pharmacological as well as other preventive and curative therapies may be developed to intercept nociceptor-induced pains at the earliest possible site, namely, the nociceptor itself.

ACKNOWLEDGMENTS

We would like to thank Mrs. C. Jansen, J. Müller, and B. Trost for expert technical assistance, Prof. W. F. Neiss and Dr. M. Pawlak for contributing some ideas and results, and Mrs. I. Laing for typing the manuscript. The work reviewed in this chapter was supported by the Deutsche Forschungsgemeinschaft.

REFERENCES

1. Andres, K. H., and von Düring, M. (1973): Morphology of cutaneous receptors. In: *Handbook of sensory physiology,* vol. II, edited by A. Iggo, pp. 3–28. Springer, Berlin.
2. Atik, O. A. (1990): Leukotriene B_4 and prostaglandin E_2-like activity in synovial fluid in osteoarthritis. *Prostaglandins Leukot. Essent. Fatty Acids,* 34:253–254.
3. Axelrod, J., Burch, R. M., and Jelsma, C. L. (1988): Receptor-mediated activation of phospholipase A_2 via GTP-binding proteins: arachidonic acid and its metabolites as second messengers. *Trends Neurosci.,* 11:117–123.
4. Beck, W., and Handwerker, O. (1974): Bradykinin and serotonin effects on various types of cutaneous nerve fibers. *Pflugers Arch.,* 347:209–222.
5. Birrell, G. J., Grubb, B. D., Iggo, A., and McQueen, D. S. (1990): Actions of PGE_2 and cicaprost on the sensitivity of high-threshold mechanoreceptors in normal and inflamed rat ankle joints. *J. Physiol. (Lond.),* 420:33.
6. Boyd, I. A. (1954): The histological structure of the receptors in the knee joint of the cat correlated with their physiological response. *J. Physiol. (Lond.),* 124:476–488.
7. Boyd, I. A., and Davey, M. R. (1968): *Composition of peripheral nerves.* E. and S. Livingstone, Edinburgh.
8. Burch, R. U. (1989): Diacylglycerol in the synergy of bradykinin and thrombin stimulation of prostaglandin synthesis. *Eur. J. Pharmacol.,* 168:39.
9. Burgess, G. M., Mullaney, I., McNeill, M., Dunn, P. M., and Rang, H. P. (1989): Second messengers involved in the mechanism of action of bradykinin in sensory neurons in culture. *J. Neurosci.,* 9:3314–3325.
10. Castagna, M., Takai, Y., Kaibuchi, K., Sano, K., Kikkawa, U., and Nishizuka, Y. (1982): Direct activation of calcium-activated, phospholipid-dependent protein kinase by tumor-promoting phorbol esters. *J. Biol. Chem.,* 257:7847–7851.
11. Coggeshall, R. E., Hong, K. A. P., Langford, L. A., Schaible, H.-G., and Schmidt, R. F. (1983): Discharge characteristics of fine medial articular afferents at rest and during passive movements of inflamed knee joints. *Brain Res.,* 272:185–188.
12. Craig, A. D., Heppelmann, B., and Schaible, H.-G. (1988): The projection of the medial and posterior articular nerves of the cat's knee to the spinal cord. *J. Comp. Neurol.,* 276:279–288.
13. Dorn, T., Schaible, H.-G., and Schmidt, R. F. (1991): Response properties of thick myelinated group II afferents in the medial articular nerve of normal and inflamed knee joints of the cat. *Somatosens. Mot. Res.,* 8:127–136.
14. Dray, A., Bettaney, J., Forster, P., and Perkinds, M. N. (1988): Bradykinin-induced stimulation of afferent fibres is mediated through protein kinase C. *Neurosci. Lett.,* 91:301–307.
15. Duggan, A. W., Morton, C. R., Zhao, Z. Q., and Hendry, J. A. (1987): Noxious heating of the skin releases immunoreactive substance P in the substantia gelatinosa of the cat: a study with antibody microprobes. *Brain Res.,* 403:345–349.
16. Duggan, A. W., Hendry, I. A., Morton, C. R., Hutchison, W. D., and Zhao, Z. Q. (1988): Cutaneous stimuli releasing immunoreactive substance P in the dorsal horn of the cat. *Brain Res.,* 451:261–273.

17. Duggan, A. W., Hope, P. J., Jarrot, B., Schaible, H.-G., and Fleetwood-Walker, S. M. (1990): Release, spread and persistence of immunoreactive neurokinin A in the dorsal horn of the cat following noxious cutaneous stimulation. Studies with antibody microprobes. *Neuroscience,* 35:195–202.

18. Edman, A., Gastrelius, S., and Grampp, W. (1986): Transmembrane ion balance in slowly and rapidly adapting lobster stretch receptor neurons. *J. Physiol. (Lond.),* 377:171–191.

19. Egg, D. (1984): Concentrations of prostaglandins D_2, E_2, F_2, 6-keto-F_{1a} and thromboxane B_2 in synovial fluid from patients with inflammatory joint disorders and osteoarthritis. *Z. Rheumatol.,* 43:89–96.

20. Ferreira, S. H., and Nakamura, M. (1979): Prostaglandin hyperalgesia, a cAMP/Ca^{2+} dependent process. *Prostaglandins,* 18:179–190.

21. Freeman, M. A. R., and Wyke, B. (1967): The innervation of the knee joint: an anatomical and histological study in the cat. *J. Anat.,* 101:505–532.

22. Gammon, C. M., Allen, A. C., and Morell, P. (1989): Bradykinin stimulates phosphoinositide hydrolysis and mobilization of arachidonic acid in dorsal root ganglion neurons. *J. Neurochem.,* 53:95–101.

23. Grigg, P., Schaible, H.-G., and Schmidt, R. F. (1986): Mechanical sensitivity of group III and IV afferents from posterior articular nerve in normal and inflamed cat knee. *J. Neurophysiol.,* 55:1–9.

24. Hanesch, U., Heppelmann, B., and Schmidt, R. F. (1991): Substance P and calcitonin gene-related peptide immunoreactivity in primary afferent neurons of the cat's knee joint. *Neuroscience (in press).*

25. Heppelmann, B. (1990): Morphologische Grundlagen peripherer und spinaler Prozesse beim Gelenkschmerz. Habilitationsschrift, Medizinische Fakultät der Universität, Würzburg.

26. Heppelmann, B., Herbert, M. K., Schaible, H.-G., and Schmidt, R. F. (1987): Morphological and physiological characteristics of the innervation of cat's normal and arthritic knee joint. In: *Effects of injury on trigeminal and spinal somatosensory systems,* edited by L. M. Pubols and B. J. Sessle, pp. 19–27. Alan R. Liss, New York.

27. Heppelmann, B., Heuss, C., and Schmidt, R. F. (1988): Fiber size distribution of myelinated and unmyelinated axons in the medial and posterior articular nerves of the cat's knee joint. *Somatosens. Res.,* 5:273–281.

28. Heppelmann, B., Messlinger, K., and Schmidt, R. F. (1989): Serial sectioning, electron microscopy, and three-dimensional reconstruction of fine nerve fibers and other extended objects. *J. Microsc.,* 156:163–172.

29. Heppelmann, B., Messlinger, K., Neiss, W. F., and Schmidt, R. F. (1990): Ultra-structural three-dimensional reconstruction of group III and group IV sensory nerve endings ("free nerve endings") in the knee joint capsule of the cat: evidence for multiple receptive sites. *J. Comp. Neurol.,* 292:103–116.

30. Heppelmann, B., Messlinger, K., Neiss, W. F., and Schmidt, R. F. (1990): The sensory terminal tree of "free nerve endings" in the articular capsule of the knee. In: *The primary afferent neuron. A survey of recent morpho-functional aspects,* edited by W. Zenker and W. L. Neuhuber, pp. 73–85. Plenum Press, New York.

31. Heyer, G., Hornstein, O. P., and Handwerker, H. O. (1989): Skin reactions and itch sensations induced by epicutaneous histamine application in atopic dermatitis and controls. *J. Invest. Dermatol.,* 93:492–496.

32. Hökfelt, T., Holets, V. R., Staines, W., et al. (1986): Coexistence of neuronal messengers—an overview. In: *Progress in brain research: coexistence of neuronal messengers: a new principle in chemical transmission,* vol. 68, edited by T. Hökfelt, K. Fuxe, and B. Pernow, pp. 33–70. Elsevier, Amsterdam.

33. Hökfelt, T., Johansson, O., Ljungdahl, A., Lundberg, J. M., and Schultzberg, M. (1980): Peptidergic neurons. *Nature,* 284:515–521.

34. Holzer, P. (1988): Local effector functions of capsaicin-sensitive sensory nerve endings: involvement of tachykinins, calcitonin gene-related peptide and other neuropeptides. *Neuroscience,* 24:739–768.

35. Hope, P. J., Jarrott, B., Schaible, H.-G., Clarke, R. W., and Duggan, A. W. (1990): Release and spread of immunoreactive neurokinin A in the cat spinal cord in a model of acute arthritis. *Brain Res.,* 533:292–299.

36. Inagaki, S., and Kito, S. (1986): Peptides in the peripheral nervous system. In: *Progress in brain research,* vol. 66, edited by P. C. Emson, M. N. Rossor, and M. Tohyama, pp. 269–316. Elsevier, Amsterdam.

37. Jackson, T. R., Hallam, T. J., Downes, C. P., and Hanley, M. R. (1987): Receptor coupled events in bradykinin action: rapid production of inositol phosphates and regulation of cytosolic free Ca^{2+} in a neural cell line. *EMBO J.,* 6:49–54.

38. Juan, H. (1977): Mechanism of action of bradykinin-induced release of prostaglandin E. *Naunyn Schmiedebergs Arch. Pharmacol.,* 300:77–85.

39. Kanaka, R., Schaible, H.-G., and Schmidt, R. F. (1985): Activation of fine articular afferent units by bradykinin. *Brain Res.*, 327:81–90.
40. Kruger, L. (1987): Morphological correlates of "free" nerve endings—a reappraisal of thin sensory axon classification. In: *Fine afferent nerve fibers and pain*, edited by R. F. Schmidt, H.-G. Schaible, and C. Vahle-Hinz. VCH, Weinheim.
41. Kruger, L., Kumazawa, T., Mizumura, K., Sato, J., and Yeh, Y. (1988): Observations on electrophysiologically characterized receptive fields of thin testicular afferent axons: a preliminary note on the analysis of fine structural specializations of polymodel receptors. *Somatosens. Res.*, 5:373–380.
42. Kupfermann, I. (1991): Functional studies of cotransmission. *Physiol. Rev. (Lond.)*, 71:683–732.
43. Langford, L. A., and Schmidt, R. F. (1983): Afferent and efferent axons in the medial and posterior articular nerves of the cat. *Anat. Rec.*, 206:71–78.
44. Larsson, J., Ekblom, A., Henriksson, K., Lundeberg, T., and Theodorsson, E. (1989): Immunoreactive tachykinins, calcitonin gene-related peptide and neuropeptide Y in human synovial fluid from inflamed knee joints. *Neurosci. Lett.*, 100:326–330.
45. Leach, K. L., and Blumberg, P. M. (1989): Tumor promoters, their receptors and their actions. In: *Inositol lipids in cell signalling*, edited by R. H. Michell, A. H. Drummond, and C. P. Downes, pp. 179–205. Academic Press, New York.
46. Leah, J. D., Cameron, A. A., and Snow, P. J. (1985): Neuropeptides in physiologically identified mammalian sensory neurones. *Neurosci. Lett.*, 56:257–263.
47. Lembeck, F., Popper, H., and Juan, H. (1976): Release of prostaglandins by bradykinin as an intrinsic mechanism of its algesic effect. *Naunyn Schmiedebergs Arch. Pharmacol.*, 294:69–73.
48. Lotz, M., Carson, D. A., and Vaughan, J. H. (1987): Substance P activation of rheumatoid synoviocytes: neural pathway in pathogenesis of arthritis. *Science*, 235:893–895.
49. Martin, H. A. (1990): Leukotriene B_4 induced decrease in mechanical and thermal thresholds of C-fiber mechanonociceptors in rat hairy skin. *Brain Res.*, 509:273–279.
50. Mayes, J. J., and Govind, C. K. (1989): Higher mitochondrial density in slow versus fast lobster sensory neurons. *Neurosci. Lett.*, 102:87–90.
51. McIntyre, A. K., Proske, U., and Tracey, D. J. (1978): Afferent fibres from muscle receptors in the posterior nerve of the cat's knee joint. *Exp. Brain Res.*, 33:415–424.
52. McMahon, S. B., and Koltzenburg, M. (1990): Novel classes of nociceptors: beyond Sherrington. *Trends Neurosci.*, 13:199–201.
53. McMahon, S. B., and Koltzenburg, M. (1990): The changing role of primary afferent neurones in pain. *Pain*, 43:269–272.
54. Melli, M. (1988): Assessment of plasma leukotriene and prostaglandin levels during adjuvant arthritis and kaolin-induced paw oedema in rats. *Prostaglandins Leukot. Essent. Fatty Acids*, 33:173–178.
55. Mense, S., and Meyer, H. (1988): Bradykinin-induced modulation of the response behaviour of different types of feline group III and IV muscle receptors, *J. Physiol. (Lond.)*, 398:49–63.
56. Miller, R. J. (1987): Bradykinin highlights the role of phospholipid metabolism in the control of nerve excitability. *Trends Neurosci.*, 10:226–228.
57. Mizumura, K., Sato, J., and Kumazawa, T. (1987): Effects of prostaglandins and other putative chemical intermediaries of the activity of canine testicular polymodal receptors studied in vitro. *Eur. J. Physiol.*, 408:565–572.
58. Moncada, S., Ferreira, S. H., and Vane, J. R. (1978): Pain and inflammatory mediators. In: *Handbook of experimental pharmacology*, vol. 5, edited by J. R. Vane and S. H. Ferreira, pp. 588–616. Springer, Berlin.
59. Moncada, S., Mullane, K. M., and Vane, J. R. (1979): Prostacyclin release by bradykinin in vivo. *Br. J. Pharmacol.*, 66:969–979.
60. Morton, C. R., Hutchison, W. D., and Hendry, I. A. (1988): Release of immunoreactive somatostatin in the spinal dorsal horn of the cat. *Neuropeptides*, 12:189–198.
61. Neugebauer, V., and Schaible, H.-G. (1988): Peripheral and spinal components of the sensitization of spinal neurons during an acute experimental arthritis. *Agents Actions*, 25:234–236.
62. Neugebauer, V., Schaible, H.-G., and Schmidt, R. F. (1989): Sensitization of articular afferents to mechanical stimuli by bradykinin. *Pflugers Arch.*, 415:330–335.
63. Novotny, V. (1973): Relation between receptor kind and afferent fibre diameter in the knee-joint capsule of the cat. *Acta Anat.*, 86:436–450.
64. Rana, R. S., and Hokin, L. E. (1990): Role of phosphoinosites in transmembrane signaling. *Physiol. Rev.*, 70:115–164.
65. Rang, H. P., and Ritchie, J. M. (1988): Depolarization of nonmyelinated fibres of rat vagus nerve produced by activation of protein kinase C. *J. Neurosci.*, 8:2606–2617.
66. Raja, S. N., Meyer, R. A., and Campbell, J. N. (1988): Peripheral mechanisms of somatic pain. *Anesthesiology*, 68:571–590.
67. Reiser, G., Walter, U., and Hamprecht, B. (1984): Bradykinin regulates the level of guanosine 3′,5′-cyclic monophosphate (cyclic GMP) in neural cell lines. *Brain Res.*, 290:367–371.

68. Schaible, H.-G., and Schmidt, R. F. (1983): Activation of groups III and IV sensory units in medial articular nerve by local mechanical stimulation of knee joint. *J. Neurophysiol.*, 49:35–44.
69. Schaible, H.-G., and Schmidt, R. F. (1983): Responses of fine medial articular nerve afferents to passive movements of knee joint. *J. Neurophysiol.*, 49:1118–1126.
70. Schaible, H.-G., and Schmidt, R. F. (1985): Effects of an experimental arthritis on the sensory properties of fine articular afferent units. *J. Neurophysiol.*, 54:1109–1122.
71. Schaible, H.-G., and Schmidt, R. F. (1988): Time course of mechanosensitivity changes in articular afferents during a developing experimental arthritis. *J. Neurophysiol.*, 60:2180–2195.
72. Schaible, H.-G., and Schmidt, R. F. (1988): Excitation and sensitization of fine articular afferents from cat's knee joint by prostaglandin E_2. *J. Physiol. (Lond.)*, 403:91–104.
73. Schaible, H.-G., Jarrott, B., Hope, P. J., and Duggan, A. W. (1990): Release of immunoreactive substance P in the spinal cord during development of acute arthritis in the knee joint of the cat: a study with antibody microprobes. *Brain Res.*, 529:214–223.
74. Schepelmann, K., Messlinger, K., Schaible, H.-G., and Schmidt, R. F. (1990): Prostaglandin I_2 enhances the mechanosensitivity of fine afferents from the knee joint of the cat. *Pflugers Arch.*, 415:suppl. 1:R107.
75. Schwerzmann, K., Hoppler, H., Kayar, S. R., and Weibel, E. R. (1988): Oxidative capacity of muscle and mitochondria: correlation of physiological, biochemical, and morphometric characteristics. *Proc. Natl. Acad. Sci. USA*, 86:1583–1587.
76. Sicuteri, F. (1967): Vasoneuroactive substances and their implication in vascular pain. In: *Research and clinical studies in headache*, vol. 1, edited by A. P. Friedman, pp. 6–45. Karger, Basel.
77. Snider, R. M., and Richelson, E. (1984): Bradykinin receptor-mediated cyclic GMP formation in a nerve cell population (murine neuroblastoma clone N1E-115). *J. Neurochem.*, 43:1749–1754.
78. Taiwo, Y. O., Bjerkenes, L. K., Goetzl, E. J., and Levine, J. D. (1989): Mediation of primary afferent peripheral hyperalgesia by the cAMP second messenger system. *Neuroscience*, 32:577–580.

Hyperalgesia and Allodynia,
edited by W. D. Willis, Jr.
Raven Press, Ltd., New York © 1992.

7

Nociceptors

Chemosensitivity and Sensitization by Chemical Agents

H. O. Handwerker and P. W. Reeh

*Institut für Physiologie und Biokybernetik, Universität Erlangen-Nürnberg,
D-8520 Erlangen, Germany*

Most fibers in peripheral nerves are unmyelinated, e.g., 80% in the saphenous nerve of the rat, a pure skin nerve, and a similar percentage in a muscle nerve of this species (4,14,24). Only about 20% of the unmyelinated units in skin nerves are sympathetic efferents; the vast majority have cell bodies in the dorsal root ganglia and hence are afferents (1). In skin, most unmyelinated afferent units can be excited by heat, mechanical, and chemical stimuli. These units often are labeled "polymodal." Although some of these polymodal or CMH (mechano-heat responsive) units have mechanical and/or heat thresholds below the pain threshold of the respective animal, they have no other known function than being nociceptors. There are strong arguments for an involvement of nociceptors, not only in stimulus-induced pain but also in pain states related to inflammation. Under model inflammation conditions, nociceptors often show reactions corresponding to inflammatory pain and hyperalgesia: they exhibit ongoing activity and are sensitized to mechanical and heat stimulation (5,9,16,17,26,27). Since both phenomena are also induced by application of substances that are released from inflamed tissue, the inflammation-induced changes in nociceptor responsiveness are presumably mediated by these agents. Hence, the selective sensitivity of CMH units (and AMH units with thin myelinated axons) to endogenous mediators provides a strong argument in favor of their involvement in inflammatory pain.

SENSITIVITY OF AFFERENT C UNITS TO ENDOGENOUS MEDIATORS OF INFLAMMATION

Apart from their unique sensitivity to capsaicin, a derivative of the red pepper (38,39), CMH and AMH units are also sensitive to a variety of substances that are released in the course of inflammation (2,6).

Traditionally, chemosensitivity of cutaneous afferents has been investigated with topical applications and injections into the tissue or afferent arteries of anesthetized animals. Unfortunately, these methods do not allow an exact control of the duration and intensity of chemical stimuli and possibly imply interference with blood-borne substances and vascular reactions. To overcome these problems several *in vitro* preparations were developed (19,28,34).

In our laboratory we have used a preparation consisting of the saphenous nerve of the rat and the skin flap innervated by that nerve. For this purpose the skin is mounted, epidermal side down, in a tissue chamber superfused with oxygenated synthetic interstitial fluid (SIF) (28). The nerve is drawn into a second chamber where small strands are dissected for single unit recording. Receptive fields are searched for by mechanically probing the skin from the corium side. Radiant heat stimuli are applied through the translucent bottom of the chamber to the epidermal surface. For selective chemical stimulation, an additional smaller chamber is placed over the receptive field in which the fluid can quickly be exchanged through push–pull cannulae (28,29).

We have found that in this preparation classic endogenous pain-producing substances, e.g., bradykinin (BK) and serotonin (5-HT) excite part of the CMH and AMH units at micromolar concentrations, but virtually no other type of cutaneous afferents (21). Hitherto on a molar base BK seems to be the most potent endogenous excitatory agent for CMH units, and thus most studies use this substance, which is generated in the tissue in the course of inflammatory reactions together with other peptides from high molecular weight precursors, the kininogens. About half of the CMH units were selectively excited by BK at concentrations of 10^{-8} to 10^{-5} M in the skin nerve preparation (21). In another *in vitro* preparation visceral nociceptors were excited even at concentrations as low as 10^{-9} M (19).

BK did not only excite CMH units but also induced sensitization to heat stimuli *in vitro* (18,21). This may be an important observation since it seems to prove that this type of sensitization is not mediated indirectly by vascular actions of BK. *In vivo* and *in vitro* BK actions on CMH units show a clear tachyphylaxis even at stimulus repetition rates of one per 15 min and less (21). A similar tachyphylaxis was also found in the pain responses of human subjects to whom this substance was applied in a blister base. This tachyphylaxis and the observation that only part of the CMH units are excited by BK make it unlikely that this agent is the unique mediator of inflammatory pain and tenderness.

However, BK may interact with prostaglandins of the E group (PGE) by activating the phospholipase A2, which supplies arachidonic acid and hence increases PG formation. PGs, in turn, may sensitize nociceptive nerve endings to BK by blocking a slow afterhyperpolarization as it does in some neurons in tissue culture. Indeed a potentiation of the BK responses by PGE_1 and PGE_2 was found in several studies, although PGEs alone usually have either no or weak excitatory effects, depending on the tissue and the species (19,20,21,26).

ARE THE ACTIVATION AND SENSITIZATION OF NOCICEPTORS BY BRADYKININ DEPENDENT ON SYMPATHETIC EFFERENTS?

It has been reported that nociceptor afferents supplying inflamed tissue may be activated by sympathetic activity (32,33; Perl, Chapter 5) and, more specifically, that the behavioral manifestations of hyperalgesia in animals after intradermal injection of BK were critically dependent on the presence of postganglionic sympathetic fibers (22). Levine and colleagues made the specific proposal that BK induces hyperalgesia by releasing PGE_2 from the postganglionic sympathetic fibers, which then was thought to sensitize nociceptive primary afferents (23).

To test this hypothesis at the level of nociceptive nerve endings, recordings of single CMH units from untreated and from chronically sympathectomized rats were compared in the skin–nerve *in vitro* preparation described above (18). Sympathectomy was performed 7 to 10 days prior to the terminal experiment under barbiturate anesthesia. To this purpose the thoracolumbar sympathetic chain was exposed retroperitoneally using a lateral approach. After segmental identification of the ganglia according to the criteria previously described (1), the left ganglia Th_{13}–L_3 containing the cell bodies of the postganglionic fibers in the saphenous nerve were excised. Because of the fusion of the lumbar ganglia, the sympathectomy in most cases involved also the contralateral part of the fused lumbar sympathetic chain to assure the complete removal of sympathetic neurons.

In preparations from intact skin, CMH units responding to superfusion of the receptive fields with 10 µM BK for 1 min were sensitized to controlled radiant heat stimuli applied 2 min later. Heat stimuli consisted of a linear temperature increase at the corium side of the preparation from 32° to 45°C in 20 sec. On average the heat threshold dropped by 5.0°C, the maximal discharge frequency increased by 34%, and the temperature eliciting this peak discharge dropped by 5.6°C. This resulted in a leftward shift and an increased slope of the stimulus response function indicating sensitization. In sympathectomized preparations, 52% of the CMH units were activated by BK, which is not different from the controls. Neither the mean threshold reduction (4.6°C), nor the increase of the peak discharge frequency (48%), nor the drop of the temperature eliciting the peak discharge differed significantly in sympathectomized rats. BK increased the heat response of CMH units by a factor of 2.14 in untreated and by 1.91 in sympathectomized preparations. This increased responsiveness was short-lived and had resolved 7 min after chemical stimulation. There was again no significant difference in the time course between units recorded from untreated and from sympathectomized rats (18). In the light of these results one has to conclude that BK can excite unmyelinated nociceptive afferents supplying the rat hairy skin and cause a short-lived sensitization for subsequent heat stimulation irrespective of the presence of sympathetic nerve fibers. Therefore, it is unlikely that the sympathetic nervous system contributes significantly to the development of nociceptor sensitization in acute inflammation via the mechanism proposed by Levine and colleagues (23).

NOCICEPTORS ARE EXCITED AND SENSITIZED BY AN "INFLAMMATORY SOUP"

Apart from BK there are numerous other mediators released in the course of inflammatory reactions, e.g., 5-HT, which is released from blood platelets as well as from sources outside the circulation. Its pharmacological effects are various, and it may in turn release other neurovasoactive agents, e.g., thromboxane A_2 from platelets. In inflammation the most prominent effect of 5-HT on the microcirculation is probably vasodilation mediated via the release of an endothelium-derived relaxation factor (for a review, see ref. 12). 5-HT was found to excite CMH units *in vivo* (2) and *in vitro* (8,10), probably mainly via $5-HT_3$ receptors (31).

In the *in vitro* skin nerve preparation in which vascular effects are absent, about 40% of the CMH units that responded to BK were also excited by 5-HT at 10-μM concentrations. However, even if CMH units were not excited by 5-HT, their subsequent responses to BK were enhanced in most cases. This potentiation of BK responses was observed even after treatment with 5-HT at 1-μM concentrations, which scarcely had an overt excitatory effect (21).

Since we observed such potentiation of BK responses also after pretreatment with PGE$_2$, we concluded that the nociceptors are excited during inflammation by varying combinations of mediators, which we have termed "inflammatory soup" (IS) (9). This hypothesis is supported by findings from several laboratories and types of preparations, indicating that probably multiple agents act at the nociceptor membrane. Individual substances excite at best part of the CMH units, and this excitation is usually prone to tachyphylaxis.

Two experiments were designed for studying synergisms of the various agents released in inflammation.

In one series of *in vitro* experiments we compared the incidence of CMH units driven by BK in skin patches of rats in which inflammation had been induced by intracutaneous carrageenan injections hours before the animal was killed with that of units from intact skin. Only about half of the units were driven in intact skin but 90% in inflamed skin. Furthermore, the tachyphylaxis of the BK responses was strikingly diminished in the skin sites that had been inflamed before excision (16). In another type of experiment we tried to imitate the influence of the multitude of agents released in an acute inflammation by applying an artificial IS consisting of BK, 5-HT, histamine, and PGE$_2$ (all at 10-μM concentrations) together with K$^+$ (7×10^{-3} M) at a pH of 7.0, applied at 38°C. This mixture usually induced a more frequent discharge in CMH and AMH units than BK alone, and more than 80% of the units responded to this kind of stimulus (15).

THE EFFECTS OF ACID pH ON NOCICEPTORS

Of course, the composition of the artificial IS described in the last paragraph is somewhat arbitrary, although similar concentrations of the different agents contained in it were found in inflammatory exudates (for review, see ref. 9). However, in inflamed and ischemic tissues, e.g., pH levels down to 5.4 were found reflecting H$^+$ concentrations far exceeding those used in our IS (7).

Therefore, in subsequent experiments on nociceptive nerve endings we studied the effects of low pH alone *in vitro* by superfusing receptive fields of isolated afferent units with carbogen-gassed SIF titrated with phosphate buffer to different acid pH levels (35,36). Low-threshold mechanosensitive A-beta and A-delta units were neither excited nor sensitized by acid pH levels. In a quarter of the CMH units irregular low-frequency discharges with poor response characteristics were induced. However, another subpopulation of about 40% of the CMHs showed stimulus-related responses to acid solutions increasing with H$^+$ concentration and encoding the time course of the pH change. Threshold levels ranged between pH 6.9 and 6.1; maximal discharges were obtained at pH 5.2 on average. Prolonged application to some units of acid pH for periods up to 30 min evoked nonadapting activity irrespective of oxygen supply. Interestingly, repeated or prolonged treatment with low pH induced a significant and sustained decrease of the mechanical (von Frey) thresholds in almost all C fibers tested, and this sensitization to mechanical stimuli was also observed in C units that were not excited by low pH. This sensitization to mechanical, in contrast to heat, stimulation was not observed with the application of the IS described above. From these results it was concluded that the sensitivity of CMH units to low pH is an important source of pain and hyperalgesia (9,36).

SYNERGISM BETWEEN ACID pH AND OTHER INFLAMMATORY MEDIATORS

The multifactorial nature of nociceptor excitation is clearly shown by the synergism of an acid pH and the mediators combined in the artificial IS described above (35). Figure 7.1 shows two units (A and B) that were first tested with a SIF solution saturated with CO_2 and thus adjusted to a pH of 6.1; 15 min later both units were tested with IS (at a pH of 7.0, see above), and finally with a combination of both solutions. The unit shown in Fig. 7.1A shows a clear additive effect of IS and low pH, whereas in unit B both the low pH and the inflammatory mediators in the IS did not exert obvious effects. However, the combination did excite this CMH unit.

Supra-additive effects were also observed with sustained superfusions that may simulate the effect of a developing inflammation more closely. An example is shown in Fig. 7.2. A CMH unit was superfused with IS for 30 min. With this treatment the initial excitation subsided after 5 min. When, however, the pH of the superfusate was lowered to 6.1 by saturation with CO_2 the unit was tonically activated.

A unifying concept of nociceptor excitation and sensitization by inflammatory agents is still lacking, since our knowledge of the processes at the nociceptor membranes is still indirect and scarce. BK, 5-HT, and other agents may change the membrane polarization via specific receptors and respective second messenger systems.

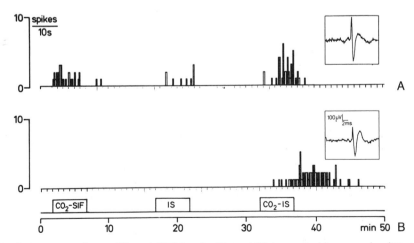

FIG. 7.1. Responses of two different CMH units (**A** and **B**) in a rat skin nerve *in vitro* preparation to superfusion of the corium side of the respective receptive field with a physiological solution buffered to pH 6.1 (CO_2-SIF) and with the artificial "inflammatory soup" (IS) described in the text. *Insets*, form of the action potential of the respective unit.

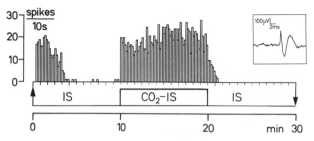

FIG. 7.2. Tonic superfusion of a CMH unit with artificial "inflammatory soup" (IS) that was buffered to pH 7.0. This solution was replaced between the 10th and 20th min of the stimulus protocol with a solution of identical composition but buffered to pH 6.1 by saturation with CO_2.

On the other hand, the H^+-induced nociceptor excitation corresponds in several aspects to a recently discovered depolarizing current in rat sensory ganglion cells that was specifically gated by downward steps in extracellular pH (3). This current occurred in about 40% of predominantly small, cultured dorsal root ganglion cells from which C fibers originate. Similar to the nociceptors, the H^+-induced sustained cation inward current was characterized by pH thresholds between 6.1 and 6.6 in individual cells, half maximal activation around pH 5.75, and a saturation between pH 5.1 and 5.4. Inactivation was very slow. Almost constant ion fluxes were observed with a whole cell patch-clamp for test periods of 1 min. This channel type could provide a molecular basis for the long-lasting nociceptor excitation described above. Bevan and Yeats (3) described some striking similarities between the actions of H^+ ions on that sustained cation current and the actions of capsaicin, suggesting that both may affect the same ion channel. Regarding the similarities of the membrane attributes of sensory ganglion cells and nociceptive nerve endings, one could expect that all pH-sensitive C-fiber endings were excited by capsaicin and vice versa. However, in our experiments only about half of the CMH units driven by low pH were also excited by capsaicin at a concentration of 10^{-6} M (36). Further experiments are needed to explain this incomplete match.

THE CONTRIBUTION OF NEUROGENIC INFLAMMATION TO NOCICEPTOR SENSITIZATION

For a long time, it has been known that unmyelinated nociceptor afferents upon stimulation release vasoactive substances, e.g., substance P, from their peripheral endings. The exact composition of the secreted agents is not yet known. However, the neurogenic vasodilation and plasma extravasation have been studied in many laboratories and in various tissues (for review, see refs. 13,37,38).

The possible biological functions of this "neurogenic inflammation" are still a matter of speculation. It has been observed that an optimal vasodilatory effect may be obtained from C fibers firing at a frequency of less than 1 spike/sec (25).

Since such low firing frequencies scarcely induce pain sensations (40), it has been conjectured that afferent C fibers have two working ranges, one for regulating the microenvironment in the respective tissue and another one for mediating pain sensations (25).

We have dealt with the question of whether substance P and other agents released from the endings of afferent C fibers can contribute to the sensitization of these C units. In an initial series of experiments, we found that *in vivo* CMH units are not sensitized but rather depressed after a train of electrical stimuli applied to the respective nerve stem (30). In contrast, clear sensitization was seen in the rat (28) and human skin (11) after application of mustard oil (allylisothiocyanate), which at low concentrations probably exerts its irritant effects exclusively by C-fiber excitation.

Since the *in vivo* experiments were not conclusive we directly tested the effects of substance P, the best-known agent of neurogenic inflammation, in the *in vitro* skin–nerve preparation (15).

In these and similar experiments of other groups (20) substance P did not excite CMH units in concentrations up to 10^{-4} M. Therefore, we tested for an interaction with the mediators of inflammation combined in the artificial IS described earlier. For this purpose the receptive fields of CMH units were superfused for 5-min periods and at 15-min intervals with IS. After assessing the baseline responsiveness of the respective unit, substance P was added 5 min before and during the IS application. In some units this type of conditioning induced a striking enhancement of the IS-induced activity.

However, the effects of substance P on a whole population of CMH units was less dramatic. A sensitizing effect became only significant at a concentration of 10^{-5} M (15). In another series of experiments we tested the tonic effects with an experimental protocol similar to that shown in Fig. 7.2. In this type of experiment substance P was completely ineffective. From these results it seems unlikely that substance P exerts more than a minor sensitizing effect on nociceptors in rat skin. However, it may well be that again a combination of neuropeptides and perhaps also other substances are effective in neurogenic inflammation.

In summary, the findings described in this chapter indicate that a variety of agents contribute to nociceptor excitation and sensitization. Hence, it is unlikely that a single kind of pharmacological agent will interfere with all instances of nociceptor sensitization and the related hyperalgesia.

ACKNOWLEDGMENTS

We wish to thank Dr. K. Steen, A. Hanisch, Dr. M. Koltzenburg, M. Kress, W. Kessler, H. Reischl, and C. Kirchhoff who participated in the experiments reviewed in this chapter. Our work was supported by the DFG.

REFERENCES

1. Baron, R., Jänig, W., and Kollmann, W. (1988): Sympathetic and afferent somata projecting in hindlimb nerves and the anatomical organization of the lumbar sympathetic nervous system of the rat. *J. Comp. Neurol.,* 275:460–468.
2. Beck, P. W., and Handwerker, H. O. (1974): Bradykinin and serotonin effects on various types of cutaneous nerve fibres. *Pflugers Arch.,* 347:209–222.
3. Bevan, S., and Yeats, J. (1991): Protons activate a cation conductance in a sub-population of rat dorsal root ganglion neurones. *J. Physiol. (Lond.),* 433:145–161.
4. Carter, D. A., and Lisney, S. J. W. (1987): The number of unmyelinated and myelinated axons in normal and regenerated rat saphenous nerve. *J. Neurol. Sci.,* 80:163–171.

5. Campbell, J. N., Raja, S. N., Cohen, R. H., Manning, D. C., Khan, A. A., and Meyer, R. A. (1989): Peripheral neural mechanisms of nociception. In: *Textbook of pain*, edited by P. D. Wall and R. Melzack, pp. 22–45. Churchill Livingstone, Edinburgh.
6. Fjällbrant, N., and Iggo, A. (1961): The effect of histamine, 5-hydroxytryptamine and acetylcholine on cutaneous afferent fibres. *J. Physiol. (Lond.)*, 156:578–590.
7. Häbler, C. (1929): Über den K- und Ca-Gehalt in Eiter und Exsudaten und seine Beziehung zum Entzündungsschmerz. *Arch. Clin. Chir.*, 156:20–42.
8. Handwerker, H. O. (1991): What peripheral mechanisms contribute to nociceptive transmission and hyperalgesia? In: *Towards a new pharmacotherapy of pain*, edited by A. I. Basbaum and J.-M. Besson, pp. 5–19. John Wiley, Chichester.
9. Handwerker, H. O., and Reeh, P. W. (1991): Pain and inflammation. In: *Proceedings of the VIth World Congress on Pain*, edited by M. R. Bond, J. E. Charlton, and C. J. Woolf, pp. 59–70. Elsevier-North Holland, Amsterdam.
10. Handwerker, H. O., Reeh, P. W., and Steen, K. H. (1990): Effects of 5HT on nociceptors. In: *Serotonin and pain*, edited by J.-M. Besson, pp. 1–16. Elsevier-North Holland, Amsterdam.
11. Handwerker, H. O., Forster, C., and Kirchhoff, C. (1991): Discharge patterns of human C-fibers induced by itching and burning stimuli. *J. Neurophysiol.*, 66:307–315.
12. Hollenberg, N. H. (1988): Serotonin and vascular responses. *Annu. Rev. Pharmacol. Toxicol.*, 28:41–59.
13. Jancso, G., Obasl, F., Toth-kasa, I., Katona, M., and Husz, S. (1985): The modulation of cutaneous inflammatory reactions by peptide-containing sensory nerves. *Int. J. Tissue Res.*, 7:449–457.
14. Jenq, C. B., and Coggeshall, R. E. (1985): Long-term patterns of axon regeneration in the sciatic nerve and its tributaries. *Brain Res.*, 345:34–44.
15. Kessler, W., Kirchhoff, C., Handwerker, H. O., and Reeh, P. W. (1989): Substance P increases nociceptor responses to mediators of inflammation in rat skin. *Pflugers Arch.*, 413:R27.
16. Kirchhoff, C., Jung, S., Reeh, P. W., and Handwerker, H. O. (1990): Carrageenan inflammation increases bradykinin sensitivity of rat nociceptors. *Neurosci. Lett.*, 111:206–210.
17. Kocher, L., Anton, F., Reeh, P. W., and Handwerker, H. O. (1987): The effect of carrageenan-induced inflammation on the sensitivity of unmyelinated skin nociceptors in the rat. *Pain*, 29:363–373.
18. Koltzenburg, M., Kress, M., and Reeh, P. W. (1992): The nociceptor sensitization by bradykinin does not depend on sympathetic neurones. *Neuroscience*, 46:465–473.
19. Kumazawa, T., Mizumura, K., and Sato, J. (1987): Response properties of polymodal receptors studied using in vitro testis superior spermatic nerve preparations of dogs. *J. Neurophysiol.*, 57:702–711.
20. Kumazawa, T., Mizumura, K., and Sato, J. (1988): Modulation of testicular polymodal receptor activities. *Prog. Brain Res.*, 74:325–330.
21. Lang, E., Novak, A., Reeh, P. W., and Handwerker, H. O. (1990): Chemosensitivity to fine afferents from rat skin in vitro. *J. Neurophysiol.*, 63:887–901.
22. Levine, J. D., Taiwo, Y., Collins, S. D., and Tam, J. K. (1986): Noradrenaline hyperalgesia is mediated through interaction with sympathetic postganglionic neurone terminals rather than activation of primary afferent nociceptors. *Nature*, 323:158–160.
23. Levine, J. D., Coderre, T. J., and Basbaum, A. I. (1988): The peripheral nervous system and the inflammation process. In: *Proceedings of the Vth World Congress on Pain*, edited by R. Dubner, G. F. Gebhart, M. R. Bond., pp. 33–43. Elsevier-North Holland, Amsterdam.
24. Lisney, S. J. W. (1989): Regeneration of unmyelinated axons after injury of mammalian peripheral nerve. *Q. J. Exp. Physiol.*, 74:757–784.
25. Lynn, B., and Shakhanbeh, J. (1988): Neurogenic inflammation in the skin of the rabbit. *Agents Actions*, 25:228–231.
26. Neugebauer, V., Schaible, H.-G., and Schmidt, R. F. (1989): Sensitization of articular afferents to mechanical stimuli by bradykinin. *Pflugers Arch.*, 415:330–335.
27. Raja, S. N., Meyer, R. A., and Campbell, J. N. (1988): Peripheral mechanisms of somatic pain. *Anesthesiology*, 68:571–590.
28. Reeh, P. W. (1986): Sensory receptors in mammalian skin in an in vitro preparation. *Neurosci. Lett.*, 66:141–146.
29. Reeh, P. W. (1988): Sensory receptors in a mammalian skin-nerve in vitro preparation. In: *Progress in brain research*, vol. 74, edited by W. Hamann and A. Iggo, pp. 271–276. Elsevier-North Holland, Amsterdam.
30. Reeh, P. W., Kocher, L., and Jung, S. (1986): Does neurogenic inflammation alter the sensitivity of unmyelinated nociceptors in the rat? *Brain Res.*, 384:42–50.
31. Richardson, B. P., and Engel, G. (1986): The pharmacology and function of 5-HT3 receptors. *Trends Neurosci.*, 9:424–428.
32. Roberts, W. J., and Elardo, S. M. (1985): Sympathetic activation of A-delta nociceptors. *Somatosens. Res.*, 3:33–44.

33. Sanjue, H., and Jun, Z. (1989): Sympathetic facilitation of sustained discharges of polymodal nociceptors. *Pain,* 38:85–90.
34. Sann, H., and Cervero, F. (1988): Afferent innervation of the guinea-pig's ureter. *Agents Actions,* 24:234–235.
35. Steen, K. H., Hanisch, A. E., and Reeh, P. W. (1991): A dominant role of acid pH in inflammatory excitation of nociceptors in rat skin. *Pflugers Arch.,* 416:R1.
36. Steen, K. H., Reeh, P. W., Anton, F., and Handwerker, H. O. (1992): Protons selectively induce lasting excitation and sensitization to mechanical stimulation of nociceptors in rat skin, in vitro. *J. Neurosci. (in press).*
37. Szolcsanyi, J. (1984): Capsaicin-sensitive chemoceptive neural system with dual sensory-efferent function. In: *Antidromic vasodilatation and neurogenic inflammation,* edited by L. A. Chahl, J. Szolcsanyi, and F. Lembeck, pp. 27–52. Akedemiai Kiado, Budapest.
38. Szolcsanyi, J. (1987): Antidromic vasodilatation and neurogenic inflammation. *Agents Actions,* 22:2–8.
39. Szolcsanyi, J., Anton, F., Reeh, P. W., and Handwerker, H. O. (1988): Selective excitation by capsaicin of mechano-heat sensitive nociceptors in rat skin. *Brain Res.,* 446:262–268.
40. Van Hees, J., and Gybels, J. (1981): C-nociceptor activity in human nerve during painful and non-painful skin stimulation. *J. Neurol. Neurosurg. Psychiatry,* 44:600–607.

Hyperalgesia and Allodynia,
edited by W. D. Willis, Jr.
Raven Press, Ltd., New York © 1992.

8

Hyperalgesic Pain: Inflammatory and Neuropathic

[*†‡§¶]Jon D. Levine, [‡]Yetunde O. Taiwo, and [‡§]Philip H. Heller

Departments of [*]Medicine, [†]Anatomy, and [‡]Oral and Maxillofacial Surgery, and Divisions of [§]Neurosciences and [¶]Rheumatology, University of California, San Francisco, California 94143

Noxious chemicals or intense mechanical or thermal stimuli activate nociceptors to produce a sensation of pain (13,40,41). In addition, following tissue injury, normally nonpainful stimuli are able to elicit pain, a phenomenon referred to as hyperalgesia or tenderness (3,9). Hyperalgesia of peripheral origin is thought to result from a sensitization of primary afferent nociceptors by inflammatory mediators released in the injured tissue. Since hyperalgesic pain is the most common type of pain seen in clinical practice, elucidation of these mediators of hyperalgesia and their cellular sources and mechanisms of action is not only of scientific interest but also of significant clinical relevance.

It is important to remember when considering mechanisms of hyperalgesia that the peripheral terminals of nociceptors are embedded in a heterogeneous matrix of cells that are capable of releasing mediators that might indirectly influence nociceptive threshold. The most specific approach employed to show an indirect hyperalgesic mechanism is the demonstration that the elimination of a specific cellular element prevents the production of hyperalgesia by the agent in question and that replacement of the deleted cellular element reconstitutes the agent's ability to produce hyperalgesia. Also, an addition of the specific element, under normal conditions, might be expected to enhance the indirect hyperalgesia. As described below, the neutrophilic leukocyte, the sympathetic postganglionic neuron (SPGN) terminal, and products of the cyclooxygenase pathway of arachidonic acid have all been implicated in indirect pathways for the production of hyperalgesia.

MECHANISMS OF INDIRECT-ACTING HYPERALGESIC AGENTS

Neutrophil-Dependent Hyperalgesia

Leukotriene B_4, a potent neutrophil attractant (10,11), produces hyperalgesia in animals (29) and humans (25). This hyperalgesia has been found to be attenuated by the depletion of circulating leukocytes (19) but re-established by the reconstitution of neutrophils by infusion. In addition, injection of glycogen, which selectively attracts neutrophils into the site to be tested, shifts the dose-dependence relationship for leukotriene B_4-induced hyperalgesia to the left by three orders of magnitude, making it the most potent hyperalgesic agent known, given in this setting, which is relevant clinically since sites of inflammation are replete with neutrophils.

The identification of the neutrophil as an important element in leukotriene B_4-mediated hyperalgesia suggested that substances that could attract and activate neutrophils would constitute a novel class of hyperalgesic agents. In fact, two such substances, C_{5a}, the anaphylactoid fragment of the fifth component of the complement cascade, and formylmethionyl-leucylphenylalanine (fMLP), the boc tripeptide bacterial cell wall fragment, have also been shown to produce neutrophil-dependent hyperalgesia (20).

Studies were, of course, directed at determining which factor(s), released by the activated neutrophils, was more directly producing hyperalgesia. Using high-pressure liquid chromatography fractionation of supernatants from activated neutrophils, one such factor has been characterized, 8R,15S-diHETE, a product of the lipoxygenation of arachidonic acid that produces a dose-dependent hyperalgesia after intradermal injection (21). Of note, 8S,15S-diHETE, a stereoisomer of 8R,15S-diHETE selectively antagonizes the hyperalgesia produced by the active agent, compatible with the hypothesis that the action of 8R,15S-diHETE to produce hyperalgesia is exerted at a stereospecific binding site or receptor.

Sympathetic Neuron-Dependent Hyperalgesia

A specific type of indirect hyperalgesia that is of considerable clinical importance is that mediated by the SPGN terminal, referred to as sympathetic-dependent (or maintained) hyperalgesia. The contribution of the SPGN terminal to hyperalgesia has been suggested in a number of clinical conditions, including reflex sympathetic dystrophy (RSD) syndromes (14,26,43), neuromal pain (6,42) following nerve injury, and inflammatory states such as rheumatoid arthritis (22).

Although the mechanism(s) by which the SPGN terminal contributes to hyperalgesia in these conditions is incompletely understood, there are promising experimental models being investigated. Based on studies of the experimentally induced neuroma, it has been proposed that injured primary afferent nociceptors develop a sensitivity to norepinephrine (NE) and that SPGNs can elicit activity in primary afferent nociceptors by action of released NE acting at alpha-adrenergic receptors (4,7,42). This hypothesis is supported by the observation that stimulation of the lumbar sympathetic chain elicits increased activity in unmyelinated afferents in neuromas (6), which is blocked by the alpha-adrenergic antagonist phentolamine (6,42). However, the location of the adrenergic receptors was not established in these studies.

Quiescent sympathetic-maintained pain (SMP) or hyperalgesia can be reactivated by iontophoresis of NE into the skin of patients with causalgia but only with a latency to onset of approximately 10 min (43), suggesting that NE might be acting as an indirect hyperalgesic agent. This hypothesis is further supported by the observation that corticosteroids, which are potent inhibitors of the release of arachidonic acid and therefore prevent subsequent formation of its metabolites, attenuate spontaneous activity in the rat neuroma (8). Experimental data also demonstrated that NE hyperalgesia can be blocked by sympathectomy (23) or cyclooxygenase inhibitors (23). SPGNs were indeed found to produce the directly acting hyperalgesic prostaglandins (PGE_2 and PGI_2) (12). Therefore, it is proposed that hyperalgesia induced by NE results from a stimulated production of prostaglandins by SPGNs, after alpha$_2$-adrenergic action (23).

The recent observation that the calcium ionophore A23187 can induce NE-sensitive hyperalgesia in normal skin has led to the further hypothesis that SPGN-dependent hyperalgesia observed in patients with nerve injury-induced pain, such as RSD syndromes and causalgia, may require another signal in addition to alpha$_2$ stimulation, namely, an increased intracellular calcium. An intracellular calcium concentration significantly in excess of that seen physiologically is a general characteristic at sites of cell injury (36).

Like NE hyperalgesia, the hyperalgesia produced by the inflammatory mediator bradykinin (BK) has also been demonstrated to be indirect and to be mediated by an SPGN terminal-dependent production of prostaglandins (23). Since BK is readily produced by a cascade of enzymes that are triggered by various types of injury including diverse inflammatory states such as that in rheumatoid arthritis or inflammatory bowel disease, sympathetically mediated pain states may be more prevalent than previously thought.

DIRECT-ACTING HYPERALGESIC AGENTS

The study of agents that act directly on the nociceptors to produce hyperalgesia will allow us to understand the mechanisms by which threshold is actually decreased in primary afferent nociceptors. Three approaches have been applied to identify a direct action of hyperalgesic agents:

1. short latency to onset of lowered nociceptive threshold,
2. persistence of hyperalgesic effects after elimination of all known indirect targets,
3. direct recording from cultured neurons.

First, the latency to onset of decreased nociceptive threshold induced by a variety of hyperalgesic substances has been evaluated in animal studies. When mechanical nociceptive threshold was sampled at 1-min intervals following intradermal injection, hyperalgesia was detectable at the time of the first measurement for PGE_2, PGI_2, 8R,15S-diHETE (33), and adenosine (35). BK and NE, which, as mentioned above, produce hyperalgesia indirectly through the SPGN, have a latency to onset of 5 min. Leukotriene B_4, which acts on neutrophils to produce hyperalgesia, does not lower threshold until 8 min after intradermal injection (33). These data support the hypothesis that the prostaglandins PGE_2 and PGI_2, 8R,15S-diHETE, and adenosine are direct-acting hyperalgesic agents.

Second, persistence of hyperalgesic effects after elimination of indirect pathways is assessed by eliminating neutrophils and sympathetic postganglionic neuron terminals, and by blocking the cyclooxygenase pathway of arachidonic acid metabolism. These studies have also provided evidence that PGE_2, PGI_2, 8R,15S-diHETE, and CV1808, an adenosine A_2-receptor selective agonist, produce hyperalgesia directly (21,34,35).

Finally, recent studies using cultured dorsal root ganglion neurons have provided more conclusive evidence for a direct hyperalgesic effect on primary afferent nociceptors by PGE_2 and PGI_2 (1,28). In these whole-cell patch-clamp electrophysiological studies, nociceptors were identified as a subpopulation of cells with diameters less than 30 μm, with a typical response to capsaicin, namely, the production of an inward current. A direct effect on these cells was demonstrated for PGE_2 and PGI_2, i.e., the magnitude of the current produced by constant capsaicin dose was increased after pre-exposure to these agents.

Second Messengers for Primary Afferent Hyperalgesia

The fact that PGE_2 and adenosine, two direct-acting hyperalgesic agents, often produce their effects on cells via the cAMP second messenger system (37) suggested that the group of direct-acting hyperalgesic compounds (PGE_2, PGI_2, 8R,15S-di-HETE, and adenosine) might all mediate hyperalgesia with cAMP as a common second messenger system. It was found that, in this regard, the membrane-permeable analogue of cAMP, 8-bromo cAMP, produced a dose-dependent hyperalgesia that is not affected by treatments that interrupt the known indirect routes of hyperalgesia production (37). Also, the phosphodiesterase inhibitors isobutylmethylxanthine (IBMX) and rolipram markedly prolong the hyperalgesic effect of 8-bromo cAMP, as well as that of the direct-acting agents PGE_2, PGI_2, 8R,15S-diHETE (37) and adenosine (35). These data, therefore, strongly suggest that the hyperalgesia produced by these agents is dependent on elevated intracellular levels of cAMP. In a variety of cell systems the action of both PGE_2 and PGI_2, as well as that of adenosine, to increase levels of the cAMP second messenger has been shown to be mediated via a stimulatory guanine nucleotide regulatory protein (G_s) (38). A contribution of stimulatory G proteins to the hyperalgesia induced by these agents is suggested by the observations that guanosine-5'-[gamma-Thio]triphosphate (GTPgammaS) and cholera toxin, which activate G_s, both increase PGE_2 hyperalgesia, whereas guanosine-5'-[beta-Thio]diphosphate (GDPbetaS), which prevents the activation of G_s, decreases PGE_2 hyperalgesia (38). The subsequent necessary events following increased intracellular cAMP to produce hyperalgesia are presently unknown. Efforts are being directed toward elucidating the (intracellular) target(s) affected by cAMP.

Antagonism of Primary Afferent Hyperalgesia

The demonstration of an important role for G-protein function in peripheral hyperalgesia suggested the possibility that a novel choice for antihyperalgesic agents would be those that either prevented G_s protein activation or those that activated inhibitory G proteins (G_i), which are known to have opposite effects. In this regard, mu opioids, which have been demonstrated to decrease intracellular cAMP via activation of inhibitory (G_i) proteins (5,18,27,30), were ideal candidates. They produce naloxone antagonizable analgesia when injected into inflamed (i.e., hyperalgesic) tissue (15,24,31). The role of G_i-protein action is demonstrated by the fact that coinjection of pertussis toxin, which irreversibly binds to and inhibits G_i (24), prevents the peripheral mu-opiate (morphine)-induced analgesia.

While mu-opioids appeared to produce their peripheral analgesic effect by a direct action on the G_i protein in primary afferent nociceptors just described, delta- and kappa-receptor–specific opioid agonists also produce antinociception in inflamed tissue (32) but, paradoxically, do not inhibit the effects of direct-acting hyperalgesic agents such as PGE_2 (24). Recent studies have demonstrated, however, that the hyperalgesia induced by BK, which is SPGN terminal dependent, is blocked by mu- as well as kappa- (U50,488H) and delta- (DPDPE) receptor–specific opioid agonists (39). Kappa and delta opioid receptors are, in fact, present on SPGN terminals (2,16,17,44). Therefore, the observed peripheral analgesic effects of kappa and delta opioid agonists appear to result from actions on these SPGN terminals.

SUMMARY

Hyperalgesic pain syndromes are still poorly treated by current therapies. This failure is due in part to the fact that multiple mechanisms contribute to hyperalgesic pain(s). Recent research in this area has allowed the elucidation of both indirect and direct mechanisms for hyperalgesic events. The knowledge gained from these studies has suggested novel approaches to the treatment of hyperalgesic pain syndromes. These include specific inhibition of direct- and indirect-acting hyperalgesic agents, inhibition of the action of cells involved in the indirect pathways, antagonism of the second messenger mediating hyperalgesia (cAMP), and use of receptor agonists that act to modulate guanine nucleotide regulatory proteins on primary afferent nociceptors. Furthermore, combinations of agents acting at these different sites may produce more potent analgesia, thereby permitting the use of lower doses of individual agents, with consequent diminution of side effects. Recognition that different hyperalgesic pain syndromes may be mediated by different combinations of these mechanisms will allow a more rational approach to the management of patients with specific painful entities.

ACKNOWLEDGMENTS

This research was supported by NIH grants NS21647, AM32634, and DE08973. JDL is a Rita Allen Foundation Fellow.

REFERENCES

1. Baccaglini, P. L., and Hogan, P. G. (1983): Some sensory neurones in culture express characteristics of differentiated pain sensory cells. *Proc. Natl. Acad. Sci. USA*, 80:594–598.
2. Berzetei, P. I., Fong, A., Yamamura, H. I., and Duckles, S. P. (1988): Characterization of kappa opioid receptors in the rabbit ear artery. *Eur. J. Pharmacol.*, 151:449–455.
3. Besson, P., and Perl, E. R. (1967): Response of cutaneous sensory unit with unmyelinated fibers to noxious stimuli. *J. Neurophysiol.*, 32:1025–1043.
4. Blumberg, H., and Janig, W. (1984): Discharge pattern of afferent fibers from a neuroma. *Pain*, 20:335–353.
5. Childers, S. R., and LaRiviere, G. (1984): Modification of guanine nucleotide-regulatory components in brain membranes. I. Relationship of guanosine 5′-triphosphate effects on opiate receptor binding and coupling receptors with adenylate cyclase. *J. Neurosci.*, 4:2764–2771.
6. Devor, M., and Janig, W. (1981): Activation of myelinated afferents ending in a neuroma by stimulation of the sympathetic supply in the rat. *Neurosci. Lett.*, 24:43–47.
7. Devor, M. J. (1983): Nerve pathophysiology and mechanisms of pain in causalgia. *J. Auton. Nerv. Sys.*, 7:371–384.
8. Devor, M. (1985): Corticosteroids suppress ectopic neural discharge originating in experimental neuromas. *Pain*, 22:127–137.
9. Dubner, R., and Bennett, G. J. (1983): Spinal and trigeminal mechanisms of nociception. *Annu. Rev. Neurosci.*, 6:381–418.
10. Goetzl, E. J., and Pickett, W. C. (1980): The human PMN leukocyte chemotactic activity of complex hydroxyeicosatraenoic acids (HETEs). *J. Immunol.*, 125:1789–1791.

11. Goldman, D. W., and Goetzl, E. J. (1982): Specific binding of leukotriene B_4 to receptors on human polymorphonuclear leukocytes. *J. Immunol.*, 129:1600–1604.
12. Gonzales, R., Goldyne, M. E., Taiwo, Y. O., and Levine, J. D. (1989): Production of hyperalgesic prostaglandins by sympathetic postganglionic neurons. *J. Neurochem.*, 53:1595–1598.
13. Handwerker, H. O. (1976): Pharmacological modulation of the discharges of C fibres. In: *Sensory functions of the skin in primate*, edited by Y. Zotterman, pp. 427–439. Pergamon Press, Oxford.
14. Hannington-Kiff, J. G. (1977): Relief of Sudek's atrophy by regional intravenous guanethidine. *Lancet*, 1:1132–1133.
15. Hargreaves, K., Joris, J., and Dubner, R. (1987): Peripheral actions of opiates in the blockade of carrageenan-induced cutaneous hyperalgesia. *Pain*, suppl. 4: S17.
16. Hughes, J. (1981): Peripheral opiate receptor mechanisms. *Trends Pharmacol. Sci.*, 2:21–24.
17. Illes, P., Pfeiffer, N., vonKugelgen, I., and Starke, K. (1985): Presynaptic opioid receptor subtypes in the rabbit ear artery. *J. Pharmacol. Exp. Ther.*, 232:526–533.
18. Lau, P. Y., Wu, J., Koehler, J. E., and Loh, H. H. (1981): Demonstration and characterization of opiate inhibition of the striatal adenylate cyclase activity. *J. Neurochem.*, 36:1834–1846.
19. Levine, J. D., Lau, W., Kwiat, G., and Goetzl, E. J. (1984): Leukotriene B_4 produces hyperalgesia that is dependent on polymorphonuclear leukocytes. *Science*, 225:743–745.
20. Levine, J. D., Gooding, J., Donatoni, P., Borden, L., and Goetzl, E. J. (1985): The role of the polymorphonuclear leukocyte in hyperalgesia. *J. Neurosci.*, 5:3025–3029.
21. Levine, J. D., Lam, D., Taiwo, Y. O., Donatoni, P., and Goetzl, E. J. (1986): Hyperalgesic properties of 15-lipoxygenase products of arachidonic acid. *Proc. Natl. Acad. Sci. USA*, 83:5331–5334.
22. Levine, J. D., Fye, K., Heller, P., Basbaum, A. I., and Whiting-O'Keefe, Q. (1986): Clinical response to regional intravenous guanethidine in patients with rheumatoid arthritis. *J. Rheumatol.*, 13:1040–1043.
23. Levine, J. D., Taiwo, Y. O., Collins, S. D., and Tam, J. K. (1986): Noradrenaline hyperalgesia is mediated through interaction with sympathetic postganglionic neurone terminals rather than activation of primary afferent nociceptors. *Nature*, 323:158–160.
24. Levine, J. D., and Taiwo, Y. O. (1989): Involvement of the mu-opiate receptor in peripheral hyperalgesia. *Neuroscience*, 32:571–575.
25. Lewis, R. A., Soter, N. A., Corey, E. J., and Austen, K. F. (1981): Local effects of synthetic leukotrienes (LTs) on monkey (M) and human (H) skin. *Clin. Res.*, 29:492A.
26. Loh, L., and Nathan, P. (1978): Painful peripheral states and sympathetic blocks. *J. Neurol. Neurosurg. Psychiatry*, 41:664–671.
27. Mankman, M. H., Dvorkin, B., and Crain, S. M. (1988): Modulation of adenylate cyclase activity of mouse spinal cord-ganglion explants by opioids, serotonin and pertussis toxin. *Brain Res.*, 445:303–313.
28. Pitchford, S., and Levine, J. D. (1991): Prostaglandin sensitize nociceptors in cell culture. *Neurosci. Lett.*, 32:105–108.
29. Rackham, A., and Ford-Hutchinson, A. W. (1983): Inflammation and pain sensitivity: effects of leukotrienes D_4, B_4 and prostaglandin E_1 in the rat paw. *Prostaglandins*, 25:588–616.
30. Sharma, S. K., Nirenberg, M., and Klee, W. A. (1975): Morphine receptors as regulations of adenylate cyclase activity. *Proc. Natl. Acad. Sci. USA*, 72:590–594.
31. Stein, C., Millan, M. J., Shippenberg, T. S., and Herz, A. (1988): Peripheral effect of fentanyl upon nociception in inflamed tissue of the rat. *Neurosci. Lett.*, 84:225–228.
32. Stein, C., Millan, M. J., Shippenberg, T. S., Peter, K., and Herz, A. (1989): Peripheral opioid receptors mediating antinociception in inflammation. Evidence for involvement of mu, delta and kappa receptors. *J. Pharmacol. Exp. Ther.*, 248:1269–1275.
33. Taiwo, Y. O., Goetzl, E. J., and Levine, J. D. (1987): Hyperalgesia onset latency suggests a hierarchy of action. *Brain Res.*, 423:333–337.
34. Taiwo, Y. O., and Levine, J. D. (1989): Prostaglandin effects after elimination of indirect hyperalgesic mechanisms in the skin of the rat. *Brain Res.*, 492:397–399.
35. Taiwo, Y. O., and Levine, J. D. (1990): Direct cutaneous hyperalgesia induced by adenosine. *Neuroscience* 38:757–762.
36. Taiwo, Y. O., Heller, P. H., and Levine, J. D. (1990): Characterization of distinct phospholipases mediating bradykinin and noradrenaline hyperalgesia. *Neuroscience*, 39:523–531.
37. Taiwo, Y. O., Bjerknes, L. K., Goetzl, E. J., and Levine, J. D. (1989): Mediation of primary afferent peripheral hyperalgesia by the cAMP second messenger system. *Neuroscience* 32:577–580.
38. Taiwo, Y. O., and Levine, J. D. (1989): Contribution of guanine nucleotide regulatory proteins to prostaglandin hyperalgesia in the rat. *Brain Res.*, 492:400–403.
39. Taiwo, Y. O., and Levine, J. D. (1991): Kappa and delta opioids block sympathetically-dependent hyperalgesia. *J. Neurosci.*, 11:928–932.
40. Torebjörk, H. E., and Hallin, R. G. (1974): Identification of afferent C units in intact human skin nerves. *Brain Res.*, 67:387–403.

41. Torebjörk, E. H., LaMotte, R. H., and Robinson, C. J. (1984): Peripheral neural correlates of the magnitude of cutaneous pain and hyperalgesia: simultaneous recordings in humans of sensory judgments of pain and evoked responses in nociceptors with C-fibers. *J. Neurophysiol.*, 51:325–339.
42. Wall, P. D., and Gutnick, M. (1974): Ongoing activity in peripheral nerves: the physiology and pharmacology of impulses originating from a neuroma. *Exp. Neurol.*, 43:580–593.
43. Wallin, G., Torebjörk, E., and Hallin, R. (1976): Preliminary observations on the pathophysiology of hyperalgesia in the causalgic pain syndrome. In: *Sensory functions of the primate skin with special reference to man*, edited by Y. Zotterman, pp. 409–502. Pergamon, Oxford.
44. Wuster, M., Schulz, R., and Herz, A. (1981): Multiple opiate receptors in peripheral tissue preparations. *Biochem. Pharmacol.*, 30:1883–1887.

Hyperalgesia and Allodynia,
edited by W. D. Willis, Jr.
Raven Press, Ltd., New York © 1992.

9

Nociceptors and Their Sensitization

Discussion

Kenneth L. Casey, Moderator

Dr. Casey: This symposium is about hyperalgesia, but we have also been introduced to the phenomenon of allodynia, and they are different phenomena. As Dr. Bonica informed us, hyperalgesia is, by the definition of the International Association for the Study of Pain, an increased response or an increased perception of pain following a noxious stimulus, whereas allodynia is the perception of pain following a stimulus that is normally not noxious. And now we have assembled before us world experts on detailed mechanisms by which nociceptors are activated and by which they are sensitized by a variety of chemicals. A simple question is whether sensitization of nociceptors, which is the term that has been used experimentally, is responsible for both allodynia and hyperalgesia, or is the phenomenon of sensitization related only to one of these?

Dr. Perl: This is known as passing the buck. Since the definition of hyperalgesia, as Dr. Bonica pointed out, has now been changed to mean something different than what was commonly the notion in the past, and now we have substituted allodynia for this, I think that, given the kind of evidence that we have seen today, you can enhance the responsiveness of a sense organ to the point where non-noxious stimuli clearly become effective, both in the skin and subcutaneous tissues. One has to consider that sensitization is contributing, whether it's in a joint or subcutaneous, to allodynia, because now nonpainful stimuli are evoking activity that the central nervous system is interpreting as pain. But at the same time, if you accept the fact that hyperalgesia means an increased reaction to a noxious stimulus or a stimulus that would provoke pain, it must also be contributing by producing more messages going to the central nervous system. So I think that, in fact, the sensitization phenomenon contributes to both of these clinically relevant phenomena.

Question: Does that mean that sensitization of mechanoreceptors occurs to produce allodynia?

Dr. Schmidt: There's no doubt about that at all in the knee joint. All types of fine afferents, even the group II afferents, are sensitized in the course of inflammation. So the peripheral input is enough to explain allodynia. My problem is how is this sorted out at the central level? We do not have good evidence that what we call specifically nociceptive neurons, which we presume are in the pain pathway, also get inflow from low-threshold afferents, which is then enhanced in such a way during inflammation that the pain pathway is being activated, producing allodynia.

Dr. Bonica: I just want to mention that in reading carefully the work of Head and of MacKenzie, Head actually determined cutaneous sensitivity or tenderness, which he later called hyperalgesia, by applying the head of the pin, and therefore he was really eliciting allodynia, whereas MacKenzie did both. He used the ball of the pin and the stick of the pin and found the same thing.

Dr. Casey: Does anyone else want to address the issue of the unity or lack thereof between hyperalgesia and allodynia?

Dr. Handwerker: I think one of the problems is that the term allodynia is still not very clear. If you speak about a pain response to a previously nonpainful stimulus, this can be a stimulus that excites sensitized nociceptors or it can be a stimulus that certainly will not do so. For example, if you look at trigeminal neuralgia and the touch-evoked pain you get there, then you certainly have a type of allodynia that cannot be explained by any kind of peripheral sensitization. So, perhaps it would be better to put the line somewhere else, and to do that, it's perhaps better to look for the characteristics of the stimuli which evoke pain. If you produce pain by a short touch which has a very dynamic component and not so much pain to a sustained pressure, even if it is non-noxious, then it is very likely that this kind of pain is not due to sensitized nociceptors, in my opinion.

Question: Dr. Walters, do the phenomena you described in invertebrates relate to this issue?

Dr. Walters: I would say we have something that looks very similar to hyperalgesia in that previously noxious stimuli will elicit greater responses and also allodynia in that the threshold for responses goes way down. I suspect that one of the things we're going to hear about later in this meeting is that it's quite likely that what we see in *Aplysia* also occurs in the mammalian nervous system, and that is that there is a synergistic interaction between the peripheral effects and the central effects. I think today we saw that allodynia might be contributed to by the activation of low-threshold afferents after sensitizing manipulations. I think Dr. Handwerker and Dr. Schmidt both showed that. If you put that together with the wide dynamic range properties of the dorsal horn neurons, you have an excellent simple mechanism that could give you allodynia. I think we'll hear later from Dr. Woolf's talk that the threshold of wide dynamic range dorsal horn neurons may go down. So you'll have complementary effects at both levels, which is similar to what we see in these simpler animals.

Dr. Casey: Now I'd like to open it up for questions from the audience.

Question: Dr. Walters, you said the purpose of pain was to reduce movement, but maybe another is to reduce the possibility of infection, since a massive bacterial infection may result from injury. Have you compared changes in animals with or without infection? Also, has Dr. Handwerker included bacterial products in his soup?

Dr. Walters: I would just say that's a very nice suggestion. In *Aplysia* we often don't worry about infection because the animal seems to be very resistant to infection, but that's a very good suggestion.

Dr. Handwerker: No, we have not done that, to say it bluntly. There are a lot of factors that could change the soup and could make it more effective. Among them may be toxins from microorganisms, but also cellular mechanisms. The cellular mechanisms are still not very well studied, and I have no hard data on that.

Dr. Bonica: Could I comment about the biologic function of pain and hyperalgesia? There's no question that with external injuries there is a very important biologic function. As was pointed out, pain imposes itself on the patient and therefore prevents activation of the pathophysiology. On the other hand, if you take a postoperative patient who has pain, he keeps quiet and as he keeps quiet, he develops atelectasis and eventually hypoxemia and pneumonia. We used to keep these patients in bed following gastrectomy for 2 to 3 weeks; now we get them up the next day. I think many pathologic processes really come too late to be a warning signal. I think the same thing really applies to the pain of childbirth. Once it serves the biologic function to tell the woman that labor is imminent, I think it really becomes a deleterious effect because, as I didn't have time to say, there are many changes—hyperventilation, which produces respiratory alkalosis and cerebral vasoconstriction, constriction of arteries in the placenta that decrease placental blood flow, and so on. While it's nice to talk about biologic function, I think once it serves the biologic function, we should try to eliminate pain and hyperalgesia.

Dr. Walters: Could I respond to that? I think that's a very interesting point. One thing we should remember in thinking about what's adaptive during evolution is that what was adaptive was selected for because it enhanced the reproductive success of whoever had it. During most of evolution we did not have modern medicine or physicians. These tremendous insults that major surgery represents would have had very little effect on evolution, so it's quite likely that what medicine is seeing today is not really adaptive, that we're producing much more severe injuries. The types of injuries that gave rise to these adaptive effects might not have been quite so extreme.

Dr. Bonica: Kellert has said that the neuroendocrine response to surgery or trauma, for that matter, is a maladaptive reaction rather than a good thing.

Question: Dr. Schmidt, do you have any data on whether most of group II or group III fibers respond to inflammation or to distention of the joint capsule?

Dr. Schmidt: We have no systematic data on that except the observation that in the beginning of the inflammation, when we carefully look at the time course of sensitization of the various types of fine afferents, the group II afferents, the thickest ones, are the first ones to become sensitized—very early, in less than half an hour. And their sensitization declines later when the group III and IV sensitization comes up and our suspicion, for which we have no proof, is that it is the edema that is forming in the early stages of inflammation that changes the tissue tension so that the forces being transmitted to the group II afferents are being increased. There are some observations from a British laboratory on discharges being produced by filling up the joint with fluid. However, they remain unsatisfactory. It's obviously very difficult in the very complicated knee joint to get a uniform type of extension, like a balloon. It's so easy to imagine it could be a balloon, but it's far from being a balloon, it's a tremendously complicated structure and it is very difficult to do such an experiment—that's why we have refrained from it. But it's quite clear that the group II sensitization begins very early and then declines when the tissue starts to relax in the course of inflammation.

Dr. Lebedev: I have two questions. One question is to Dr. Walters. You talked about the role of trauma and possible retrograde inflammation from this trauma. What's your point of view? First, what is the real messenger for this inflammation, and second, is it possible to imagine that there is a transsynaptic inflammation of the next neuron? How does the trauma produce inflammation of all systems that are used for ascending nociception?

Dr. Walters: I have to say we don't know very much about either question. I think your second comment is a very interesting possibility. As far as the signal that is carried by the axon after axonal injury, we don't know what it is. It could be one or more of several things, including a negative signal; that is, we could be interrupting the supply of trophic factors that are continually being returned back to the cell body, and there's some evidence for that contributing to hyperexcitability after axotomy in several other animals. But there have been other suggestions like adenylate cyclase builds up and begins to go back to the cell body—there are many, many possible signals.

Dr. Lebedev: Another question is for Dr. Handwerker. Professor Ayuken of Moscow studied C fibers and suggested that synchronization of their impulses was important in spinal cord function. It is a very important thing that synchronization of impulses forms, for example, on dorsal horn neurons because if they are desynchronized, they don't excite dorsal horn neurons, but if they are synchronized, they can excite.

Dr. Handwerker: Perhaps I was a bit short in my lecture. I have shown one slide with a schema on what happens in the central nervous system when the input from the periphery increases. There are two factors, which probably combine. One factor is that the number of impulses from the known nociceptors increases with sensitization, and this causes what neurophysiologists call temporal summation in the central nervous system, in particular, when you have EPSPs that have a very long duration at the synapse. And, on the other hand, it really could be, as has been shown by Dr. Schmidt and myself, that in inflammation, formerly unresponsive nociceptive units are recruited. Then you get in addition another mechanism and that is that at the same time impulses arrive on several additional terminals on the neuron. This is called in physiology spatial summation. Probably you have both effects.

Question: Dr. Schmidt, if silent nociceptors really exist, I wonder if you'd be willing to speculate for us what biological function they might serve under conditions other than inflammation?

Dr. Schmidt: Speculations are cheap. You can talk of trophic functions and things like that, efferent functions of such units, and they may have them, but the evidence is rather limited. But mind you, maybe we are surprised by these sleeping nociceptors, but on second thought, remember that if you have healthy teeth, none of your thousands of fine afferents in the tooth pulp will ever send a single impulse into your nervous system for all your life. So it's nothing so special, as we at first had thought. I think they are actually very common. And if you look at the innervation of the viscera, which is numerically very small, things like ureter or human bladder, innervated not by thousands or hundreds, but by dozens of fine afferents; nevertheless, the pain of a kidney stone can be excruciating. And the only explanation I have now is that there is a tremendous sensitization of these fine afferents. Jänig in Kiel, for instance, was always fighting my concept because he couldn't find specific nociceptors in the cat bladder, for instance, or in the cat colon. In their very careful work, they either found afferents that had only low thresholds or that had low thresholds and increased their discharges in the course of extending the stimulation into the noxious range. And I kept telling him, you have to inflame the tissue, then you will see them, and he does see them now when he inflames the bladder. So I think the concept of sleeping nociceptors is a very important one and maybe they just have mainly a pathophysiological function and not a physiological one.

Dr. Perl: Let me make a comment on this. One of the things that Dr. Schmidt has shown very nicely is that not only that there are quiet sense organs that become unquiet under certain circumstances, but he's also shown that low-threshold sense organs alter their characteristics and their responses. That immediately raises the possibility and everybody jumps in and says, well, they must be contributing to the allodynia. That's not at all sure. We don't know that. What we do know is that they increase their discharges, but you can increase their discharges or do things equivalent to that in the normal animal, in the normal creature, in the normal person, without necessarily evoking pain. You don't get allodynia until perhaps some of the other nociceptors are active, until you have the regular nociceptors sensitized, and then there is something else happening. I believe at that stage we are correct in thinking that this something else is happening in the central nervous system, and there is, in fact, now convergence of increased nociceptive information from sense organs whose main job is to tell the difference between noxious and innocuous circumstances; one noxious circumstance is inflammation, and once they are going and once they are putting their input in, then perhaps some of the other inputs may modify it, but we don't know that. What we really know is that the sense organs are increasing their discharges, as a consequence of tissue damage, of damaging circumstances, and inflammation.

Question: Do psychogenic factors change during inflammation?

Dr. Handwerker: Psychological effects. Well, I personally believe, and this may be the belief of most neurobiologists, that psychologic effects work on a central nervous level, but they may also act on a peripheral level, but this has never been proven. I don't know a mechanism for that.

Question: I was wondering if anybody on the panel could comment on a possible role of sensitization of a large number of so-called visceral receptors in the so-called functional bowel disorder. There is recent evidence that a balloon distention of the esophagus or colon produces allodynia and hyperalgesia. Could you speculate on the mechanisms involved in allodynia and hyperalgesia?

Dr. Bonica: I think Cervero made a very good point in thinking about what is the adequate stimulus for the viscera. And it's not electrical stimulation, but distention, and a lot of people, as far back as 50 or 60 years ago, put balloons down the esophagus in the upper or lower part and showed that there was referred pain in the upper part of the chest or the lower part of the chest. Jones in 1938 published a book on the gastrointestinal tract showing referred pain that he incidentally said he was able to eliminate by infiltrating the skin. I think this was because the nociceptive input was very mild. But, I think that the issue is that if you have inflammation, then this changes things. In the famous study by Wolf and his group on a subject with a gastric stoma, they were able to grasp the inside of the stomach with a firm stimulus that would in the skin produce excruciating pain, but the patient didn't have any pain. But when they stimulated an inflamed area, the patient had referred pain.

Question: May I ask about the absence of any inflammation on the role of sleeping nociceptors?

Dr. Perl: There is another possibility. There are at least two other things that I think ought to be figured in. I must say the evidence is very slim, but one of the circumstances that may be involved is an actual change in the characteristics over time of sensory neurons that are, let's say, in the normal, intact creature, nociceptors of either the sleeping or the waking type. But in the presence of a chronic change in the tissues, in fact there is an induction of altered responsiveness. Now, it is not necessarily a direct result of the usual type of inflammatory change; that's a possibility, and I think it's becoming a more real one. But there is another factor that I think is extremely important. The unmyelinated visceral afferent fibers have a uniquely different distribution, according to Sugiura, in terms of their terminals within the spinal cord and therefore the nature of the neurons that they are going to contact, than the somatic afferent fibers. The visceral afferent fibers, presumably nociceptive to the extent that fibers running through the sympathetic system are nociceptive, have a very diffuse set of connections, almost as if they have the capacity to produce synaptic activation of a much larger group of neurons. If you wake up nociceptors under those circumstances, well, you could see that there may be a spread of effect and enhancement of activity over a much greater range of cells than you would see from similar kinds of circumstances in the somatic system.

Dr. Levine: I would like to make one comment in relationship to the question in terms of a different system. I think the kind of pain syndromes you are referring to occur in multiple organ systems and variously relate to cardiopulmonary problems, to musculoskeletal problems, and to gastrointestinal problems. As rheumatologists, probably the largest percentage of patients we see fit into this class of "functional pain syndromes of musculoskeletal origin," for which there are a large number of pejorative terms used in the diagnosis, but it's true that in the vast majority of these patients there's a clear-cut antecedent trauma and that most of these patients have had some form of injury, prior to the onset of their symptoms, which is relatively significant. In most individuals that particular response would have been over in some reasonable period of time, and it somehow seems to have persisted or even been amplified in these patients. It may be that there is in these individuals some former primary lesion that is otherwise amplified by a central phenomenon, whether it be psychological or not, but there may, at least within the musculoskeletal syndromes, actually even be some evidence for continued injury.

Question: I would like to ask Dr. Walters about the pharmacology of sensitization in *Aplysia* and about any possible role of opioids.

Dr. Walters: It seems that during evolution, receptors have changed much more dramatically than mediators, and one of the problems is that many molluscan receptors don't respond very well to many of the standard blocking agents and agonists. Serotonin is very effective, but we can't say much about the pharmacology. As I say, the serotonin system is very important; there are some peptides that also seem to have changed quite a bit during evolution that are probably important as well. Interestingly enough, there are several reports that naloxone can block certain responses in *Aplysia* and that leu-enkephalin and met-enkephalin, I believe, are able to produce neurophysiological responses, but there's no good evidence that I've seen yet that the enkephalins or other opiates are actually in molluscs. Some people think that another peptide that has similar effects called FMRF-amide might be related to the opioids and play an "analgesic-like role" in some of these defensive responses similar to what the opioids do in the mammals.

Question: For Drs. Perl and Handwerker. Have you any data on the role of bradykinin antagonists? Further, have you looked at other peptides?

Dr. Handwerker: We have tested substance P and also CGRP, which do not have a profound sensitizing action. We have used tachykinins, but not other analogs of the bradykinin molecules, and we have not yet used selective bradykinin antagonists. There are some available and work is underway, but we have not finished that yet.

Question: Were you able to test the effects of neurokinins?

Dr. Handwerker: Neurokinins? We have only tested substance P and CGRP, as I mentioned, not the other ones.

Dr. Perl: In part, your question was about how suitable were the tachykinin agonists and antagonists. Well, if substance P is a reasonable agonist for substance P, we certainly tried it, and we used the antagonist that Lembeck specifically suggested blocked vasodilation and the fluid extravasation. There are other analogs, but we used the ones that he had specifically chosen and therefore whatever was blocking the effect was the one that did not produce any marked effect upon sensitization of the polymodal nociceptors in the rabbit ear preparation.

Dr. Handwerker: I didn't get to the second part of your question. We have used, of course, substance P and agonists, including spantide and also some synthetic nonpeptide substance P agonists, but as I mentioned in my lecture, our substance P effects were very small and so it was very hard to see if there's any specific antagonism in these *in vitro* experiments. When we tested an antagonist against our soup without substance P, we didn't see any effect. We looked also for the effect on the plasma extravasation and vasodilation with laser Doppler flowmetry, but there another problem arises and that is that at least spantide is a partial agonist and induces vasodilation itself. This makes it very hard to test if there is any true antagonism in this mechanism.

Dr. Basbaum: Two methodological questions. One is that people tend to mix up mechanical hyperalgesia and thermal hyperalgesia. Dr. Levine pointed out that the patients complain about mechanical hyperalgesia; they rarely complain about thermal hyperalgesia, and the question is are we working with different fiber systems? Do they always go together or not? And the other question relates to the use of *in vitro* versus *in vivo* systems. Particularly, Dr. Perl pointed out that since prostaglandin sensitized afferents *in vitro*, one can conclude that circulating blood elements are not relevant, but when you don't get an effect with leukotrienes, one cannot conclude that they are not relevant under those circumstances.

Dr. Perl: Well, the first thing is, I didn't say what you said I said, Allan. What I said was that in the *in vitro* situation, in the absence of blood, the unit sensitized, which meant that the white blood cells and the constituents of blood were not essential for the sensitizing process. I did not say that that had anything to do with the leukotrienes or the prostaglandins. What I did show is that a relatively effective leukotriene-inhibiting substance, BW755C, did not produce any difference in the sensitization pattern compared to the cyclooxygenase blocker, specifically indomethacin. And from that I concluded that in the *in vitro* preparation, the leukotriene effects were minimal, or at least not evident. I didn't say that the blood or the leukotrienes were not effective because they were absent in the blood-free perfusion. I'll let Dr. Handwerker take the question of mechanical versus heat.

Dr. Handwerker: It's an old problem. With our models we found it very difficult to induce mechanical hyperalgesia; for example, bradykinin superfusion or bradykinin bolus injection in the *in vivo* preparation does not induce profound mechanical hyperalgesia. It is sometimes marginal and sometimes not statistically significant. The heat hyperalgesia, on the other hand, is very pronounced; it is very clear and is to be seen in all units. We have now recently, by checking everything through, found that you get a profound mechanical hyperalgesia in the *in vitro* system by lowering the pH, but this is the only measure by which we can get a true mechanical hyperalgesia. When comparing now our *in vitro* and *in vivo* single-fiber experiments in behavioral experiments like Dr. Levine has done, you have always to take into account that perhaps part of the effect may be recruitment of silent nociceptors, and this we would not see easily in single-unit studies.

Dr. Perl: As long ago as 1969 we reported that heat sensitization was associated with mechanical sensitization but was much more difficult to quantitate and to analyze. Part of the problem is that the nociceptors, even the not-so-silent ones, have such high thresholds that it's hard to deliver mechanical stimuli that do not physically destroy the tissue at the receptive site on repeated application and therefore it's very hard to get a baseline. However, many observers have reported that mechanical sensitization is a regular feature under such circumstances. There may be some differences in the processes, just as there is a difference in the processes of the ongoing activity that seems to be evoked as a consequence of noxious stimuli, and the changes in threshold. We have clear indications that these things can be separated because there are circumstances in which you can lose the reaction to the effective stimulus and still have persisting ongoing activity in nociceptors. This is very easy to demonstrate and it's fairly regularly seen. The real problem is the quantification of the mechanical nociceptive responses in noninflamed tissue. If you go through the process of inflaming tissue, as Dr. Levine's lab has done and as Dr. Schmidt and Dr. Handwerker have all shown, you then get responses that can be evoked by stimuli that are controllable and reproducible.

Hyperalgesia and Allodynia,
edited by W. D. Willis, Jr.
Raven Press, Ltd., New York © 1992.

10

Nociceptors and Primary Hyperalgesia

Overview

*John C. Liebeskind and †William D. Willis, Jr.

*Department of Psychology, University of California, Los Angeles,
Los Angeles, California 90024; †Department of Anatomy and Neurosciences,
Marine Biomedical Institute, University of Texas Medical Branch,
Galveston, Texas 77550-2772

The characteristics of human nociceptors are described by Torebjörk, based on recordings from C and A delta fibers in human peripheral nerve using microneurography. Human C nociceptors behave like those described in animals. They sensitize following a mild burn injury, and their lowered threshold and enhanced responsiveness correlate well with the primary hyperalgesia in the same subject. A patient is described in whom chronic sensitization of C nociceptors seemed to underlie his hyperalgesia and allodynia. Experimental studies in human subjects involving intradermal capsaicin injections provide a means for investigating primary and secondary hyperalgesia. Activation of C fibers by capsaicin helps to account for the painful nature of such injections and sensitization of such nociceptors for the primary hyperalgesia. On the other hand, secondary hyperalgesia appears to depend on the activation of A fibers.

In Chapter 5, Perl described the induction of sensitivity of C nociceptors in the rabbit ear to catecholamines following nerve injury. Pharmacological experiments indicate that this sensitivity was due to the appearance of alpha$_2$ receptors in the nerve endings. Campbell and colleagues have been interested in sympathetically maintained pain following either nerve or tissue injury. Operating on the hypothesis that the pathogenesis of sympathetically maintained pain depends on peripheral release of norepinephrine, Campbell's group investigated the effects of systemic administration of phentolamine, as well as those of sympathetic blockade with a local anesthetic, on suspected sympathetically maintained pain. Patients that had a placebo response to intravenous saline were excluded from the study. There was a good correlation between the amount of pain relief produced by the sympathetic block and that by phentolamine. Propranolol had no effect, indicating that alpha receptors were likely to have been involved. The local administration of pharmacological agents indicated that the alpha receptor subtype involved is likely to be the alpha$_1$ receptor. Thus, there may be a species difference in the alpha receptor subtype that undergoes upregulation following nerve or tissue damage.

Ochoa has been examining patients with different varieties of hyperalgesia. He uses quantitative tests, such as the Marstock thermotest, to evaluate sensation in these patients. He and others have shown that the sensation of burning pain is associated with excessive activity in C nociceptors. In addition to peripheral mechanisms, it is likely that central changes also contribute to hyperalgesia. However, in some patients disease affecting primary afferent fibers induces a peripherally based hyperalgesia. One such group of patients have the "ABC syndrome" caused by angry backfiring C nociceptors. In these patients, the skin is hot and has heat hyperalgesia. The vasodilation is hypothesized to result from antidromic neurosecretion from C fibers. A different syndrome in another group of patients is characterized by cold hyperalgesia. In addition, they have cold hypoesthesia and cold skin, and so the condition is called the "triple cold syndrome." Many patients with long-standing hyperalgesia are placebo responders. It is therefore difficult to assess the value of sympathetic blockade in this group of patients.

Hyperalgesia and Allodynia,
edited by W. D. Willis, Jr.
Raven Press, Ltd., New York © 1992.

11

Nociceptive and Non-nociceptive Afferents Contributing to Pain and Hyperalgesia in Humans

Erik Torebjörk

*Department of Clinical Neurophysiology, University Hospital,
S-75185 Uppsala, Sweden*

This chapter reviews advances in our knowledge of the physiological properties of human nociceptors and their capacity to signal pain. Reference will be made to work showing that nociceptors in the skin become sensitized following tissue injury and that such sensitization largely accounts for hyperalgesia to heat and possibly to sustained pressure (static mechanical hyperalgesia) at the site of the lesion (primary hyperalgesia). In addition, evidence is provided to support the notion that hyperalgesia to gently moving tactile stimuli (dynamic mechanical hyperalgesia) both within and around the injury (secondary hyperalgesia) is due to an altered sensory processing of signals in non-nociceptive, probably low-threshold mechanoreceptive afferents that, in the presence of an ongoing input from nociceptive fibers, evoke unpleasant sore sensations described as pain.

METHODS

Two principal techniques have been used. Microneurography (30) involves microelectrode recordings of impulses in single myelinated or unmyelinated nerve fibers in intact peripheral nerves in awake human subjects. Intraneural microstimulation (26) takes advantage of the same type of electrodes, which can be used alternately for recording impulses from identifiable nerve fibers and for stimulating these fibers electrically in the same intraneural site. The great advantage of these techniques is that the subjects are able to report what they feel when their peripheral nerve fibers are stimulated. Thus, not only can the receptive properties of various types of sensory units be studied, but the perceptual consequences of their activation under a variety of experimental conditions as well. This approach has yielded useful information on somatosensory processing in general and on mechanisms related to pain and hyperalgesia in particular.

Details of these techniques and the psychological methods have been given elsewhere (12,20,31).

RESULTS

Nociceptors in Human Skin

Numerous microelectrode recordings from human peripheral nerves have shown that our skin is richly innervated by C-polymodal nociceptors, which respond in a graded fashion to mechanical, heat, and chemical stimuli in the near-painful or painful intensity range (24). These nociceptors have receptor characteristics similar to those of the C-polymodal nociceptors identified in the cat (4) and monkey (3,11,13). Intraneural microstimulation of bundles of human C-nociceptive fibers typically evokes painful sensations, described as dull or burning (21), or rarely as itch (27). Pain from C-nociceptor stimulation is projected with an accuracy on the order of 2 cm relative to the receptive fields of the stimulated units in the skin on the dorsum of the foot (9), and in the glabrous skin of the hand, the error is even less, about 1 cm (21).

A-delta nociceptors found in both hairy and glabrous skin in humans preferentially respond to mechanical stimuli of high intensity (1,25), whereas another type found only in hairy skin responds to mechanical, heat, and/or chemical stimuli (1). These nociceptors resemble type I and II A-delta nociceptors in monkey skin (18). Intraneural microstimulation of type I A-delta nociceptors innervating the glabrous skin in the human hand gives rise to sharp pricking pain that is accurately projected to the receptive fields (25).

Sensitization of Nociceptors

After a mild heat injury, C-polymodal nociceptors in hairy skin have lowered thresholds to heat stimuli and enhanced responses to suprathreshold stimuli (28). Such sensitization of C-nociceptors correlates with hyperalgesia to heat (12,28). The situation seems to be different in glabrous skin, where neurophysiological experiments in monkeys suggest that sensitization of A-delta rather than C-nociceptors accounts for hyperalgesia after burn lesions (19).

Sensitization of nociceptors by release of algogenic substances is an important peripheral mechanism for primary hyperalgesia in inflamed tissue. That chronic sensitization of C-nociceptors can occur in patients has been documented by microneurography in one case (6). Results from psychophysical experiments with topical application of capsaicin (7,10) or mustard oil (10) indicate that sensitization of C-nociceptors accounts not only for heat hyperalgesia but also for hyperalgesia to sustained pressure (static mechanical hyperalgesia) in inflamed hairy skin.

Altered Signal Processing in the Central Nervous System

Intracutaneous injection of capsaicin activates C-nociceptors and is severely painful (15). It is accompanied by hyperalgesia to gentle stroking, spreading to a wide skin area surrounding the injection site, and lasting for an hour or two after the injection (14). Recordings from nociceptors with receptive fields in the hyperalgesic surrounding area in monkeys (2) and humans (15) have failed to show any signs of sensitization that could account for the tactile hypersensitivity. Instead, experiments with selective nerve blocks indicate that the tactile hyperalgesia is demonstrable only in the presence of intact conduction in large myelinated nerve fibers (29). Furthermore, intraneural stimulation of non-nociceptive probably mechanoreceptive fibers innervating the hyperalgesic skin area gives rise to abnormal sensations of pain, a reversible phenomenon that disappears when the hyperalgesia is gone (29). These observations in humans are consistent with neurophysiological demonstrations of increased excitability to A-fiber input in nociceptive neurons in the spinal cord in monkeys following capsaicin injections (23). Recent psychophysical experiments with topical mustard oil and capsaicin suggest that the dynamic mechanical hyperalgesia to gentle stroking in both the injured area (the zone of primary hyperalgesia) and the surrounding area (the zone of secondary hyperalgesia) is critically dependent on ongoing afferent input from nociceptive C-fibers, and is quickly relieved when this input is abolished, for instance, by cooling (10). Taken together these findings indicate that the dynamic mechanical hyperalgesia to gentle stroking, typically demonstrable in the presence of background pain, is due to reversible changes in central processing of non-nociceptive mechanoreceptor signals, caused by ongoing input from nociceptive fibers.

CLINICAL IMPLICATIONS

The present results obviously challenge both the specificity theory (8) and the gate control theory of pain (17). Not only do nociceptive afferents signal pain, and more so when sensitized, but their activation leads to reversible changes in central processing of non-nociceptive input to the extent that signals from low-threshold mechanoreceptors, normally evoking tactile sensations and inhibiting pain, instead give rise to pain. If such disinhibition can occur under experimental conditions in normal subjects, similar mechanisms probably apply also in patients with chronic pain. Indeed, several clinical observations support the notion that low-threshold mechanosensitive afferents with large-diameter fibers signal the brush-evoked pain in neuralgia (5,16,22). It appears that allodynia to gentle touch and vibration is a common symptom in various forms of neuralgia, regardless of whether the pain condition is relieved by sympathetic blockade (32,33), suggesting that the dynamic mechanical hyperalgesia is a consequence of the ongoing pain but not necessarily linked with its pathophysiological cause. The reversible character of the tactile hyperalgesia observed under experimental conditions has its clinical counterpart in the rapid relief of tactile allodynia sometimes observed after sympathetic blockade in patients with sympathetic reflex dystrophy. It is rewarding from the therapeutic viewpoint that the central changes in signal processing can be reset very quickly in these patients, even if the pain syndrome has lasted for more than a decade (32).

Another point of clinical interest is that there are different forms of mechanical hyperalgesia, here described as dynamic or static, and that they have distinctly different underlying mechanisms. While most patients with neuralgia complain of hyperalgesia to gentle touch (dynamic mechanical hyperalgesia), others are bothered by firm, steady pressure (static mechanical hyperalgesia), and both forms may coexist (Koltzenburg, Wahren, and Torebjörk, *unpublished observations*). Whereas the dynamic type depends on sensitization of central neurons, the static component is probably the consequence of an increased response of primary nociceptive afferents to mechanical stimuli (6,7,10).

ACKNOWLEDGMENT

This work was supported by the Swedish Medical Research Council, Project no. 14X-05206.

REFERENCES

1. Adriaensen, H., Gybels, J., Handwerker, H. O., and van Hees, J. (1983): Response properties of thin myelinated (A-delta) fibers in human skin nerves. *J. Neurophysiol.,* 49:111–122.
2. Baumann, T. K., Simone, D. A., Shain, C., and LaMotte, R. H. (1991): Neurogenic hyperalgesia: the search for the primary cutaneous afferent fibers that contribute to capsaicin-induced pain and hyperalgesia. *J. Neurophysiol.,* 66:212–227.
3. Beitel, R. E., and Dubner, R. (1976): The response of unmyelinated (C) polymodal nociceptors to thermal stimuli applied to the monkey's face. *J. Neurophysiol.,* 39:1160–1175.
4. Bessou, P., and Perl, E. R. (1969): Response of cutaneous sensory units with unmyelinated fibers to noxious stimuli. *J. Neurophysiol.,* 32:1025–1043.
5. Campbell, J. N., Raja, S. N., Meyer, R. A., and Mackinnon, S. E. (1988): Myelinated afferents signal the hyperalgesia associated with nerve injury. *Pain,* 32:89–94.
6. Cline, M. A., Ochoa, J. L., and Torebjörk, H. E. (1989): Chronic hyperalgesia and skin warming caused by sensitized C nociceptors. *Brain,* 112:621–647.
7. Culp, W. J., Ochoa, J., Cline, M., and Dodtson, R. (1989): Heat and mechanical hyperalgesia induced by capsaicin. *Brain,* 112:621–647.
8. Frey, M. von. (1985): Beiträge zur Sinnesphysiologie der Haut. *Königliche Sächsische Gesellschaft der Wissenschaften. Leipzig. Berichte über die Verhandlungen Matematische Physische Classe,* 47:166–184.
9. Jorum, E., Lundberg, L. E. R., and Torebjörk, H. E. (1989): Peripheral projections of nociceptive unmyelinated axons in the human peroneal nerve. *J. Physiol. (Lond.),* 416:291–301.
10. Koltzenburg, M., Lundberg, L. E. R., and Torebjörk, H. E. Dynamic and static components of mechanical hyperalgesia in human hairy skin *(submitted).*
11. Kumazawa, T., and Perl, E. R. (1977): Primate cutaneous sensory units with unmyelinated (C) afferent fibers. *J. Neurophysiol.,* 40:1325–1338.
12. LaMotte, R. H., Thalhammer, J. G., Torebjörk, H. E., and Robinson, C. J. (1982): Peripheral neural mechanisms of cutaneous hyperalgesia following mild injury by heat. *J. Neurosci.,* 2:765–781.
13. LaMotte, R. H., Torebjörk, H. E., Robinson, C. J., and Thalhammer, J. G. (1984): Time-intensity profiles of cutaneous pain in normal and hyperalgesic skin: a comparison with C-nociceptor activities in monkey and human. *J. Neurophysiol.,* 51:1434–1450.
14. LaMotte, R. H., Shain, S. N., Simone, D. A., and Tsai, E.-F. (1991): Neurogenic hyperalgesia: psychophysical studies of underlying mechanisms. *J. Neurophysiol.,* 66:190–211.
15. LaMotte, R. H., Lundberg, L. E. R., and Torebjörk, H. E. Pain, hyperalgesia and activity in nociceptive C units in humans after intradermal injection of capsaicin. *J. Physiol. (Lond.) (in press).*
16. Lindblom, U., and Verillo, R. T. (1979): Sensory functions in chronic neuralgia. *J. Neurol. Neurosurg. Psychiatry,* 42:422–435.
17. Melzack, R., and Wall, P. D. (1965): Pain mechanisms: a new theory. *Science,* 150:971–979.
18. Meyer, R. A., Campbell, J. M., and Raja, S. N. (1985): Peripheral neural mechanisms of cutaneous hyperalgesia. In: *Advances in pain research and therapy, vol. 9,* edited by H. L. Fields, R. Dubner, F. Cervero, and L. E. Jones, pp. 53–71. Raven Press, New York.
19. Meyer, R. A., and Campbell, J. N. (1981): Myelinated nociceptive afferents account for the hyperalgesia that follows a burn to the hand. *Science,* 213:1527–1529.
20. Ochoa, J. L., and Torebjörk, H. E. (1983): Sensations evoked by intraneural microstimulation of single mechanoreceptor units innervating the human hand. *J. Physiol. (Lond.),* 342:633–654.
21. Ochoa, J., and Torebjörk, E. (1989): Sensations evoked by intraneural microstimulation of C nociceptor fibres in human skin nerves. *J. Physiol. (Lond.),* 415:583–599.
22. Price, D. D., Bennett, G. J., and Rafii, A. (1989): Psychophysical observations on patients with neuropathic pain relieved by a sympathetic block. *Pain,* 36:273–288.

23. Simone, D. A., Sorkin, L. S., Oh, U., Chung, J. M., Owens, C., LaMotte, R. H., and Willis, W. D. (1991): Neurogenic hyperalgesia: central neural correlates in responses of spinothalamic tract neurons. *J. Neurophysiol.*, 66:228–246.

24. Torebjörk, H. E. (1974): Afferent C units responding to mechanical, thermal and chemical stimuli in human non-glabrous skin. *Acta Physiol. Scand.*, 92:374–390.

25. Torebjörk, E. (1985): Nociceptor activation and pain. *Philos. Trans. R. Soc. Lond. [Biol.]*, 308:227–234.

26. Torebjörk, H. E., and Ochoa, J. L. (1980): Specific sensations evoked by activity in single identified sensory units in man. *Acta Physiol. Scand.*, 110:445–447.

27. Torebjörk, H. E., and Ochoa, J. L. (1981): Pain and itch from C fiber stimulation. *Soc. Neurosci. Abstr.*, 7:228.

28. Torebjörk, H. E., LaMotte, R. H., and Robinson, C. J. (1984): Peripheral neural correlates of magnitude of cutaneous pain and hyperalgesia: simultaneous recordings in humans of sensory judgements of pain and evoked responses in nociceptors with C-fibers. *J. Neurophysiol.*, 51:325–339.

29. Torebjörk, H. E., Lundberg, L. E. R., and LaMotte, R. H. Central changes in processing of mechanoreceptor input in capsaicin-induced secondary hyperalgesia in humans. *J. Physiol. (Lond.) (in press)*.

30. Vallbo, Å. B., and Hagbarth, K.-E. (1968): Activity from skin mechanoreceptors recorded percutaneously in awake human subjects. *Exp. Neurol.*, 21:270–289.

31. Vallbo, Å. B., Olsson, K. A., Westberg, K. G., and Clark, F. (1984): Microstimulation of single tactile afferents from the human hand: sensory attributes related to unit type and properties of receptive fields. *Brain*, 107:727–749.

32. Wahren, L.-K., Torebjörk, E., and Nyström, B. (1991): Quantitative sensory testing before and after regional guanethidine block in patients with neuralgia in the hand. *Pain*, 46:23–30.

33. Wahren, L.-K., and Torebjörk, E. Quantitative sensory tests in patients with neuralgia 11 to 25 years after injury. *Pain (in press)*.

Hyperalgesia and Allodynia,
edited by W. D. Willis, Jr.
Raven Press, Ltd., New York © 1992.

12

Sympathetically Maintained Pain

A Unifying Hypothesis

*‡James N. Campbell, *‡Richard A. Meyer, *Karen D. Davis, and
†Srinivasa N. Raja

*Departments of *Neurosurgery and †Anesthesiology, and ‡Applied Physics
Laboratory, Johns Hopkins University School of Medicine,
Baltimore, Maryland 21205*

It has been recognized for decades that pain may in certain instances be dependent on sympathetic innervation of the area afflicted with pain. We will refer to this condition as *sympathetically maintained pain* (SMP). SMP is recognized by many to be an aspect (or even a defining characteristic) of causalgia and reflex sympathetic dystrophy (RSD). Causalgia refers to the burning severe pain that may complicate nerve injury. RSD refers to a similar pain problem that occurs as a complication of soft tissue or bony injury. Whether SMP is a requisite part of RSD or causalgia is disputed.

The mechanism of SMP has long puzzled clinicians and scientists alike. Leriche (12) first brought attention to the linkage between pain and the sympathetic nervous system. He reported that high periarterial "sympathectomy" relieved pain in certain soldiers injured in World War I. As noted by Gybels and Sweet (9), resection of the sympathetic chain as a treatment of SMP was reported in 1930 by three separate investigators (6,16,23). It was later realized that in many instances merely performing a series of anesthetic blocks of the sympathetic chain could in fact suffice to establish long-term or even permanent relief of pain in patients with SMP (2).

NOREPINEPHRINE IS THE CULPRIT IN SYMPATHETICALLY MAINTAINED PAIN

Could afferent fibers that course with the sympathetic fibers account for SMP? Walker and Nulson (25) and White and Sweet (27) stimulated the sympathetic chain in patients both with and without SMP. In patients without SMP such stimulation did not cause pain, whereas stimulation in patients with SMP did in fact induce pain. Moreover, Walker and Nulson (25) noted that stimulation of the peripheral but not central cut end of the sympathetic chain reproduced pain in SMP patients. This observation suggests that events in the periphery account for the capacity of the sympathetic nervous system to evoke pain.

What are these events? Sympathetic terminals release many substances, one of which is norepinephrine. Three observations suggest that norepinephrine is crucial in the maintenance of SMP. (a) Hannington-Kiff (10) noted that regional infusion of guanethidine relieved pain temporarily in patients with SMP, and in some cases on a long-term basis. Guanethidine is thought to achieve this effect via depletion of norepinephrine from the sympathetic terminals. (b) A second line of evidence emerges from observations made initially by Wallin et al. (26). In patients whose pain had been relieved by either a sympathetic block or surgical sympathectomy, an intracutaneous injection of norepinephrine into the previously painful area rekindled the pain and hyperalgesia. (c) Finally, oral administration of the alpha-adrenergic receptor blocking agents phenoxybenzamine and prazosin confer pain relief in patients with SMP (1,8).

SYMPATHETICALLY MAINTAINED PAIN IS A RECEPTOR DISEASE

If the pathogenesis of SMP resides in the peripheral nervous system, is the abnormality on the efferent side or the afferent side? The answer is suggested by the experiments of Wallin et al. (26). Unlike with SMP patients, norepinephrine injected intracutaneously into normal subjects induces very mild pain that is short-lived and not associated with the development of hyperalgesia (5). Thus, the release of norepinephrine is not likely the basis of SMP. In addition, microneurographic recordings from SMP patients indicated that there was no gross increase in sympathetic efferent activity to the affected limb (24). These experiments suggest that the disease is on the afferent side, i.e., it is the response to norepinephrine that is abnormal.

THE PHENTOLAMINE TEST

Norepinephrine activates both alpha- and beta-adrenergic receptors. Which receptor is involved? The clinical reports on the usefulness of phenoxybenzamine and prazosin suggest that the alpha receptor is the culprit. To investigate this and to explore better techniques with which to diagnose SMP, we compared the relief of pain induced by systemic intravenous phentolamine, a short-acting alpha-adrenergic receptor antagonist, with the pain relief imparted by an anesthetic blockade of the sympathetic ganglia (18). Patients suspected of having SMP were entered into the study. All had touch-evoked pain (mechanical hyperalgesia) and hyperalgesia to cooling stimuli. The sympathetic ganglion block and the phentolamine block were done on separate days, and the order of the blocks was randomized. Ongoing pain and pain to mechanical and cooling stimuli were rated on a visual analogue scale.

In pilot studies it was determined that 25 mg of phentolamine delivered intravenously over a 20-min period induced nasal stuffiness, an indication of alpha-receptor blockade. In the initial phase of the study, reflex tachycardia to a pulse rate of 150 beats per minute was typically noted. To block this effect, patients were routinely pretreated with propranolol (1–2 mg) in a second phase of the study.

Prior to delivery of phentolamine or propranolol, patients were given intravenous saline for 20 to 30 min. Patients were not told when drug would be delivered. Three patients had a striking reduction of pain during the infusion of saline. This was considered to be a placebo response, and these patients were excluded from further analysis.

As shown in Fig. 12.1, the pain relief induced by the local anesthetic block of the sympathetic ganglia was highly correlated ($r = 0.84$) to the pain relief induced by the phentolamine block. Propranolol had no effect on the correlation. Thus, the pain relief induced by local anesthetic block of the sympathetic ganglia is likely due to the decrement of alpha-receptor activation.

Our experience with intravenous phentolamine has led us to conclude that this test should replace other tests to diagnose SMP. The ideal diagnostic test in medicine is characterized by the following features: sensitivity, specificity, and safety. Sensitivity can be a problem with the administration of local anesthetics to the sympathetic ganglia. When fluoroscopy is used as an adjunct to performance of the ganglia blocks, the likelihood of missing the ganglia is lessened. However, there still may be problems with target localization. It is well to recall that in doing a stellate block, the real target is the T2 ganglion, since the T2 ganglion supplies the sympathetic innervation to the hand. The only sensitivity issue with the phentolamine test is achieving an adequate dose. The ideal dose of phentolamine has not been established as yet, although with coadministration of propranolol, higher doses would likely be well tolerated.

There is a problem of specificity with the local anesthetic block of the sympathetic ganglia and with the regional infusion of guanethidine. There is no ready mechanism for interpretation of a placebo response in either test. Also, with the ganglion block it is well to keep in mind that lidocaine and its analogues may, via a systemic effect, attenuate neuropathic pain (20). Similarly, lidocaine is usually given with the regional infusion of guanethidine to decrease pain from the initial norepinephrine release. This compromises interpretation of the test. Likewise, the tourniquet inflation, applied during the regional infusion of guanethidine, blocks conduction in sensory fibers and may, in and of itself, reduce pain (3). An important and frequent problem with local anesthetic blockade of the sympathetic ganglion is that the somatic roots that serve the painful area are very near the sympathetic chain. It may be difficult to determine whether the pain relief that is achieved from ganglion block is a result of the sympathetic block or a somatic block.

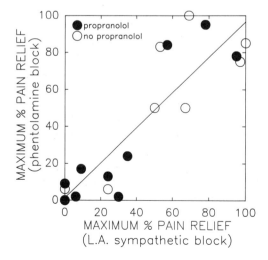

FIG. 12.1. Comparison of the pain relief obtained from a local anesthetic sympathetic ganglion block with that obtained from intravenous administration of phentolamine. Each point represents a different patient ($n = 18$). Ten patients were pretreated with propranolol. The pain relief obtained with the two different types of sympathetic blocks was highly correlated ($r = 0.84$). (From ref. 18.)

Safety comparisons between the different procedures are premature. To date more than 60 phentolamine blocks have been performed at Johns Hopkins, and no untoward effects have been observed. Patients greatly prefer the phentolamine test because the test is essentially painless. Both the local anesthetic block of the sympathetic ganglia and the regional infusion of guanethidine have been associated with complications. These include injury to the recurrent laryngeal nerve, pneumothorax, inadvertent vascular injection, puncture of the kidney, and leakage of guanethidine into the systemic circulation with attendant hemodynamic changes. In addition, the pain associated with these tests is often not well tolerated by the patients.

ALPHA-1 OR ALPHA-2 ADRENERGIC RECEPTOR?

There are two principal subgroups of alpha-adrenergic receptors: alpha-1 and alpha-2. The alpha-1 receptors are found in peripheral tissues. The alpha-2 receptors are located on the postsynaptic sympathetic terminals and are thought to be autoreceptors. Which is responsible for SMP? To determine this we applied locally the alpha-2 agonist clonidine to the painful area in patients with SMP (5). Six patients were studied, four with SMP and two with sympathetically independent pain (SIP). Clonidine is supplied as a patch for cutaneous application (Catapress-TTS, Boehringer). The patch is 10.5 cm^2 and provides programmed delivery of 0.3 mg/day. If presynaptic alpha-2 receptors mediate SMP, the patch should aggravate pain locally. If alpha-1 receptors are the culprit in SMP, clonidine should locally relieve pain, since the release of norepinephrine from the sympathetic terminals would be decreased.

The four patients with SMP all had complete relief of hyperalgesia in the clonidine-treated area, whereas no pain relief was obtained for the two patients with SIP. The effect was localized to the vicinity of the patch. Ongoing pain was not affected, as the area of relief from the hyperalgesia was small compared to the entire affected region. However, in two subsequent patients with a small area of SMP, clonidine also attenuated the ongoing pain.

We determined that clonidine patches conferred no local anesthetic effect. Detection thresholds in a control subject, in uninvolved areas in patients with SMP, in the painful area of SMP patients, and in the painful area of patients with SIP were not altered by application of clonidine. The skin was never rendered analgesic; rather, pain thresholds were normalized in the SMP patients.

These data with clonidine implicate the alpha-1 receptor as being the mediator of pain in SMP in humans. Moreover, the locus for this alpha–1-mediated effect is likely in the painful tissues themselves, since pain to light touch persisted in the untreated areas adjacent to the patch site. To test this further we injected intracutaneously norepinephrine as well as the alpha-1 agonist phenylephrine into the skin of normal subjects and patients with SMP. The patients with SMP were injected in the area rendered free of hyperalgesia by application of clonidine. As shown in Fig. 12.2, norepinephrine caused little pain when injected into normal subjects, and hyperalgesia to mechanical stimuli did not develop. In the clonidine-treated area of patients with SMP, norepinephrine evoked substantial pain. Hyperalgesia to mechanical and cooling stimuli developed within 10 to 15 min in the patch site, analogous to the findings presented earlier of Wallin et al. (26). Similar results were obtained following injection of phenylephrine.

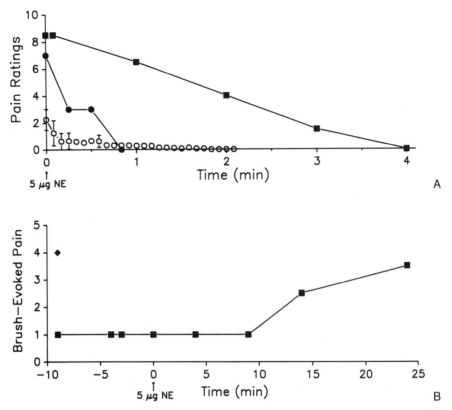

FIG. 12.2. Pain and hyperalgesia evoked by an intradermal injection of norepinephrine (5 μg in 10 μl saline). **A:** Norepinephrine evoked more pain in an SMP patient than in normal subjects. Pain was rated as a function of time on a scale from "0" (no pain) to "10" (most intense pain). Injections were made into a clonidine patch site (*filled squares*) and a contralateral site (*filled circles*) for an SMP patient and into the lateral leg of four normal subjects (*open circles*) (mean ± SEM are indicated). **B:** The norepinephrine injection rekindled the hyperalgesia to mechanical stimuli at the patch site in the patient. The pain evoked by light brushing at the patch site (*filled squares*) approached that reported before the injection at a site adjacent to the patch (*filled diamond*). (From ref. 5.)

PAIN AND THE LOW-THRESHOLD MECHANORECEPTOR

These data taken together provide evidence that SMP is a disease wherein the alpha-1 receptor develops the capacity, when activated, to evoke pain. The next question is, therefore, how does this happen? One explanation (19) is that central neurons concerned with pain sensation become sensitized to peripheral inputs, such that activity in low-threshold mechanoreceptors becomes capable of evoking activity in central–pain-signaling neurons. There is evidence that sympathetic efferents may evoke activity in low–threshold mechanoreceptors. Thus, it is reasoned that SMP results from sympathetically mediated activation of low-threshold mechanoreceptors. This explanation, however, does not account for the prompt relief of pain invoked by a sympathetic block. Pain evoked by stroking the skin quickly disappears with onset of the block, despite the fact that low-threshold mechanoreceptors can still be activated by touching the skin.

A MODEL OF SYMPATHETICALLY MAINTAINED PAIN

A schema that illustrates a more likely explanation of SMP is shown in Fig. 12.3. The core of this explanation rests with three postulates: (a) activity in nociceptors has the capacity to evoke pain, (b) nociceptive input into the spinal cord may sensitize central neurons such that inputs from low-threshold receptors (mechanoreceptors) impart pain (3,11,22), (c) sympathetic efferent activity gains the capacity to activate nociceptive fibers via an alpha–1-adrenergic receptor mechanism.

How reasonable are these postulates? The substantial evidence for postulate a will not be reviewed here, as other reviews cover this topic (4). Postulate b has been given credence in a recent study by Price et al. (17) in which peripheral nerves that served the painful area were electrically stimulated at low intensities in patients with SMP. Under conditions of a sympathetic block, when pain was relieved, stimulation evoked sensations of tingling only. The same stimulus applied when the patients were not under the influence of the block evoked pain and a tingle sensation concurrently. Thus, whether stimulation of low-threshold mechanoreceptors evoked pain depended on whether the patient was under the influence of a sympathetic block. The site of interaction is most likely in the painful tissues, i.e., peripheral. For reasons given above, sympathetically mediated activation of low-threshold mechanoreceptors is not a likely mechanism of action. This suggests that the critical interaction must be between nociceptors and sympathetic efferent fibers (postulate c).

We can put this model together in the following way to show the chain of events that occurs in SMP following injury. An injury results in a barrage of activity in nociceptors that leads to the sensitization of central–pain-signaling neurons such that input from low-threshold mechanoreceptors now has the capacity to evoke pain. Sympathetic efferent fibers activate nociceptive fibers via an alpha–1-adrenergic re-

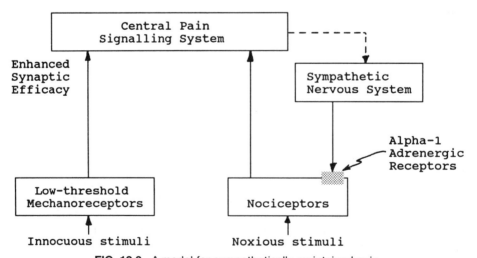

FIG. 12.3. A model for sympathetically maintained pain.

ceptor that develops in the nociceptive afferent. Aside from evoking pain, this nociceptor activation serves to maintain the central–pain-signaling neurons in a sensitized state. A sympathetic block eliminates activation of the nociceptors, the central sensitization is eliminated, and thus ongoing pain and touch-evoked pain are eliminated.

HOW DO ALPHA–1-ADRENERGIC RECEPTORS BECOME INVOLVED IN SYMPATHETICALLY MAINTAINED PAIN?

How does activation of the alpha-1 receptor become linked to the production of action potentials in nociceptors? Loh and Nathan (14) demonstrated that guanethidine delivered regionally distal to the area of nerve injury still conferred pain relief. Thus, even in cases of nerve injury the interaction with the alpha-1 receptor is likely to be in the tissues innervated by the injured nerve. Is the interaction with the nociceptor itself, or is the activation of the nociceptor indirect? As an example of the latter, Levine et al. (13) suggested an alpha-adrenergic mechanism wherein sympathetic terminals are activated by alpha-adrenergic agonists and induced to release prostaglandins, which in turn activate and sensitize nociceptors. Alpha-1 receptors could also be upregulated on other cellular elements (e.g., platelets or mast cells) such that norepinephrine released by the sympathetic terminals induces release of inflammatory mediators from these cells, leading again to nociceptor activation. Psychophysical studies in humans provide evidence against this explanation. Inflammatory mediators such as prostaglandins and bradykinin injected into the skin induce hyperalgesia to heat stimuli (15). Although hyperalgesia to mechanical and cooling stimuli are consistent features of SMP (7), hyperalgesia to heating stimuli is not always a part of SMP (17). Given these psychophysical findings, it is unlikely that alpha–1-mediated pain results from actions on non-neural cells.

The more likely explanation is that alpha-1 receptors are expressed on the peripheral terminals of nociceptors themselves. It may be that a barrage of activity in nociceptive fibers produces a genetic signal, such that the production of alpha-1 receptors is upregulated. In patients with SMP this production may be excessive, such that nociceptive fibers develop sensitivity to the norepinephrine that is released by the sympathetic efferent fibers. Now the ingredients for a vicious cycle are in place. Nociceptive inputs to the spinal cord trigger sympathetic efferent activity normally. The sympathetic efferent activity increases the activity in the nociceptive fibers via activation of the alpha–1-adrenergic receptor. The activity in the nociceptive fibers induces further production of alpha-1 receptors and more activity in the sympathetic fibers. Now a series of sympathetic blocks is done. Let it be supposed that the original injury that initially incited the activity in the nociceptive fibers is gone. The sympathetically mediated activation of the nociceptive fibers is eliminated by the sympathetic blocks. The neural–activity-based production of alpha-1 receptors in nociceptors is downregulated. The nociceptor-dependent activation of sympathetic efferent fibers is eliminated. The patient obtains a sustained period of pain relief.

A variation of this hypothesis is that alpha-1 receptors are in place in the terminals of the nociceptors, but in an inactive form. Neural activity in the nociceptors could invoke expression of these receptors. The hypothesis that SMP involves a phenotype alteration in nociceptors is testable in animal models if there is some up- and downregulation of alpha-receptor expression normally. One caveat here is that Sato and

Perl (21) found in rabbit that nerve injury induced expression of alpha–2-receptor sensitivity in the terminals of nociceptors (these animals apparently did not have any behavioral signs of neuropathic pain). This result is clearly different from what we would expect based on experience in humans, primarily since the alpha-2 agonist clonidine applied to the painful area in patients with SMP locally relieved pain (see discussion above). There may be species variations therefore in the involvement of different types of adrenergic receptors. Also, both the alpha-1 and alpha-2 receptors have subtypes. Nothing to date has been done to clarify which subtype may be involved in SMP.

In the above scenario it is stated that downregulation of alpha–1-receptor synthesis accompanies the sympathetic block. This need not always be the case. It is well-known clinically that there are some patients in whom the pain relief invoked by sympathetic blockade lasts consistently only for the period of the pharmacological block. These may be the patients that require a surgical sympathectomy in order to achieve sustained pain relief. Patients with SMP may also have a component of sympathetically independent pain. The production of action potentials in the nociceptors may be based partly on a SMP mechanism and partly on an independent problem such as nerve entrapment.

SUMMARY AND CONCLUSIONS

1. Release of norepinephrine from terminals of sympathetic fibers in certain patients after injury induces pain.
2. The norepinephrine induces pain by activating alpha–1-adrenergic receptors.
3. The alpha-1 receptors are most likely expressed on the terminals of nociceptive fibers.
4. Nociceptors when active induce central sensitization such that inputs of other receptor types may induce pain. This sensitization is dynamic, such that when the nociceptor input to the spinal cord is eliminated, the central sensitization disappears.
5. It is hypothesized that action potential activity in nociceptors triggers expression of alpha–1-adrenergic receptors in the terminals of the nociceptor. This could be a result of upregulation in synthesis, i.e., a phenotypic change.
6. In certain patients this upregulation is excessive and results in a pathological state (SMP) sometimes referred to as RSD or causalgia.

ACKNOWLEDGMENTS

We wish to thank Dr. R.-D. Treede for many helpful discussions. This research was supported by NIH grants NS-14447 and NS-26363.

REFERENCES

1. Abram, S. E., and Lightfoot, R. W. (1981): Treatment of long-standing causalgia with prazosin. *Reg. Anaesth.*, 6:79–81.
2. Bonica, J. J. (1979): Causalgia and other reflex sympathetic dystrophies. *Adv. Pain Res. Ther.*, 3:141–166.

3. Campbell, J. N., Raja, S. N., Meyer, R. A., and Mackinnon, S. E. (1988): Myelinated afferents signal the hyperalgesia associated with nerve injury. *Pain*, 32:89–94.
4. Campbell, J. N., Raja, S. N., Cohen, R. H., Manning, D. C., Khan, A. A., and Meyer, R. A. (1989): Peripheral neural mechanisms of nociception. In: *Textbook of pain*, edited by P. D. Wall and R. Melzack, pp. 22–45. Churchill Livingstone, London.
5. Davis, K. D., Treede, R.-D., Raja, S. N., Meyer, R. A., and Campbell, J. N. (1991): Topical application of clonidine relieves hyperalgesia in patients with sympathetically-maintained pain. *Pain*, 47:309–317.
6. Flothow, P. G. (1930): Relief of pain from a neurologic viewpoint. *N.W. Med.*, 29:69–76.
7. Frost, S. A., Raja, S. N., Campbell, J. N., Meyer, R. A., and Khan, A. A. (1988): Does hyperalgesia to cooling stimuli characterize patients with sympathetically maintained pain (reflex sympathetic dystrophy)? In: *Proceedings of the Vth World Congress on Pain*, edited by R. Dubner, G. F. Gebhart, and M. R. Bond, pp. 151–156. Elsevier, Amsterdam.
8. Ghostine, S. Y., Comair, Y. G., Turner, D. M., Kassell, N. F., and Azar, C. G. (1984): Phenoxybenzamine in the treatment of causalgia. *J. Neurosurg.*, 60:1263–1268.
9. Gybels, J. M., and Sweet, W. H. (1989): *Neurosurgical treatment of persistent pain*. Karger, London.
10. Hannington-Kiff, J. G. (1974): Intravenous regional sympathetic block with guanethidine. *Lancet*, 2:1019–1020.
11. LaMotte, R. H., Shain, C. N., Simone, D. A., and Tsai, E. P. (1991): Neurogenic hyperalgesia: psychophysical studies of underlying mechanisms. *J. Neurophysiol.*, 66:190–211.
12. Leriche, R. (1939): *The surgery of pain*. Bailliere, Tindall & Cox, London.
13. Levine, J. D., Taiwo, Y. O., Collins, S. D., and Tam, J. K. (1986): Noradrenaline hyperalgesia is mediated through interaction with sympathetic postganglionic neurone terminals rather than activation of primary afferent nociceptors. *Nature*, 323:158–160.
14. Loh, L., and Nathan, P. W. (1978): Painful peripheral states and sympathetic blocks. *J. Neurol. Neurosurg. Psychiatry*, 41:664–671.
15. Manning, D. C., Raja, S. N., Meyer, R. A., and Campbell, J. N. (1991): Pain and hyperalgesia after intradermal injection of bradykinin in humans. *Clin. Pharmacol. Ther.*, 50:721–729.
16. Pieri, G. (1930): Contributi clinici alla chirurgia del sistema nervoso vegetativo: la cura della nevrite ascendente. *Arch. Ital. Cir.*, 27:288–298.
17. Price, D. D., Bennett, G. J., and Rafii, A. (1989): Psychophysical observations on patients with neuropathic pain relieved by a sympathetic block. *Pain*, 36:273–288.
18. Raja, S. N., Treede, R-D., Davis, K. D., and Campbell, J. N. (1991): Systemic alpha-adrenergic blockade with phentolamine: a diagnostic test for sympathetically maintained pain. *Anesthesiology* 74:691–698.
19. Roberts, W. J. (1986): A hypothesis on the physiological basis for causalgia and related pains. *Pain*, 24:297–311.
20. Rowbotham, M. C., and Fields, H. L. (1989): Post-herpetic neuralgia: the relation of pain complaint, sensory disturbance, and skin temperature. *Pain*, 38:129–144.
21. Sato, J., and Perl, E. R. (1991): Adrenergic excitation of cutaneous pain receptors induced by peripheral nerve injury. *Science*, 251:1608–1610.
22. Simone, D. A., Sorkin, L. S., Oh, U., et al. (1991): Neurogenic hyperalgesia: central neural correlates in responses of spinothalamic tract neurons. *J. Neurophysiol.*, 66:228–246.
23. Spurling, R. G. (1930): Causalgia of the upper extremity. Treatment by dorsal sympathetic ganglionectomy. *Arch. Neurol. Psychiatr.*, 23:784–788.
24. Torebjörk, E. (1990): Clinical and neurophysiological observations relating to pathophysiological mechanisms in reflex sympathetic dystrophy. In: *Reflex sympathetic dystrophy*, edited by M. Stanton-Hicks, W. Janig, and R. A. Boas, pp. 71–80. Kluwer, Boston.
25. Walker, A. E., and Nulson, F. (1948): Electrical stimulation of the upper thoracic portion of the sympathetic chain in man. *Arch. Neurol. Psychiatr.*, 59:559–560.
26. Wallin, B. G., Torebjörk, E., and Hallin, R. G. (1976): Preliminary observations on the pathophysiology of hyperalgesia in the causalgic pain syndrome. In: *Sensory functions of the skin in primates*, edited by Y. Zotterman, pp. 489–499. Pergamon Press, Oxford.
27. White, J. C., and Sweet, W. H. (1969): *Pain and the neurosurgeon. A forty-year experience*. Charles C. Thomas, Springfield, IL.

Hyperalgesia and Allodynia,
edited by W. D. Willis, Jr.
Raven Press, Ltd., New York © 1992.

13

Thermal Hyperalgesia as a Clinical Symptom

José Ochoa

Departments of Neurology and Neurosurgery, Good Samaritan Hospital and Medical Center, Oregon Health Sciences University, Portland, Oregon 97210

A definition of "hyperalgesia," as offered by the Subcommittee on Taxonomy of the International Association for the Study of Pain (IASP), namely, "an increased response to a stimulus which is normally painful" (*Pain,* suppl. 3, S219, 1986) invites debate. It excludes "allodynia" (pain in response to stimuli which are *not* normally painful) as a separate category, thus assuming that subthreshold and suprathreshold abnormalities of pain perception commonly dissociate from one another. In our experience, the separation is in part artificial. Patients who express "pain in response to stimuli which are normally not painful" usually also have "increased response to normally painful stimuli" (although the reverse is not true; indeed, patients with abnormally exaggerated pain response may have elevated pain thresholds). Therefore, the IASP definition will not be applied during the conceptual treatment of the present subject. Instead, classical concepts will be honored for good tradition and on the grounds of their being better in keeping with clinical reality. In the late 19th century, a great neurologist wrote, "increased sensitiveness to pain, or *hyperalgesia*" (13). Just earlier, it was written by another master: "A painful sensation is often felt more acutely than normal; this is called *hyperaesthesia* or, more correctly, *hyperalgesia*" (12). At the turn of the century, the patron Déjérine (8) stated: "L'hyperesthésie (l'exagération de la sensibilité) porte rarement sur l'une des qualités spécialisées de la sensibilité tactile (tact, pression, localisation). L'hyperesthésie ne consiste donc pas en une augmentation des facultés tactiles, mais en une tendance à la transformation rapide des sensations tactiles en sensations douloureuses et en une exagération de la sensibilité douloureuse; elle est synonyme d'hyperalgésie." This translates: "Hyperaesthesia rarely relates to any of the specialized qualities of tactile sensibility (touch, pressure, localization). Hyperaesthesia does not result from augmentation of tactile faculties, but from a tendency towards rapid transformation of tactile sensations into painful sensations and towards an exaggeration of painful sensibility: it is synonymous with *hyperalgesia*."

These classical statements did not separate subthreshold from suprathreshold abnormalities of pain perception.

A common and intriguing variety of hyperalgesia is expressed in response to stimulation with thermal energy. Gentle elevation of temperature that normally evokes a sensation of warmth may, under abnormal circumstances, induce a pain response: *heat hyperalgesia.* Gentle reduction of temperature that normally evokes a sensation of cold may, under abnormal circumstances, induce a pain response: *cold hyperalgesia*. Thermal hyperalgesias may occur concurrent with, or independent of, spontaneous pains and mechanical hyperalgesias, of which two types have been discriminated: static and dynamic mechanical hyperalgesia (21). In turn, *heat and cold hyperalgesias* may be expressed concurrently or independent of each other. Although much experimental research on animals and humans has addressed heat hyperalgesia, there are few rigorous animal experimental studies on cold hyperalgesia and few clinical studies on either type of thermal hyperalgesia in human patients.

Multidisciplinary investigation of pathophysiological mechanisms in chronic neuropathic pain patients indicates that, like spontaneous pains and mechanical hyperalgesias, the subjective expression of thermal hyperalgesias probably recognizes multiple pathogeneses: peripheral, central, and psychological. "Every patient with chronic neuropathic pain harbors a personal mosaic of multiple abnormal mechanisms which include customized mixtures of peripheral, central, and psychogenic phenomena" (19). Contribution of *peripheral* mechanisms is currently supported by fair evidence for heat hyperalgesia and weakly so for cold hyperalgesia in humans. *Peripheral-central* mechanisms are strongly suspected: release phenomena (at least) for cold hyperalgesia and *central* hyperexcitability for either type of thermal hyperalgesia. *Primary psychological* mechanisms are seldom considered in scientific studies on chronic painful syndromes following peripheral neurological disease or injury, and yet they appear to account for a significant incidence of spontaneous pains, mechanical hyperalgesias, and thermal hyperalgesias in the clinic (8,32).

TEST METHODS

In order to properly document the presence of thermal hyperalgesias, it becomes necessary to test quantitatively subjective magnitude of thermal pains. Quantitative measurement of subjective magnitude of thermal pains should be supplemented with correlative measurement of cold and warm sensory functions. This is desirable for the sake of comprehensiveness in probing small-caliber afferent channel function and also because of the existence of clinical conditions in which disturbed modulatory interactions between thermal specific and thermal pain afferent channels are instrumental in determining painful status. But, of course, measurements of sensory intensity functions should not be restricted to warm and cold specific functions, since these may be intact in skin expressing either heat or cold hyperalgesia (15,33). It is a mistake to attempt to draw conclusions about pain function and dysfunction based solely on measurement of warm and cold specific functions, because cold pain is not the hyperbole of cold sensation and heat pain is similarly unrelated to warm sensation. As recommended by an expert panel, all four functions should be included in the testing: warm and cold specific plus heat pain and cold pain sensory thresholds (1).

Threshold measurements are more practical than suprathreshold estimates and have become the established routine in the clinical laboratory. Different methods for testing thermal perception thresholds are currently in use in different somatosensory clinical laboratories. Due to operation of the reaction time artefact, the threshold signaled by the subject may become deceptively elevated, particularly for sensations evoked by slowly conducted afferent signals (35). Methods that do not include reaction time in the measurement of threshold are not liable to the artefact. All these methods depart from real measurement of absolute thresholds, but, to the extent they provide a useful analog value, they are as useful as they are comprehensive and simple to apply. In this regard the quantitative Marstock (Marburg-Stockholm) sensory thermotest method is unsurpassed (10). The sensory thermotest provides information about function of four separate somatosensory channels serving warm sensation, cold sensation, heat pain, and cold pain, each wired by a specific apparatus served by small-caliber myelinated or unmyelinated fibers, which may break down in dissociated fashions. Notably, the test may detect abnormal deviation of small-caliber afferent functions in the direction of irritative positive phenomena, specifically, thermal hyperalgesias. This is critical in the study of neurological painful syndromes featuring thermal hyperalgesias, because such somatosensory abnormalities may exist in the absence of warm or cold specific dysfunction (Fig. 13.1).

Quantitative documentation of equivalents of function of small-caliber afferent channels make available a missing piece in clinical evaluation of somatosensory status. It should be emphasized that conventional electrophysiology explores the status of only large-caliber channels through measurement of sensory nerve action potentials and somatosensory evoked potentials (18).

The quantitative thermotest probes function of somatosensory afferents between cutaneous receptor and brain-mind, without specifying the precise locus of dysfunc-

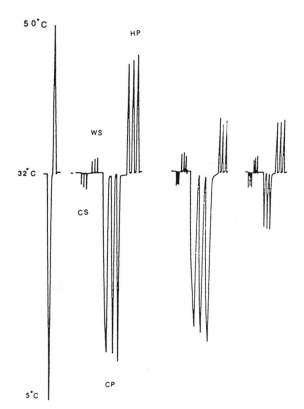

FIG. 13.1. Normal and abnormal profiles of quantitative sensory thermotest from control subjects and patients with chronic neuropathic painful syndromes. Thermal stimulation was given in skin of the palm. **Left,** Normal control profile; **middle,** heat hyperalgesia; **right,** heat and cold hyperalgesia without associated warm or cold hypoesthesia. CS, cold sensation; WS, warm sensation; CP, cold pain; HP, heat pain.

tion along the channels. However, the feature may be advantageous in that the profile and its degree of consistency along time may indicate a possible psychological
basis for the anomaly.

THE SUBJECTIVE QUALITY OF THERMAL HYPERALGESIAS

The subjective quality of heat hyperalgesia is familiar. Gentle elevation of temperature to a degree that normally evokes a sensation of warmth will abnormally evoke
a burning sensation when in the state of heat hyperalgesia. Cold hyperalgesia is less
of a common experience in normal everyday life, and perhaps for this reason, there
is a tendency to assume that the subjective quality of cold hyperalgesia involves
reduced threshold for, and exaggeration of, natural cold pain sensation. Often, however, if not usually, the subjective description of individuals expressing reduced
threshold to pain induced by low temperature features a *burning* pain. Furthermore,
the subjective denominator "burning" is common not only to thermal hyperalgesias,
but, as is well-known, it often applies to mechanical hyperalgesias as well. Thus the
expression "It feels like a burn" or "It feels like fire," verbalized by patients or
experimental pain volunteers, points to a subjective experience that is commonplace
enough to be described not with a specific term, but essentially through naming the
nature of the stimulus. What is special about a burn injury is that it excites nociceptor discharge and that it may desensitize and sensitize nociceptors.

BURNING SENSATION AND C-NOCICEPTORS

"Burning" is one of the primary sensations in the somatosensory repertoire. Together with touch, tickle, itch, cold, warm, stinging pain, and dull pain, "burning
pain" is a distinctive sensation. The specific primary somatosensory apparatus
whose excitation triggers afferent input that evokes a sensation of "burning" or
"fire" is served by unmyelinated C-nociceptor fibers. Early evidence for this was
gathered three-quarters of a century ago, when Zotterman (38) had to scald the
tongue of his experimental animals in order to discover the minute C afferent signals
in nerves. In other words, only when intense stimuli that cause burning pain in humans were applied to animals did the C fibers respond (Fig. 13.2). To follow the
Swedish tradition, Torebjörk and Hallin (27) pioneered the equivalent experiment in
humans by applying noxious thermal stimuli to skin, while recording the afferent
input with intraneural microelectrodes. Indeed, a noxious heat stimulus activates
high-threshold, slowly conducting C unmyelinated units (Fig. 13.3).

Through application of the technique of intraneural microstimulation (28,29) it was
demonstrated that selective microstimulation of identified human C-nociceptors
evokes sensations of dull or burning pain precisely projected to the unitary receptive
fields (20,30). This pain expresses a long reaction time between intraneural stimulus
and perception, in keeping with conduction along slow C unmyelinated fibers. The
pain does not disappear during selective blockade of myelinated afferent fibers by
means of compression–ischemia. In contrast, the pain evoked by selective microstimulation of A-delta myelinated nociceptors is sharp rather than burning, has a
short reaction time, and disappears during myelinated fiber block (31).

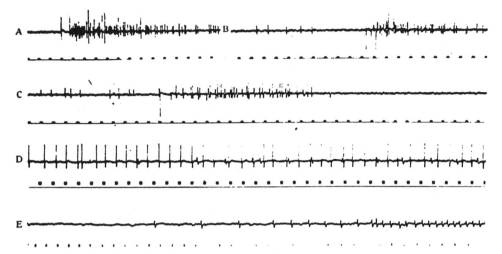

FIG. 13.2. Afferent spike potentials from different sensory fibers of a fine strand of the lingual nerve of the cat when applying different stimuli to the tongue. **A:** The effect of a drop of water of 14°C falling on the tongue. **B:** First, the effect of a faint puff of air that does not cause any visible deformation of the surface, followed by the effect of a stronger puff of air that makes a definite deformation. **C:** A drop of water of 80°C falling on the tongue. **D:** The effect of pressing a pointed rod into the tongue. **E:** Squirting hot water (60°C) over the tongue. (From ref. 39.)

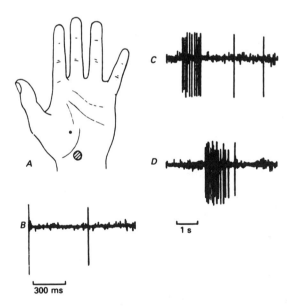

FIG. 13.3. A: Projected field of dull pain (*hatched area*) and mismatching receptive field (•) of recordable C polymodal nociceptor unit. **B:** Long latency to unitary response, conduction distance 45.5 cm. Calculated conduction velocity = 0.83 msec^{-1}. **C:** Intermediately adapting response to stroking unitary receptive field with blunt stick. Note two afterdischarges. **D:** Unitary receptor response to heat applied to receptive field. (From ref. 20.)

HYPERALGESIAS AND C-NOCICEPTORS

By design, human C-nociceptors have a high receptor threshold, with notable exceptions (16). Nevertheless, a burn injury is typically characterized by "increased sensitiveness to pain" (13). In other words, a burn characteristically causes hyperalgesia. Following a burn injury, the abnormal development by nociceptors of lowered threshold to their adequate stimuli, i.e., "sensitization," was strikingly demonstrated in the 1960s by directly recording abnormal receptor–response characteristics of C-nociceptors in experimental animals (3) (see also Perl, Chapter 5).

Similar to those in many animal species, C-nociceptors in humans are polymodal in that they respond to several different types of adequate stimulus energies (20,27). On these grounds it would be anticipated that any kind of adequate stimulus sufficient to activate normal polymodal nociceptors should be able to activate, at reduced thresholds, nociceptors that are sensitized. The mere examination of the psychophysical characteristics of a burn injury immediately points to a significant exception. Indeed, whereas human C-nociceptors are normally excitable by intense mechanical stimuli, heat, and noxious cold (26), a burn expresses hyperalgesia to mechanical and heat stimuli, but not to low-temperature stimuli. On the contrary, low temperature tends to soothe the mechanical hyperalgesia and the spontaneous

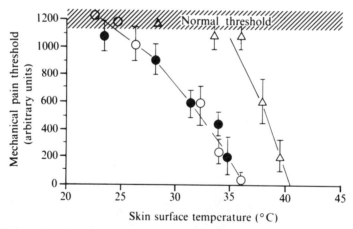

FIG. 13.4. Effect of selective A-fiber block induced by compression–ischemia and of the postischemic period on capsaicin-induced mechanical hyperalgesia. A skin region on the palm was treated with 3.3×10^{-3} M capsaicin. Approximately 3 hr after application, pressure algometry measurements were carried out at the indicated skin surface temperatures (○). A selective A-fiber block was then established. Pressure algometry was then repeated over a similar range of temperatures at a time when touch, sharp pain, and cold sensation were abolished while warm sensation and dull pain were preserved (●). Each point represents the mean of at least five measurements in a single representative experiment. Bars = range. Pressure algometry measurements were repeated at a range of skin temperatures in the postischemic period immediately following the release of the sphygmomanometer cuff (△). Because of the need to work rapidly during this period, temperature equilibration prior to pressure algometry was limited to approximately 2 min. Each point represents the mean of at least four determinations over a 2-min period. Bars = range. The five determinations in the postischemic period were made, in order of increasing temperature, at 4, 11, 19, 25, and 36 min following cuff release. This postischemic effect is abolished within approximately 45 min. (From ref. 7.)

pains. This puzzling dichotomy is also expressed in very pure fashion for the case of the acute lesion caused by capsaicin, a neurotoxin known to sensitize nociceptors in experimental animals (25) (see also Torebjörk, Chapter 11, for sensitization of human nociceptors by capsaicin). As has become well-known, this neurotoxin lends a useful experimental model in which spontaneous burning pain, burning hyperalgesia to mechanical stimuli, and burning hyperalgesia to gentle elevation of temperature are consistently reproduced. The (primary) hyperalgesia that develops near the site of capsaicin application in humans resists A-fiber block. It is therefore C-fiber mediated (7) (Fig. 13.4).

The observation that thermal hyperalgesia related to malfunctioning of C-nociceptors may remain selective to heat raises the question of whether these biological injuries induced by noxious heat, the neurotoxin capsaicin, and other agents selectively damage subclasses of nociceptors with polymodality restricted to heat (and mechanical) responsiveness. The alternative is whether those injuries selectively affect specific biophysical transducers for heat and for mechanical energy, while sparing transducers for noxious low temperature in the excitable membrane of conventional, broadly polymodal nociceptors. This question becomes more significant when it is taken into consideration that, in the clinical patient setting, cold hyperalgesia may also occur in pure form, dissociated from heat hyperalgesia, and that sensitization to low temperatures has also been observed as a fairly selective phenomenon in response to cold injury in animal nociceptors that, under normal circumstances, are mechano-cold responsive (24; P. W. Reeh, 1990, *personal communication*).

HEAT HYPERALGESIAS IN PATIENTS

Central Dysfunction

Among clinicians and scientists interested in pain related to peripheral injury or neurological disease, there is growing awareness of the idea that, like spontaneous neurological pains, mechanical hyperalgesias may be a result of primary dysfunction of peripheral sensory units or secondary dysfunction in central somatosensory stations (21). As discussed below, there is persuasive evidence that a similar duality may apply to mechanisms behind cold hyperalgesia in the context of peripheral neurological disease or injury. It is therefore conceivable that, in the same context, heat hyperalgesia, which can be a clear consequence of dysfunction of peripheral sensory units, may also develop as a result of secondary pathophysiological change in the central nervous system. To date, the issue of secondary central heat hyperalgesia appears to have been approached preliminarily in a single study that applied rigorous scientific methods to human patients. Indeed, Fruhstorfer and Lindblom (11) concluded that heat hyperalgesia following (nerve) injury is probably the consequence of abnormal central processing of primary non-noxious input carried by warm specific receptors.

Peripheral Dysfunction

There is a subgroup of patients who have not had a burn and have not been exposed to capsaicin or other nociceptor-sensitizing agents but who have clear-cut

disease of primary sensory units and express burning pain as the cognitive experience associated with heat hyperalgesia, coexistent or not with mechanical hyperalgesia. In these patients, a diagnostic compression–ischemia block, selective to myelinated fiber input, does not abolish the hyperalgesia (at least the mechanical type).
Thus far, there is only one report in the literature directly demonstrating sensitized
human C-nociceptors supplying the area of symptomatic expression of heat and mechanical hyperalgesia. Indeed, direct microneurographic recordings of single identified C polymodal nociceptors from symptomatic skin confirmed the presence of
units with pathologically enhanced receptor responses: lowered threshold and very
prolonged afterdischarges (Fig. 13.5). While bypassing skin receptors, strong intraneural microstimulation in fascicles supplying symptomatic or contralateral skin
evoked equivalent magnitudes and temporal profiles of pain from both sides in the
patient. Thus, secondary CNS dysfunction need not be postulated to explain such a
painful syndrome. The finding of sensitized C polymodal nociceptors was consistent
with the clinical features, namely, the reduced threshold for pain evoked by non-
noxious stimuli, the exaggerated pain magnitude, and the abnormally prolonged aftersensation of pain (6).

One remarkable feature is that in a good number of these patients with heat hyperalgesia and regularly in the acute capsaicin model, the skin that "burns" is physically hot (7,17). Moreover, it only hurts where it is objectively hot. In other words,
the skin needs to be hot for it to be hyperalgesic (Fig. 13.6). In the context of C-
nociceptor sensitization, the hot skin is most likely due to antidromic neurosecretion
of vasoactive substances from C-nociceptors. That is why this syndrome was called

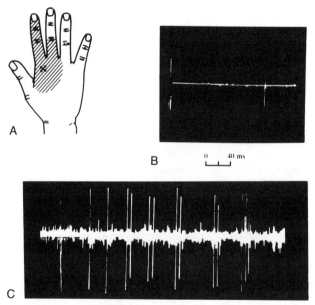

FIG. 13.5. A: Receptive field (RF) for identified C unit (five squares) within the area of hyperalgesia (*hatched area*). **B:** Intradermal electrical stimulation in the RF evoked a slowly conducted unitary response (conduction velocity = 1.25 msec^{-1}). **C:** Intraneural recording of
C-unit response to nine repetitive light mechanical stimulation of the RF with a wisp of cotton.
(From ref. 6.)

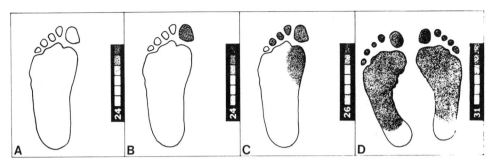

FIG. 13.6. Sequential liquid crystal contact thermograms of the feet of a diabetic boy. Spontaneous development of pain and mechanical hyperalgesia paralleled progressive warming of the skin, beginning in the right big toe. The painful sequence exactly replicated the thermographic spread in time and space. **A:** Pain-free baseline state induced by cold immersion minutes prior to thermographic examination. The left foot was colder than the "coldest" detector (24°C). **B** and **C:** Pain, hyperalgesia, and skin warming expand beyond the big toe. **D:** Patient is experiencing burning pain in both feet. Note bilateral cutaneous temperature elevation. (Modified from ref. 17.)

the angry backfiring C-nociceptor (ABC) syndrome (4,17). Direct evidence is awaited for the thesis that the regional warming, which obviously reflects vasodilation, is due to antidromic neurosecretion. Indeed, direct micromeasurement of pertinent substances in the skin remains to be carried out in these patients. Tentative affirmation of this possibility is based on its being in harmony with the general concept of sensitization of nociceptors and antidromic discharge and also the fact that, when tested for, the alternative dysfunction is not encountered, namely, vasoparalysis due to sympathetic vasoconstrictor denervation.

Another fascinating feature of some of these patients, and of the acute capsaicin model of hyperalgesia, is *cross-modality receptor threshold modulation* (7,17). In both the natural disease state and experimental model, passive cooling abolishes the hyperalgesia (Figs. 13.6 and 13.7). Although by definition heat hyperalgesia cannot be tested while the symptomatic part is passively cooled, mechanical hyperalgesia obviously can, and it may be shown to spectacularly disappear when the symptomatic skin is passively cooled. The interpretation of this concrete observation is that one stimulus, in this case low temperature, changes the threshold for pain induced by another stimulus energy, in this case mechanical energy. This is clearly not because the applied low temperature may have "anesthetized" cutaneous receptors (14), since at that time pinprick sensation remains viable. Further, the effect is not due to the possibility that low-temperature stimuli may activate cold specific A-delta afferents and that such input might "shut" central modulatory gates, because the phenomenon of cross-modality receptor threshold modulation definitely persists during A-fiber block (7,17). The modulatory effect of low temperature on mechanical hyperalgesia and spontaneous pain must therefore be resolved at the very level of the sensitized peripheral nociceptors that generate those painful symptoms.

If the primary molecular injury in ABC patients affects intramembrane heat transducers, then heat hyperalgesia is readily explained. The associated (polymodal) mechanical hyperalgesia (17) is also explained if the C-nociceptor functions under a principle of *cooperative membrane threshold*, whereby either thermal or mechanical (or chemical) adequate stimuli may depolarize the membrane to a level close to

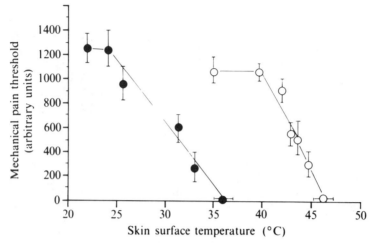

FIG. 13.7. Temperature dependence of capsaicin-induced mechanical hyperalgesia. A skin region on the palm was treated with 3.3×10^{-3} M capsaicin. Three hours following capsaicin application, a series of measurements were carried out at the indicated skin surface temperatures to determine the amount of vertical sustained pressure adequate to elicit burning pain (●). Similar measurements were carried out on untreated skin at a homologous site on the contralateral palm (○). Each point represents the mean of at least five measurements in a representative single experiment. Bars = range. (From ref. 7.)

threshold for discharge. In this state, a small quota of complementary mechanical energy would bring the polymodal membrane to threshold, thus firing afferent messages for mechanically evoked pain sensation at hyperalgesic standards. A detailed analysis of another alternative is given by Culp et al. (7). In the present communication it is again proposed that the beneficial influence of cooling on the symptom mechanical hyperalgesia, and, for that matter, also on the symptom spontaneous pain, is due to rectification, or unloading, by action of reduced temperature of leaky heat transducers in the excitable polymodal C-nociceptor membrane (17).

COLD HYPERALGESIAS IN PATIENTS

The same as neurologically based spontaneous pains, mechanical hyperalgesias (22), and perhaps heat hyperalgesias, cold hyperalgesia seems to be a plural matter in terms of underlying pathophysiology.

Central Versus Peripheral Dysfunction?

Clinical or animal experimental evidence is available to entertain the hypotheses that (a) cold hyperalgesia might be the expression of sensitization of C-nociceptors to low temperature and (b) at least in humans the phenomenon of cold hyperalgesia may be a consequence of central disinhibition of low–temperature-triggered nociceptor input, due to loss of the normal modulatory cold specific input, which is naturally coactivated by the low-temperature stimulus. In addition, on the basis of psychophysical reaction times it has been hypothesized that, in the context of peripheral

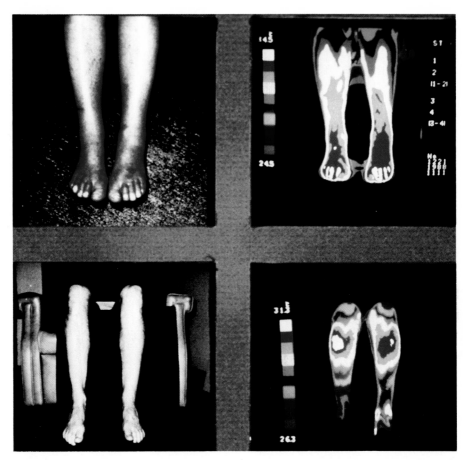

FIG. 13.8. Top: Red, swollen, painful feet of patient (age 72) with chronic small fiber neuropathy. On the right, electronic thermography displays pathological elevation of temperature in symptomatic areas, typical of ABC syndrome. **Bottom:** Lower extremities of 70-year-old patient with chronic painful small fiber neuropathy, expressing clinical characteristics of triple cold syndrome. Appropriately, the thermogram on the right shows abnormally low temperature in the symptomatic skin.

neurological disease or injury, cold hyperalgesia may result from true secondary central abnormalities (distinct from natural disinhibition due to lack of peripheral modulatory input) pertaining to the realm of neuronal hyperexcitability. This concept is based on the recording of reaction time values, which suggest that the primary input triggered by low temperature and leading to cold hyperalgesia is probably transmitted by cold specific rather than nociceptor channels. Therefore, this would be a form of secondary central cold hyperalgesia (11).

Cold hyperalgesia is a fairly common symptom in patients who, on the grounds of associated complaints of *chronic* spontaneous pains, hyperalgesias, and transient response to diagnostic "sympathetic" blocks, are given the variable diagnosis of "*causalgia–reflex sympathetic dystrophy–sympathetically maintained pain.*" To the extent that there are solid reasons to question the scientific basis for the concept that sympathetic neural transmission is a critical anomaly that determines the pains in these patients, the idea largely inbred among clinicians that cold hyperalgesia signals sympathetic pathogenesis for pains should be questioned. Furthermore, to the extent that such an idea carries an invasive therapeutic connotation, it should be rigorously revised. Under no circumstances should this symptom, which has been rated as "a sensitive but not specific sign of sympathetically maintained pain" (9), be regarded as a useful predictor to recommend therapeutic sympathectomy (23).

A Particular Subgroup of Patients with Cold Hyperalgesia and Cold Skin

There exists a fascinating syndrome, the reverse of the ABC syndrome, in which cold hyperalgesia is associated with cold skin (Fig. 13.8). There is also cold hypoesthesia. Afferent events related to function of primary cold specific thermoreceptors and C-nociceptors are postulated as crucial in determining the painful component in this syndrome. In the context of human painful polyneuropathy, expression of this cold syndrome is associated with a small-caliber fiber neuropathy with critical dropout of unmyelinated somatic and sympathetic fibers and cold specific A-delta myelinated fibers. In view of the fact that the full-blown syndrome includes cold hyperalgesia, cold hypoesthesia, and cold skin, the term "triple cold syndrome" was coined to define the condition of these patients (22).

These patients have paradoxically "burning" cold hyperalgesia, and they have loss of cold sensation. In addition, and significantly, A-fiber block does not abolish the cold hyperalgesia. Clearly, this paradoxical cold hyperalgesia is C-fiber mediated. These patients probably have what a normal volunteer has after provoking experimental blockade of A-fiber input, for example, by application of compression–ischemia or direct nerve compression for a suitable period of time. At the stage of A-fiber block, application of gentle mechanical stimuli fails to evoke a sensation of touch; application of pinprick fails to evoke a sharp pain, evoking instead a burn; application of low temperature fails to evoke a cold sensation and, at a certain threshold, evokes a paradoxical sensation of burning. It is important to emphasize that low temperature tends to evoke a sensation of "burning" and not a "cold pain," because normally, "cold pain" may be accepted to be a modulated blend of cold specific and C-nociceptor input (36). There is reasonable experimental evidence to support the concept that, normally, myelinated input (probably cold specific input, since patients may express the syndrome in absence of significant loss of tactile myelinated function) suppresses the burning component of the blend cold–pain

(34,36). Furthermore, the paradoxical burning sensation in response to low-temperature stimulation is felt at reduced thresholds; in other words, it becomes hyperalgesic because not only does the modulatory input alter the subjective quality of the pain sensation, but such specific input also inhibits the magnitude of C-mediated pain, at least when induced by low temperature (Fig. 13.9).

The cold skin of these patients serves as an abnormal and unwanted adequate stimulus for the probably disinhibited C-nociceptors. The mechanism behind the abnormally cold state of the symptomatic skin is proposed to relate to the degeneration of unmyelinated sympathetic vasoconstrictor nerve fibers, as part and parcel of the nerve injury or polyneuropathy and as proposed for the second stage of the rat model of painful nerve injury (2). Under those circumstances, the smooth muscle of arterioles would develop sympathetic denervation supersensitivity, leading to a degree of vasospasm and consequent cutaneous hypothermia (5). It will be asked: Why should individuals in whom sympathetic C fibers have dropped out continue to have afferent C–fiber-mediated painful input? A reasonable explanation for this apparent inconsistency lies in the observation that these patients obviously do not have total ablation of small-caliber fibers, but degrees of denervation supersensitivity might be critically sufficient to cause the hypothermic phenomenon. At the same time, the minimal requirement of spatial summation by nociceptor channels (20,37) continues to render surviving C-nociceptors able to evoke pain.

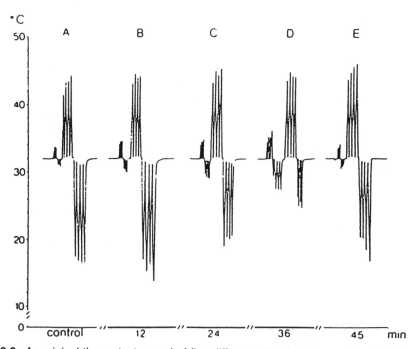

FIG. 13.9. An original thermotest record of five different trials from one subject. Trial A is the control situation, trials B, C, and D during nerve compression block, and trial E control of recovery from conduction block of myelinated fibers. (Note cold hyperalgesia in D.) Solid bar indicates the time course of compression block. (From ref. 34.)

THERMAL HYPERALGESIA AS EXPRESSION OF PSYCHOLOGICAL DYSFUNCTION

Like spontaneous pains and mechanical hyperalgesias, thermal hyperalgesia may recognize nonorganically based psychological genesis. Déjérine (8) stated:

Dans l'hystérie, il existe souvent des zones d'hyperesthésie superficielle ou profonde qui atteignent, soit les téguments sous forme de plaques plus ou moins étendues ou de points limités comme le vertex, soit des régions anatomiques comme les régions mammaire, cardiaque, rachidienne, soit des organes, l'ovaire, le testicule. Ces points d'hyperesthésie apparaissent spontanément, mais, très souvent aussi, ils sont le résultat d'une suggestion inconsciente de l'observateur qui les recherche. La pression au niveau de ces régions détermine parfois des crises convulsives et c'est pour cette raison qu'on les appelle zones hystérogènes. On rencontre chez les hystériques un trouble encore plus singulier que Pitres a nommé *l'aphalgésie.* Des sensations ordinairement indifférentes, comme celles qui résultent du contact de corps neutres, produisent chez ces sujets des impressions douloureuses très pénibles; mais ici on est en présence de faits suggérés inconsciemment et, pour ma part, il ne m'a pas encore été donné de les observer. Du reste, les troubles de la sensibilité des hystériques défient toute description complète et précise; ils peuvent varier à l'infini sous l'influence de la suggestion et on ne s'est pas toujours assez méfié de l'influence de cette dernière, dans l'étude des troubles de la sensibilité chez ces malades. *Généralement l'hyperesthésie est totale, c'est-à-dire qu'elle atteint tous les modes de la sensibilité;* elle peut cependant être inégale chez un même malade pour des excitations de même nature mais d'intensités différentes.

It is relatively common for patients expressing chronic combinations of negative and positive sensory symptoms, with or without associated negative and positive motor phenomena, and in the absence of evidence of organic impairment of nerve impulse generation or propagation functions, to complain of cold (or heat) hyperalgesia. It is remarkable that a huge proportion of these patients are placebo responders during diagnostic test blocks (32). In these patients, skilled clinical and laboratory neurological investigation may raise explicit evidence that the sensory or the sensorimotor complaints are, by their nature, nonorganic, psychogenic in origin (J. Ochoa, *unpublished observations*).

Because psychologically based and organically based dysfunction leading to neuromuscular symptoms coexist fairly commonly, a diagnostic statement on the psychological basis for the syndrome cannot be made solely based on the presence of psychiatric dysfunction. Neither can absence of clinically recognized psychological dysfunction be construed by default in support of organic basis for the sensorimotor phenomena. Moreover, since most psychiatrists are not qualified to test for explicit neurological signs to document that the syndrome is nonorganic in origin, these specialists cannot effectively assist in clarifying the difficult and highly specialized question of whether neuromuscular complaints are organically or psychologically based.

REFERENCES

1. Asbury, A. K., Porte, D., Genuth, S. M., et al. (1988): Report and recommendations of the San Antonio conference on diabetic neuropathy. *Diabetes Care,* 11:592–597.
2. Bennett, G. J., and Ochoa, J. L. (1991): Thermographic observations on rats with experimental neuropathic pain. *Pain,* 45:61–67.
3. Bessou, P., and Perl, E. R. (1969): Response of cutaneous sensory units with unmyelinated fibers to noxious stimuli. *J. Neurophysiol.,* 32:1025–1043.

4. Bonica, J. J. (1990): *The management of pain*, vol. I. Lea & Febiger, Philadelphia.
5. Cannon, W. B., and Rosenblueth, A. (1949): *The supersensitivity of denervated structures: a law of denervation*. Macmillan, New York.
6. Cline, M. A., Ochoa, J. L., and Torebjörk, H. E. (1989): Chronic hyperalgesia and skin warming caused by sensitized C nociceptors. *Brain*, 112:621–647.
7. Culp, W. J., Ochoa, J. L., Cline, M., and Dotson, R. (1989): Heat and mechanical hyperalgesia induced by capsaicin: cross modality threshold modulation in human C nociceptors. *Brain*, 112:1317–1331.
8. Déjérine, P. J. (1901): Sémiologie du système nerveux. In: *Traité de pathologie générale*, pp. 559–1168, Masson, Paris.
9. Frost, S. A., Raja, S. N., Campbell, J. N., Meyer, R. A., and Kahn, A. (1988): Does hyperalgesia to cooling stimuli characterize patients with sympathetically maintained pain (reflex sympathetic dystrophy)? In: *Proceedings of the Vth World Congress on Pain: pain research and clinical management*, vol. 3, edited by R. Dubner, G. F. Gebhart, and M. R. Bond, pp. 151–156. Elsevier, Amsterdam.
10. Fruhstorfer, H., Lindblom, U., and Schmidt, W. G. (1976): Method for quantitative estimation of thermal thresholds in patients. *J. Neurol. Neurosurg. Psychiatry*, 39:1071–1075.
11. Fruhstorfer, H., and Lindblom, U. (1984): Sensibility abnormalities in neuralgic patients studied by thermal and tactile pulse stimulation. In: *Wenner-Gren International Symposium Series. Somatosensory mechanisms*, vol. 41, edited by C. Von Euler, O. Franzén, U. Lindblom, and D. Ottoson, pp. 353–361. Macmillan, London.
12. Gowers, W. R. (1886): *A manual of diseases of the nervous system, vol. I, disease of the spinal cord and nerves*. J. & A. Churchill, London.
13. Head, H. (1893): On disturbances of sensation with especial reference to the pain of visceral disease. *Brain*, 16:1–132.
14. Kunesch, E., Schmidt, R., Nordin, M., Wallin, U., Hagbarth, K.-E. (1987): Peripheral neural correlates of cutaneous anaesthesia induced by skin cooling in man. *Acta Physiol. Scand.*, 129:247–257.
15. Lindblom, U., and Ochoa, J. L. (1986): Somatosensory function and dysfunction. In: *Disease of the nervous system*, vol. I, edited by A. K. Asbury, G. M. McKhann, and W. I. McDonald, pp. 283–298. Ardmore, Philadelphia.
16. Nordin, M. (1990): Low-threshold mechanoreceptive and nociceptive units with unmyelinated (C) fibres in the human supraorbital nerve. *J. Physiol. (Lond.)*, 426:229–240.
17. Ochoa, J. L. (1986): The newly recognized painful ABC syndrome: thermographic aspects. *Thermology*, 2:65–107.
18. Ochoa, J. L. (1987): Mechanisms of symptoms in neuropathy. *The London Symposia*, EEG suppl. 39:121–127.
19. Ochoa, J. L. (1991): Scientific clinical evaluation of chronic neuropathic painful syndromes. American Academy of Neurology Annual Meeting, "Pain" course no. 421, pp. 15–31.
20. Ochoa, J. L., and Torebjörk, H. E. (1989): Sensations evoked by intraneural microstimulation of C nociceptor fibres in human skin nerves. *J. Physiol. (Lond.)*, 415:583–599.
21. Ochoa, J. L., Roberts, W. J., Cline, M. A., Dotson, R., and Yarnitsky, D. (1989): Two mechanical hyperalgesias in human neuropathy. *Soc. Neurosci. Abstr.*, 15:472.
22. Ochoa, J. L., and Yarnitsky, D. (1990): Triple cold ("CCC") painful syndrome. *Pain*, suppl. 5:S278.
23. Ochoa, J. L., Marchettini, P., and Cline, M. (1991): Lessons from human research on the pathophysiology of neuropathic pains in limbs. In: *Management of pain in the hand and wrist*, edited by C. B. Wynn-Parry. Churchill Livingstone, London, Edinburgh.
24. Reeh, P. (1986): Sensory receptors in mammalian skin in an in vitro preparation. *Neurosci. Lett.*, 66:141–146.
25. Szolcsanyi, J. (1977): A pharmacological approach to elucidation of the role of different nerve fibers and receptor endings in mediation of pain. *J. Physiol. (Paris)*, 73:251–259.
26. Torebjörk, H. E. (1974): Afferent C units responding to mechanical, thermal and chemical stimuli in human non-glabrous skin. *Acta Physiol. Scand.*, 92:374–390.
27. Torebjörk, H. E., and Hallin, R. G. (1970): C-fibre units recorded from human sensory nerve fascicles in situ. *Acta Societatis Medicorum Upsaliensis*, 75:81–84.
28. Torebjörk, H. E., and Ochoa, J. L. (1980): Specific sensations evoked by activity in single identified sensory units in man. *Acta Physiol. Scand.*, 110:445–447.
29. Torebjörk, H. E., Vallbo, A. B., and Ochoa, J. L. (1987): Intraneural microstimulation in man: its relation to specificity of tactile sensations. *Brain*, 110:1509–1529.
30. Torebjörk, H. E., and Ochoa, J. L. (1990): New method to identify nociceptor units innervating glabrous skin of the human hand. *Exp. Brain Res.*, 81:509–514.
31. Torebjörk, H. E., and Ochoa, J. L. Receptor characteristics and sensory attributes of nociceptors with myelinated (A) fibres innervating the glabrous skin of the human hand *(submitted)*.

32. Verdugo, R., and Ochoa, J. (1991): High incidence of placebo responders among chronic neuropathic pain patients. *Ann. Neurol.*, 30:229.
33. Verdugo, R., and Ochoa, J. L. Quantitative somatosensory thermotest. A key method for functional evaluation of small caliber afferent channels. *Brain (in press)*.
34. Wahrén, L. K., Torebjörk, H. E., and Jørum, E. (1989): Central suppression of cold-induced C fibre pain by myelinated fibre input. *Pain*, 38:313–319.
35. Yarnitsky, D., and Ochoa, J. L. (1990): Studies of heat pain sensation in man: perception thresholds, rate of stimulus rise and reaction time. *Pain*, 40:85–91.
36. Yarnitsky, D., and Ochoa, J. L. (1990): Release of cold-induced burning pain by block of cold specific afferent input. *Brain*, 113:893–902.
37. Yarnitsky, D., and Ochoa, J. L. (1991): Differential effect of compression–ischaemia block on warm sensation and heat-induced pain. *Brain*, 114:907–913.
38. Zotterman, Y. (1933): Studies in the peripheral nervous mechanism of pain. *Acta Med. Scand.*, 80:185–242.
39. Zotterman, Y. (1936): Specific action potentials in the lingual nerve of cat. *Scand. Arch. Physiol.*, 75:105.

Hyperalgesia and Allodynia,
edited by W. D. Willis, Jr.
Raven Press, Ltd., New York © 1992.

14

Nociceptors and Primary Hyperalgesia

Discussion

John C. Liebeskind, Moderator

Dr. Casey: This question relates to the role of cholinergic sympathetic fibers that are known to form a significant percentage of the sympathetic efferent fibers going to the skin. I wonder, in view of the fact that there appears to be a dissociation between the vasoactive effects of the sympathetic activity and the presence or absence of sympathetically maintained pain, if this explains the difference between the vasoactive effects you see in the cold limb versus the warm limb and the presence or absence of pain. In other words, do the cholinergic sympathetics play any role in this?

Dr. Campbell: I can say something about that. I think it's good for us to remain aware that there are perhaps different types of sympathetically maintained pain. Sympathetic terminals also release other things, like substance Y, and it may be that there is a syndrome related to that, and a syndrome related to cholinergic mechanisms, and a syndrome related to norepinephrine release. The tendency for us has always been to think of the efferent limb as being the culprit. I think the evidence emerging from Dr. Perl's work and perhaps from the things that we and other people are doing is that the culprit is on the receptor side. The fact is that development of a cold limb is a very common problem in neuropathic pain. Of course, we see the opposite occur, as Dr. Ochoa emphasized in terms of developing a hot limb in certain pathologic states, but with nerve injury problems, developing a cold limb is, in fact, seen very commonly. What we have to fight is the tendency to equate that with a sympathetically maintained pain state. The fact is that when nociceptors discharge, there is a tendency for that to cause vasoconstriction (if you will, a sympathotone), and so the mere presence of decreased temperature doesn't mean that there's an abnormal interaction between the sympathetic fibers and nociceptive fibers.

Dr. Handwerker: My question is similar to that of Dr. Casey. You need to take into account that you very often have edema in the skin in SMP. The other variable is the effect of temperature.

Dr. Perl: Well, it depends on whose hypothesis. The observations that I reported really show something that's a bit unusual. The neurons that change their characteristics were essentially normally behaving neurons—they had not degenerated, so they were normal, residual neurons. What I was postulating was that, in fact, this was secondary to a loss of sympathetic innervation of the region. There is some evidence in favor of that. Drummond has just completed a study in Australia that has measured sympathetic outflow on the two sides of persons with causalgia or no causalgia (sympathetically maintained pain or no sympathetically maintained pain), and what he found fit the observations of Wallin and Torebjörk and Hallin some years ago. On the side that was abnormal, that had the sympathetically maintained pain, whether or not it was adequately treated, there was less sympathetic activity than on the normal side, suggesting less mediator was being liberated, so this was not a case of overactivity of the sympathetics. So this would, in part, deal also with Dr. Casey's question. There may be other mediators, as Dr. Campbell has said, causing several different kinds of sympathetically maintained pain, but the interesting thing is that there is evidence now that sympathetic activity is decreased. This might fit with the edema question, and there is increased reactivity, which would fit with the upregulation idea.

Question: I'd like to ask Dr. Torebjörk and Dr. Perl if you had looked thermographically at the hand in the capsaicin experiments, and the entire ear in Dr. Perl's experiments as well as the ear on the other side. Dr. Ochoa and I did an experiment on his daughter by putting in a nerve stimulator, and the most remarkable thing that occurred was that when he made it painful and then stopped, the hand we worked on got totally hot, and not just in the ulnar nerve territory. But the more amazing thing was that the normal hand shut down, almost 4° and was still cold the next day, although it wasn't painful.

Dr. Torebjörk: Well, to the extent that you ask me whether I have used thermography, the answer is no, I haven't. But obviously, if you apply capsaicin topically to the skin, you get reddening, as shown, for instance, by Dr. Ochoa.

Dr. Perl: To the extent that the question referred to the rabbit ear, we did not do thermography. We did sample the drop in temperature at several different places on the ear, and we always sampled it in all of the experiments in the receptive field of the unit that we were studying. So we knew that there were changes going on in terms of vasoconstriction at that particular locus.

Dr. Perl: I have a question for Dr. Torebjörk. I wanted to get clear exactly what happened in that block experiment where you were inducing secondary hyperalgesia with capsaicin. As I understood it, and I want you to correct me if this is wrong, block of the small-diameter fibers prevented the occurrence of the secondary hyperalgesia, but once it had taken place, block of the small fibers did not. Leaving the large fibers intact caused the large fiber activity to initiate that secondary hyperalgesia. I just wanted that clarified.

Dr. Torebjörk: In order for secondary hyperalgesia to develop, I think a massive input in C fibers is necessary, and that evokes rather intense pain. Whether it is the input in C polymodal nociceptors that is critical, or perhaps in other types of chemosensitive nociceptors, is not known. Dr. LaMotte favors the idea of activation of specific C chemonociceptors as critical for inducing these central changes. The central changes are contingent upon input from C fibers of some sort, but the phenomenon of secondary hyperalgesia to touch can only be detected clinically and perceived if you have intact conduction in myelinated fibers.

Dr. Besson: Is there any morphological evidence of alpha-adrenergic receptors on primary afferent fibers?

Dr. Perl: I don't think there's any solid evidence one way or the other that's been published.

Dr. Campbell: No, but the experiments can be done, and I think it will be valuable to apply an injury and look for upregulation of alpha-1 and alpha-2 receptors to see if there is a neurally mediated production of the cDNA for either of those receptors.

Dr. Lebedev: I want to ask Dr. Perl a question. Tell me, if you produce a model of causalgia by partial lesion of a peripheral nerve, or by stretching the nerve, then in 11 to 20 days, is the most expressed effect of the lesion a degeneration of C fibers? My question is: is there degeneration of C fibers or are these normal C fibers?

Dr. Perl: I'm sorry if I didn't make that clear. They were essentially normal. I can't say they are normal; I can say that they had not had time to degenerate and regenerate because that takes, given the place of the lesion, at least 30 days, based upon our past evidence, and their behavior in terms of threshold, responsiveness, and sensitization in the absence of sympathetic stimulation made them look exactly like the normal population. I cannot tell you anything about the receptive field changes because we did not study that, and it would have been very difficult, since receptive fields of the rabbit C-fiber nociceptors are very small.

Dr. Guilbaud: A question for Dr. Perl. At 10 to 20 days after a nerve lesion, I see exactly the same thing. We have maximal degeneration of the afferent fibers also at the same time. It is difficult to assess if all of the sensitization that we are seeing is only due to supersensitivity of the sympathetic system since the sensitization is not seen for all types of stimuli. It is seen for cold and heat, but not mechanical stimuli, at least in the model we are studying, which in some aspects is comparable to causalgia.

Dr. Perl: We know how long it takes for the fibers to regenerate; the fibers had normal qualities, and regenerating fibers don't show up in less than 30 days. The distance for degeneration and regeneration is an important factor in the time for regeneration. Given the time we had and the distance, it is very unlikely that any of the fibers had regenerated. Now, I'm absolutely sure that it requires the combination of afferent fiber injury plus probably sympathetic nerve injury. Both the afferent and the sympathetic supply to the ear are partially through that same nerve that we were injuring, and that is probably the case in almost all instances of sympathetically maintained pain. There is a real probability that sympathetic fibers are involved in the tissues, in the distribution of the nerves injured.

Dr. Campbell: I want to make just one comment about that. In patients it's not at all clear that a nerve injury is prerequisite to development of sympathetically maintained pain. In fact, in a good many patients, the development of this syndrome is after, for example, hairline fracture of a navicular bone in the wrist or an ankle sprain, and it's impossible to detect in many of these patients any signs of nerve injury. One can make sensory measurements after the pain is completely relieved with a surgical sympathectomy, for example, and find no alterations of cutaneous sensibility with normalization of the pain sensibility from this sympathectomy. So I think, along the lines of what Dr. Levine has postulated with his chloroform injury that what may be the signal for upregulation and production of alpha-1 or alpha-2 receptors may be neural activity itself. What may happen in the patients is that this neural activity-modulated upregulation gets out of whack.

Dr. Torebjörk: I wonder about the production of allodynia in SMP patients, because you said usually they don't have hyperalgesia or allodynia to heat. How well have you tested for it? The reason I'm questioning you is that in our hands with rather carefully conducted thermal test data, we have seen allodynia to heat in these patients, which is consistent and which persists in follow-up studies over 10 years. This is, I think, a feature in this condition.

Dr. Campbell: Well, we haven't done the careful testing that you have done and your observations actually fit with those of Dr. Price, with whom I was talking about this earlier. What I said, though, was not how usual it is to have heat hyperalgesia; what I said was that there are many patients who have sympathetically maintained pain in whom we can't demonstrate heat hyperalgesia. I think you probably agree with that and I think Dr. Price agrees with that, and that's been our observation also.

Dr. Ochoa: I am a clinician and I'm a scientist, and I should say that I believe absolutely everything that has to do with experimental animal studies on mechanisms of afferent dysfunction and relationships between the sympathetic activity and afferent function. But having spent many years looking very critically at the concept that the sympathetic system is instrumentally involved in determining pains in chronic painful syndromes in humans following injury, we have become very wary about this for a number of reasons. If one looks at the history of the idea that the sympathetic system is involved in pain, one is appalled by its simplicity. Initially it was simply that the limb looked different in terms of color or temperature, and somehow the idea of a vasomotor dysfunction developed. It is true, of course, that most of the time the pale limb, the red limb, the hot limb, or the cold limb has a vasomotor disturbance. But concluding that the sympathetic system is abnormal and is involved in the pain is a big jump. Now somehow that idea became reinforced by the clinical studies whereby patients given diagnostic blocks responded "yes, doctor, your injection took my pain away." If one looks at that criterion and if one takes into account that having studied 100 consecutive patients with chronic neuropathic pain that fit the diagnosis of causalgia RSD, one finds, and I mentioned this in my talk, that amazingly twice as many as expected are placebo responders. Now, if one looks at what the classic studies using sympathetic blocks did in terms of placebo response, well, one is shocked by finding that they have not been placebo controlled. I asked a colleague in the Academy of Neurology a few weeks ago how many of his 800 patients treated with anywhere between 20 and 60 blocks followed by sympathectomy had placebo control, and he acknowledged that none did. Another colleague in Australia said that none of his several hundred patients had a placebo control. Yet another colleague in London a few weeks ago said that none of his 300-odd patients have ever been placebo controlled. In a new series presented from the Mayo Clinic a few weeks ago in the Academy of Neurology, none of the 407 patients were placebo controlled. Now you put those things together and you start wondering. The last time we did a sympathectomy was in a young man who absolutely had causalgia or RSD. The sympathectomy was done after five successful sympathetic blocks that transiently took the pain away, the thoracic sympathectomy took the pain away completely, pain and hyperalgesia, and the limb warmed up and after 2 months he came back with exactly the same symptoms. He was given a local anesthetic block in the T2 root, hoping that perhaps there may have been some sympathetic fibers left, and lo and behold he was cured of pain for 2 weeks, and then he came back. He wanted another block, and I gave him an injection of saline and he was cured completely for 2 weeks, and he came back again and again until I reported that to the insurance company, and they didn't know what to do with the patient, so they sent him back to have more sympathetic blocks, and he's currently having sympathetic blocks and being cured for 2 weeks after each of the $600 sympathetic blocks. We started doing phentolamine blocks about a year ago, and we followed the prescription by Dr. Raja. We have done 47. We were going to do 50, but we got curious and we broke the code. We find that if the placebo stage is extended to half an hour from the first injection of saline rather than half an hour from the moment the patient starts having tests for baseline, then either patients don't respond to anything or they respond to saline, and when you add the phentolamine half an hour later nothing changes. So, I think that, although it makes tremendous sense and is very attractive to put together an *ad hoc* overall theory which is based on early clinical observations, which is apparently endorsed by brilliant and real experimental animal results and which is heavily endorsed by the results of blocks not placebo controlled, we must face the possibility that perhaps we're getting it wrong, and that's something that we simply must, as people who treat patients, consider and I may well be wrong, but if I am right, then we're hurting patients and for that reason I have a duty to raise this question.

Dr. Liebeskind: Dr. Ochoa, may I take the chairman's prerogative and ask how you would relate your comments to those made earlier today by Dr. Bonica that there's a timing factor in relation to the efficacy of sympathectomy and sympathetic blocks and that if you catch the problem early on, then blocks can be efficacious, but if you wait too long they are not? Do you have any experience that relates to that point?

Dr. Ochoa: I have no doubt that Dr. Bonica must have cured many early patients with RSD by injections or by recommending sympathectomy. But what we're talking about here is those who come with chronic pain and nevertheless do respond to sympathetic blocks; those patients are not cured by sympathectomy. I haven't seen a single person cured by sympathectomy, and Dr. Richard Payne, who has a tremendous amount of experience on the subject, volunteered a few weeks ago in his session on pain in the American Academy of Neurology that after 5 years, having recommended many sympathectomies, he has to admit he has seen one single patient improved after sympathectomy. So those of you who get these magnificent results following sympathectomy are lucky. Your patients are lucky.

Dr. Liebeskind: Dr. Perl, I think we'll go to you for the last question.

Dr. Perl: At one time in my life I did see patients and I have to agree with what Dr. Ochoa just said. I have yet to see a case of so-called causalgia, reflex sympathetic dystrophy, that was chronic, at least 6 to 8 months, that was cured permanently by sympathectomy. What I really wanted to raise a question about was Dr. Campbell's argument that there had to be some special kind of process going on that would dissociate mechanical and thermal hyperalgesia. The reason for raising this question is that there are at least four or five very sound experimental studies in primate and carnivore clearly indicating that there is a pathway for mechanical nociceptors that is independent of a pathway that has input from heat nociceptors or from a more generic type, as well as the ubiquitous multireceptive type of neuron. So that I'm not surprised that there's a dissociation between hyperalgesia of mechanical and heat origin. I think there's good indication there could be theoretically. Not every nociceptor goes through the same central projection pathway. There's clear evidence that there are multiple pathways and that some of them are relatively more selective than others.

Dr. Campbell: I think any one experiment by itself has pitfalls and you've identified one pitfall. But I think when taken with other evidence such as the work of Eric Torebjörk, the fact that you have a combination of thermal hypalgesia with mechanical hyperalgesia, and the fact that you can't with a burn injury demonstrate mechanical sensitization of nociceptors regardless of what you do, I think when you take all of those things into account that there is a quite compelling case for a new channel opening that allows the neurons centrally related to pain sensation to be activated.

Dr. Perl: I don't disagree with that at all. That was not the question. It was just a question of the dissociation between mechanical and thermal hyperalgesia because I do think there's evidence suggesting that that could easily happen given the connections that exist.

Dr. Campbell: I think that is a worthwhile point.

Hyperalgesia and Allodynia,
edited by W. D. Willis, Jr.
Raven Press, Ltd., New York © 1992.

15

Role of Central Changes in Secondary Hyperalgesia

Overview

Howard L. Fields

*Department of Neurology, University of California Medical School,
San Francisco, California 94143*

Sensitization of the peripheral terminals of nociceptive primary afferents is a well-established phenomenon that certainly contributes to the prolonged tenderness associated with tissue damage. The chapters in this section clearly establish that input from nociceptive primary afferents enhances the responses of CNS neurons beyond what can be attributed to sensitization of primary afferents.

LaMotte, in important human psychophysical studies, shows that capsaicin, which activates only small-diameter afferents, produces a secondary hyperalgesia that is spatially distant from the region of sensitized primary afferents. Human subjects report an enhanced subjective response to proximal stimulation of the trunk of the nerve that supplies the region of secondary hyperalgesia, demonstrating that this process is primarily, if not exclusively, central. Parallel studies in primates confirm this conclusion. These studies set the stage for the other chapters in this section that address the mechanisms of the central changes induced by intense peripheral stimuli.

Although there are many gaps and contradictions in the available data, there are enough consistencies to suggest a preliminary outline of the central changes. Interestingly, although the human data have so far revealed only a limited, strictly unilateral, spatial spread of hyperalgesia, several of the investigations reported in this section demonstrate an enhanced efficacy of contralateral inputs to spinal neurons. The data of Guilbaud et al., in fact, show what amounts to a generalized enhancement of CNS responses to noxious stimuli from anywhere on the body. The evidence for this "arousal" state has to be reconciled with Schaible's observations of an enhanced tonic descending inhibition. It is important that these widespread central changes are produced by a variety of acute and chronic pain models, including mono- and polyarthritis and neuropathic pain models.

Woolf and Schaible have begun to address the cellular mechanisms underlying the spinal facilitation produced by noxious input. The neuropeptide substance P, which is only present in small-diameter primary afferents, is released in relatively large amounts by input from an inflamed joint. This peptide produces prolonged depolarization of spinal neurons and enhances their responses to other excitatory neurotransmitters. There is also consistent and convincing evidence that excitatory amino acids, which are present in small-diameter primary afferents, act through *N*-methyl-D-aspartate (NMDA) receptors to mediate long-lasting depolarization of spinal neurons. This depolarization of dorsal horn neurons would obviously enhance their response to subsequent stimuli (noxious or innocuous). As Woolf shows, depolarization would also permit activation of the neuron by inputs constituting a subliminal fringe (e.g., contralateral inputs). It is important that simple depolarization of the spinal neuron by current passed through the recording electrode does not produce the long-lasting changes produced by "natural" stimulation. This suggests that there is something unique about the input pathway activated by nociceptive afferents. One possibility could be selective activation of NMDA receptors by nociceptive afferents. This would allow the entry of Ca^{2+} into the activated neurons and could serve as a trigger to long-lasting intracellular metabolic changes.

The studies reported in this section represent important pioneering work. However, there are still critical pieces of the puzzle that are missing. Perhaps the most glaring problem is our uncertainty about the precise spinal circuitry that links primary afferents with nociceptive transmission neurons that project to supraspinal sites. Although there is no question that primary afferents directly contact projection neurons, especially in lamina I, these contacts represent only a tiny fraction of the total dorsal horn input to these projection cells. There are huge numbers of interneurons activated by primary afferents. Some of these interneurons are excitatory and some are inhibitory; many contain neuropeptides such as dynorphin and substance P, which have been implicated in hyperalgesic mechanisms. It seems likely that connections between spinal neurons play a major and as yet unexplored role in the enhancement of activity produced by nociceptive input. Similar arguments apply to the role of descending inputs from brain stem, diencephalic, and cortical regions.

Despite the complexities of the CNS, it is obvious that significant progress has been made in understanding the prolonged changes induced by nociceptor input. The studies reported in this section represent a very important and fertile new area of pain research.

Hyperalgesia and Allodynia,
edited by W. D. Willis, Jr.
Raven Press, Ltd., New York © 1992.

16

Neurophysiological Mechanisms of Cutaneous Secondary Hyperalgesia in the Primate

Robert H. LaMotte

Department of Anesthesiology and Section of Neurobiology, Yale University School of Medicine, New Haven, Connecticut 06510

The cutaneous hyperalgesia that can develop in a wide area of normal skin surrounding a local injury is called secondary (2°) hyperalgesia as opposed to the primary hyperalgesia within the region of injury (2). The first detailed and systematic studies of experimentally produced 2° hyperalgesia in humans were carried out by Lewis (6). Lewis concluded that the hyperalgesia spread away from a site of injury by means of a peripheral axon reflex: To paraphrase his ideas with our own terminology, nerve impulses travel not only orthodromically along a parent axon supplying the injured skin but also antidromically along branches to remote areas of skin thereby triggering the release of a chemical substance that increases the responsiveness ("sensitizes") other cutaneous receptors (e.g., nociceptors), thereby causing the remote hyperalgesia.

Many of Lewis's experiments were repeated by Hardy et al. (2) who concluded that the neurons responsible for the spread of hyperalgesia away from the site of injury and the neurons that became sensitized were located in the spinal cord and were not peripheral nerve fibers as hypothesized by Lewis.

In order to study the peripheral and central mechanisms of 2° hyperalgesia, a parallel series of sensory psychophysical and neurophysiological experiments were performed. The hyperalgesia was produced by an intracutaneous injection of capsaicin, a potent algesic ingredient in hot chili peppers. This "chemical injury" was deemed more useful than the physical injuries produced by Lewis and by Hardy's group because (a) its magnitude could be easily graded by the concentration injected (7), (b) it produced no scarring or other long-lasting visible effects, and (c) its ability to induce sensory changes, e.g., hyperalgesia, appeared to be transient (about an hour) relative to that of a physical injury (4).

Sensory measurements of pain and hyperalgesia in humans were made under a variety of experimental conditions in order to repeat many of the experiments of Lewis and of Hardy et al. that were designed to uncover candidate neural mechanisms of cutaneous 2° hyperalgesia (4). Then, in order to investigate the roles of different types of cutaneous receptors, the sensory measurements were correlated with electrophysiological recordings from single peripheral nerve fibers in both the anesthetized monkey and awake humans using the same experimental stimuli (1,5). Finally, in order to identify central neurons contributing to 2° hyperalgesia, a correlative study was undertaken of evoked responses in spinothalamic neurons in the spinal cord of the anesthetized monkey (8). In each set of experiments, the same experimental stimuli were used. Only a brief summary of the methods and results of these experiments is presented in the following. Complete details are available in the cited publications.

PSYCHOPHYSICAL MEASUREMENTS OF THE PAIN AND SECONDARY HYPERALGESIA FROM CAPSAICIN INJECTION

A dose of 100 μg of capsaicin in 10 μl of a tween-saline vehicle was injected intracutaneously into the hairy skin, typically the volar forearm. Immediately upon injection, an intense burning pain was accompanied by the presence of hyperalgesia (lower than normal pain thresholds and enhanced pain to normally painful cutaneous stimuli) in surrounding skin (Fig. 16.1). The pain reached a maximum within about 15 sec after injection and then decreased until finally disappearing in 10 to 30 min. The bleb produced by the injection was analgesic to pinprick. A careful mapping of the skin with heat and mechanical stimuli revealed three areas of hyperalgesia surrounding the bleb: a small area of hyperalgesia to heat stimuli, a larger area of tenderness (allodynia) to stroking the skin with a cotton swab, and a still larger area of hyperalgesia to punctate stimulation with a nylon filament (von Frey type). Based on indirect evidence that the capsaicin remained within the bleb (1), most or all of the hyperalgesia was believed to be of the secondary type and very little if any to be primary hyperalgesia, defined as that existing within the area of injury. The areas of hyperalgesia to heat and stroking gradually decreased and disappeared after 1 to 3 hr. In contrast, the area of hyperalgesia to punctate stimuli shrank more gradually and was gone after 13 to 24 hr.

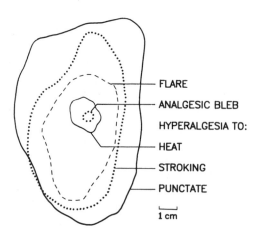

FLARE

ANALGESIC BLEB

HYPERALGESIA TO:

HEAT

STROKING

PUNCTATE

1 cm

FIG. 16.1. Areas of analgesia and hyperalgesia and the flare produced by an intradermal injection of 100 μg of capsaicin in the middle volar forearm of a human subject. The bleb produced by the injection was analgesic. (From ref. 4.)

PSYCHOPHYSICAL STUDIES OF THE NEURAL MECHANISMS RESPONSIBLE FOR SECONDARY HYPERALGESIA

Since the area of hyperalgesia to heat was small, most of the following experiments applied only to the 2° hyperalgesia to mechanical stimuli (henceforth "2HM"). However, some of the conclusions may be applicable to the heat hyperalgesia as well.

The results of experiments carried out in both male and female human volunteers (4) supported two main hypotheses: (a) 2HM depends on the presence of neural activity that originates at the site of injury and spreads radially away within a special class of chemosensitive intracutaneous nerve fibers and (b) the sensory neurons whose response properties are altered as a result of the activity in these peripheral nerve fibers are in the CNS.

There are five experimental results on which the statements in the first hypothesis are based. (i) The 2HM remote to the capsaicin injection site depends on neural activity originating at that site because no hyperalgesia developed around skin that was first infiltrated with local anesthetic and then injected with capsaicin. (ii) 2HM does not depend on the transport of capsaicin through blood or lymph vessels: 2HM spreads across a tight elastic band that blocked venous return and lymph flow and was not prevented from occurring by a circulatory block produced by a pressure cuff. (iii) 2HM spreads away from the injury via neural activity within intracutaneous nerve fibers: 2HM did not cross a narrow mediolateral strip of locally anesthetized skin (Fig. 16.2) or, if it did (which, we suggest, may have occurred when the block was not completely effective), its magnitude on the crossed side of the barrier was reduced. (iv) It is speculated that these intracutaneous nerve fibers are "chemospecific" because it was found that an algesic chemical (10-µg dose of capsaicin) was more effective in producing 2HM than an equally painful but relatively noninjurious physical stimulus (heat). It is suggested that for heat or mechanical stimuli to produce as large an area of 2HM as the injection of 100 µg or capsaicin, these stimuli must cause the release of endogenous chemical stimuli (e.g., certain mediators of the inflammatory response to acute injury) that can then activate the chemospecific nerve fibers responsible for initiating the development of 2HM. (v) After 2HM develops, it continues to be maintained to some degree by neural activity originating

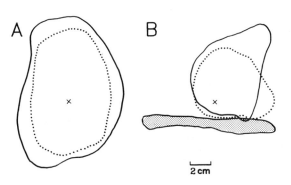

FIG. 16.2. Hyperalgesia was prevented from spreading away from the capsaicin injection site by a "barrier" of local anesthetic. **A:** Normal development of hyperalgesia to stroking (*dotted line*) and punctate stimulation of the skin (*solid line*). The "x" marks the site of injection. **B:** When a mediolateral strip of skin was anesthetized (*stippled area*) before capsaicin was injected on the distal side, the hyperalgesia failed to develop on the proximal side. (From ref. 4.)

2 cm

at the site of injury and transmitted away from that site via intracutaneous nerve fibers: (a) Anesthetizing the site of injury (e.g., cooling, to 1°C, a 1-cm diameter area of skin centered on the capsaicin injection site) reduced the area of 2HM to stroking the skin after which warming brought it back and (b) anesthetizing a mediolateral strip of skin reduced the area of 2HM to stroking on the side opposite the capsaicin injection site.

The results of another series of experiments on 2HM in humans supported the second major hypothesis: that the neurons that become "sensitized" to mechanical and heat stimulation of the skin surrounding a local cutaneous injury are located in the central and not the peripheral nervous system. A nerve block was produced by infiltrating a peripheral nerve (lateral antebrachial or superficial radial) with a local anesthetic. Capsaicin was then injected into the anesthetic skin distal to the nerve block. After complete recovery from the anesthesia 2 to 3 hr later, there was no hyperalgesia nor did any hyperalgesia subsequently develop. In cases in which the anesthesia lasted only a short time (e.g., 0.5–1.5 hr), the hyperalgesia to heat or mechanical stimuli was absent or significantly reduced in area (Fig. 16.3) in comparison to that produced by a control injection of capsaicin, on the other arm, that had

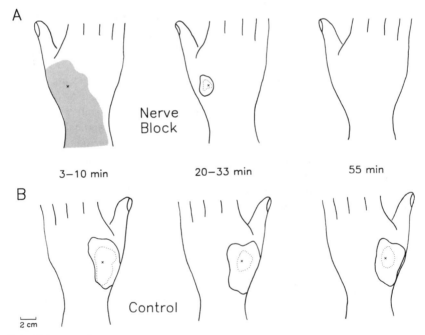

FIG. 16.3. The area of hyperalgesia was small and transient after recovery from a short-lasting proximal anesthetic block of nerve conduction given just before injection of capsaicin. **A:** Capsaicin was injected (x) into an area of anesthetized skin (*shaded region*) after a proximal block of the superficial radial nerve. After recovery from the anesthetic, the areas of 2HM and hyperalgesia to heat (not shown) were smaller and shorter lasting than normal. There was no hyperalgesia after anesthetic blocks that lasted 1 to 2 hr. **B:** Normal areas of hyperalgesia to stroking and punctate stimuli (*dotted* and *solid lines*, respectively) surrounded the injection of capsaicin on the control hand. At 55 min, 2HM and hyperalgesia to heat (not shown) were still present on the control hand but not on the hand that had received the nerve block. (From ref. 4.)

been given without prior anesthesia. The nerve block would not have interfered with the sensitization of peripheral nerve terminals, had sensitization occurred, and the hyperalgesia would be fully developed upon recovery from the anesthetic. But since hyperalgesia did not fully develop or, in the case of sufficiently long-acting anesthetics, was totally absent, the sensitization must have occurred in the CNS. Thus, the nerve block acted to "protect" central neurons from receiving the sensitizing effects of evoked responses in capsaicin-activated primary afferent peripheral nerve fibers.

NEUROPHYSIOLOGICAL STUDIES OF PERIPHERAL NEURONS THAT CONTRIBUTE TO CAPSAICIN-EVOKED PAIN AND SECONDARY HYPERALGESIA

Responses to the same heat and mechanical stimuli used in the psychophysical experiments were recorded in both low- and high-threshold primary afferent nerve fibers in the anesthetized monkey (1). The most common fibers studied were the C- and A-fiber mechanoheat nociceptive afferents (CMHs and AMHs). But a small number of nociceptive fibers responsive only to heat, cold, or mechanical stimuli were also included as well as a few low-threshold mechanoreceptive and thermoreceptive afferents. Parallel experiments were carried out in a study of CMHs in humans, using microneurography (5).

Usually capsaicin was first injected outside 5 to 7 mm away from the border of the fiber's receptive field. This distance was sometimes greater for human subjects. The main purpose was to see whether or not any fiber could be remotely sensitized, i.e., develop lowered response thresholds or enhanced suprathreshold responses to mechanical or thermal cutaneous stimuli. Then, after appropriate testing, another injection was given adjacent to or inside the receptive field. After each injection, any evoked responses to capsaicin were recorded in order to determine which population of afferents contribute to the pain from capsaicin, a pain that human subjects estimated to be, at its maximum, about 2.5 times greater than that produced by a 5-sec 51°C heat stimulus.

Peripheral Nerve Fibers Contributing to Capsaicin-Evoked Pain

Only heat-sensitive and/or chemically sensitive afferent fibers responded to an injection of capsaicin. These fiber types included (a) CMHs, (b) type II AMH (which behaves like a CMH), but not type I AMH, (which is commonly unresponsive to stimulus temperatures of less than 51°C), (c) C-fiber heat nociceptors (CHs) (fibers responsive to heat but not to cold or to mechanical stimuli), (d) warm receptors, and (e) putative chemonociceptors (fibers that were unresponsive to heat or mechanical stimuli). Fibers that were insensitive to heat including those with high- or low-threshold mechanoreceptors, cool receptors, or cold nociceptors were unresponsive to capsaicin. In both monkeys and humans, the mean discharge rates of CMHs, while changing in a manner roughly parallel to the time course of magnitude estimates of pain in humans, were very low. In monkey, maximum discharge rates to capsaicin of CMHs and those of any other nociceptive fibers, except CHs, were less than those evoked by a 5-sec 51°C heat stimulus. In contrast, maximum discharge rates of CHs were two to three times greater to capsaicin than to heat in correspondence with human estimates of the magnitude of pain elicited by these two stimuli. It is likely that CHs and, to a lesser extent, CMHs and AMH II fibers contribute most to the pain from a capsaicin injection.

Peripheral Nerve Fibers Contributing to Secondary Hyperalgesia

Aside from a very transient change in sensitivity of a few fibers, there was no definitive sensitization to either mechanical stimuli (stroking or punctate) or heat stimuli of CMHs in humans or CMHs, AMHs, or any other type of afferent fiber studied in the monkey. This was true regardless of the locus of the injection. In fact, the most common effect of capsaicin injected close to or within a receptive field was an elevation of threshold and a reduced (or abolished) response to cutaneous stimulation. This "desensitization" of fiber responses probably accounts for the analgesia experienced by humans to pinprick in the bleb at the capsaicin injection site (4).

The absence of peripheral sensitization is consistent with the hypothesis that certain capsaicin-activated peripheral nerve fibers can bring about the sensitization of nociceptive neurons in the CNS. It is unlikely that these peripheral nerve fibers belong to any of the well-studied classes of fibers such as CMHs or AMHs. Noninjurious heat and mechanical stimuli that produce pain but no flare and little or no hyperalgesia are more effective in exciting these fibers than an injection of capsaicin that is capable of producing both a flare and a large area of hyperalgesia. However, our speculation that the missing nociceptors might be a class of chemonociceptors (3,4) has yet to be tested. A concentrated search is required for peripheral afferents, particularly in humans, that respond better to algesic chemicals than to heat or mechanical stimuli. For our hypothesis to be correct, these fibers must then have sufficiently broad receptive fields, or have receptive fields that are functionally (chemically or electrically) linked together to (a) account for the large area of 2HM obtained in humans after a localized cutaneous injury and (b) explain why a barrier of anesthetic blocks the spread of hyperalgesia away from the site of injury.

CENTRAL NEURAL CORRELATES OF CAPSAICIN-EVOKED PAIN AND SECONDARY HYPERALGESIA

Capsaicin-Evoked Changes in the Central Neuronal Processing of Tactile Information

Torebjörk et al. (9) used the technique of intraneural microstimulation to investigate whether or not there is a change in the central neuronal processing of tactile information after the development of 2HM. Human subjects judged the quality of cutaneous sensation referred to an area of skin during intraneural electrical stimulation of myelinated mechanoreceptive peripheral nerve fibers before and after capsaicin was injected 7 to 20 mm outside the area. Before capsaicin, the electrical stimulus evoked a sensation of touch without pain. But once 2HM developed in the area of referred sensation, a sensation of pain, in addition to touch, was evoked by the same electrical stimulus—a pain that had the same quality of "soreness" as that elicited by stroking the hyperalgesic skin. Touch, without pain, returned to the area of referred sensation after the disappearance of 2HM. These observations support the hypothesis that certain neurons in the CNS had become sensitized to the normally painless peripheral neural activity evoked by stroking the skin.

Experiments to Investigate the Role of Spinothalamic Tract Neurons in Capsaicin-Evoked Pain and Secondary Hyperalgesia

Electrophysiological responses of identified spinothalamic tract (STT) neurons to the same stimuli used in the psychophysical studies were recorded in anesthetized monkeys (8). Neurons were classified as wide dynamic range (WDR) or high-threshold (HT) cells according to responses elicited by graded cutaneous mechanical stimulation. Responses to punctate and stroking mechanical stimuli were recorded before and after an intracutaneous injection of vehicle at one locus and, subsequently, capsaicin at another locus, within the receptive field on the hairy skin of the postaxial surface of the leg. In addition, 5-sec heat stimuli of 30° to 50°C were delivered before and after each injection by a Peltier thermode centered on versus 2 cm away from the injection site. Last, a new series of psychophysical measurements was carried out in which magnitude estimates of pain evoked by the punctate mechanical stimuli and the heat stimuli were obtained from human subjects before and after injections of vehicle and capsaicin. The purpose of these experiments was to determine whether there was a correlation between the sensory measurements of pain and hyperalgesia in humans and the responses of STT neurons in monkeys using the same experimental stimuli. Such a correlation would suggest a contribution of these neurons to capsaicin pain and 2° hyperalgesia.

Comparison of Capsaicin-Evoked Discharge Rates of Spinothalamic Tract Neurons with Magnitude Estimates of Pain

An injection of the vehicle evoked neither pain in humans nor significant discharges in STT neurons. In contrast, the intense burning pain elicited upon the injection of capsaicin was paralleled by a vigorous discharge rate in all but one of the WDR neurons and more than half of the HT cells (Fig. 16.4). Both the mean magnitude estimates of pain and the maximum mean discharge rates of the WDR and HT cells reached peak values in the first 15 sec after injection. The rapid decrease in pain over the next 5 min was roughly paralleled by a similar decrease in the mean discharge rates of the STT neurons, averaged for HT and WDR cells. Analyzed separately, the discharges of WDR cells correlated better with the magnitude judgments of pain than did the discharges of the HTs.

The peak mean discharge rate evoked in the WDRs by capsaicin was approximately three times greater than the mean discharge rate evoked by the 5-sec heat stimulus of 50°C. Approximately the same ratio was found in the magnitude estimates by humans of the pain from capsaicin versus the pain from noxious heat (51°C, 5 sec). (The HT neurons in our sample were generally unresponsive to the heat stimuli.) This result, together with the parallel time course of WDR discharges and magnitude judgments of pain after capsaicin injection, suggests an important contribution of STT neurons, particularly WDR cells, to the pain from capsaicin.

Heat Hyperalgesia and the Sensitization of Spinothalamic Tract Neurons

The mean magnitude estimates by humans of pain evoked by heat stimuli of 30° to 50°C increased significantly after capsaicin injection but only when the thermode was centered on the capsaicin injection site and not when it was placed on the test

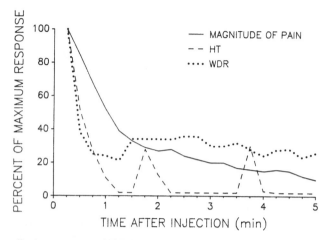

FIG. 16.4. Mean discharge rates of WDR and HT neurons, recorded from monkey, compared with mean magnitude estimates of pain obtained from humans after an intradermal injection of capsaicin. The magnitude of pain is the mean of the magnitude estimates expressed as a percentage of the maximum for each subject. Discharge rates are expressed as a percentage of the maximum obtained averaged separately for WDRs and HTs. (Replotted data from ref. 8.)

site located 2 cm away. Injection of the vehicle alone had no significant effect on heat pain. The mean pain threshold (lowest stimulus temperature evoking a sensation of pain) decreased at the capsaicin injection site from about 45°C before to 34°C after the injection. Similarly, most of the WDR cells in the monkey responded to the same heat stimuli. Most of these neurons became greatly sensitized to heat delivered to the capsaicin injection site and not, with the exception of one neuron, at the test site located 2 cm away (Fig. 16.5). (Although a few of the HT cells also became sensitized to heat, most in our sample were generally unresponsive to heat after as well as before the injections.) The mean response threshold (lowest stimulus temperature eliciting a response) of the WDR cells to heat delivered to the capsaicin injection site

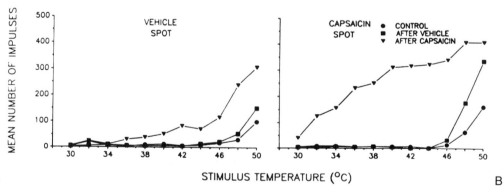

FIG. 16.5. The mean responses of WDR neurons to heat stimuli of different temperatures delivered to the vehicle (**A**) and capsaicin (**B**) injection sites before and after each injection (see text). (From ref. 8.)

decreased from about 49°C before capsaicin to 34°C after. Discharges to suprathreshold heat stimuli were significantly increased after capsaicin injection but not after the vehicle (Fig. 16.5). Thus, the location of the area of hyperalgesia on the skin and the magnitude of the hyperalgesia in humans were paralleled by a similar cutaneous locus and magnitude of heat sensitization of the WDR neurons as studied in the monkey.

Mechanical Hyperalgesia and the Sensitization of Spinothalamic Tract Neurons

The injection of capsaicin, but not the vehicle alone, significantly increased the responses of the HT and WDR neurons to stroking the skin within the receptive field. After capsaicin, the mean number of impulses elicited by each stroke increased about ninefold in HT cells and approximately twofold in the WDR cells (Fig. 16.6). The enhanced responses to stroking in these neurons were observed at each trajectory site within the receptive field. Thus, the sensitization of these STT neurons provides a physiological substrate for the 2HM (allodynia) to gentle mechanical stimulation of the normal skin surrounding a cutaneous injury.

Magnitude estimates by humans of the pain to punctate stimulation of the skin with the nylon filament increased after an injection of capsaicin and increased significantly more than after an injection of the vehicle alone. The pain increased about sixfold for punctate stimulation of each test site located 1, 2, or 3 cm away from the injection site. No increase was found for stimulations at the capsaicin injection site. Similarly, the responses of both HT and WDR neurons were enhanced after capsaicin, but not after the vehicle alone, to punctate stimulation of the test sites located 1 to 3 cm away from, but not on, the injection site. The mean number of impulses evoked per stimulus (at the 1-, 2-, and 3-cm test sites) increased by an average of ninefold for HT cells and 2.5-fold for the WDR cells. Many of the HT and WDR neurons also exhibited afterdischarges that lasted several seconds after the stimulus was terminated. These STT neurons are therefore likely to contribute to the en-

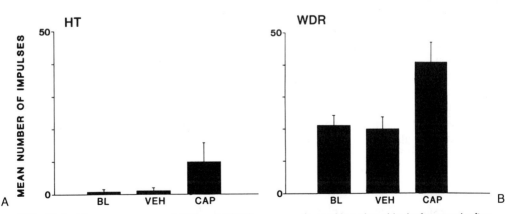

FIG. 16.6. Mean responses of HT and WDR neurons to stroking the skin before and after injections of vehicle and capsaicin. **A:** Mean number of impulses/stroke (±SE) evoked in HT neurons before (BL) and after injections of vehicle (VEH) and capsaicin (CAP). **B:** Mean number of impulses/stroke evoked in WDR neurons. (From ref. 8.)

hanced and abnormally prolonged pain produced when a normally painful punctate stimulus is delivered to the hyperalgesic skin surrounding a cutaneous injury.

Effect of Capsaicin in Increasing the Excitability of Spinothalamic Tract Neurons

Injury-induced changes in central excitability were tested by recording, in an additional group of STT neurons, the responses evoked by electrical stimulation of the proximal end of a cut dorsal rootlet before and after an injection of capsaicin. It was found that after capsaicin, the mean number of impulses elicited increased significantly above preinjection values for most of these cells. This result indicates that the hyperalgesia to natural stimulation of the skin surrounding an injury is due, at least partly, to an increase in the excitability of STT neurons. This is consistent with three findings already described: (a) a nerve block delivered prior to a capsaicin injection prevents 2° hyperalgesia from developing, (b) intraneural electrical stimulation that evokes only tactile sensation referred to a cutaneous projection field before injection of capsaicin elicits an additional component of pain after the injection but only when the projection field is included in the area of hyperalgesia, and (c) the absence of the sensitization of primary afferent fibers after capsaicin injection.

It seems unlikely that the changes in excitability are confined to the STT neuron itself because if this were true, one would expect that there would be an increase in responses, after capsaicin, to heat delivered anywhere within its receptive field and not, as was commonly observed, only to heating the skin within a small area around the capsaicin injection site. Thus, it is possible that the increased excitability is mediated by sensitized interneurons that interface between the primary afferents and the STT neurons. The idea would be that chemically sensitive nociceptive afferent peripheral nerve fibers release neurochemicals, for example, certain neurokinins, in the dorsal horn that enhance the responses of these interneurons. The hyperalgesia resulting from the sensitization of one set of neurons by activity in another was called "neurogenic hyperalgesia" (4). Two kinds are hypothesized to occur after a capsaicin injection: (a) capsaicin-activated C-heat nociceptive afferents sensitize interneurons that receive a converging input from low-threshold "warm fibers" (giving rise to neurogenic heat hyperalgesia) and (b) chemonociceptive primary afferent fibers with broad receptive fields release a neurochemical that sensitizes two types of mechanoreceptive interneurons—one receiving input primarily from low-threshold mechanoreceptive afferents (responsive to innocuous stroking), the other activated by high-threshold mechanonociceptive afferents responsive to noxious punctate stimulation (giving rise to mechanical hyperalgesia). These three sets of interneurons are hypothesized to converge onto, and facilitate the responses of, STT neurons in different ways in order to account for the differences in sensory characteristics (e.g., spatial distribution, time courses) of the hyperalgesias to heating, stroking, and punctate stimulations of the skin after the capsaicin injection.

CONCLUSION

The results of these psychophysical and neurophysiological experiments suggest that the 2° hyperalgesia surrounding a cutaneous injury is a consequence of an increase in the excitability of neurons in the dorsal horn of the spinal cord, as hypothesized by Hardy et al. (2) and not the result of the sensitization of peripheral nerve fibers as proposed by Lewis (6). However, the fact that a strip of anesthetized skin can act as a barrier to prevent the spread of hyperalgesia away from the site of injury confirms the observation originally made by Lewis and is consonant with a generalized statement of his hypothesis: Stated in general terms, Lewis hypothesized that a special class of "nocifensor" afferent nerve fibers can transmit nerve impulses through the skin away from an injury and, as a result, somehow enhance the responses of sensory neurons to innocuous and noxious mechanical stimulation of the surrounding uninjured skin. We propose that the mechanism for this enhancement is the release of a sensitizing neuromodulator, from a special class of nerve fibers with large cutaneous receptive fields, that acts centrally and not, as Lewis proposed, peripherally via an axon reflex. If this idea proves correct, it would go a long way toward resolving a controversy that has existed for more than half a century.

ACKNOWLEDGMENTS

This research was carried out in collaboration with C. Shain, D. Simone, E. Tsai, T. Baumann, L. Sorkin, U. Oh, J. Chung, C. Owens, and W. Willis and supported by National Institute of Neurological Disorders and Stroke grants NS-14624 (LaMotte), NS-11255, NS-09743 (Willis), and NS-21266 (Chung), a National Research Service Award (Simone), and a National Institutes of Health Training Grant (Shain).

REFERENCES

1. Baumann, T. K., Simone, D. A., Shain, C. N., and LaMotte, R. H. (1991): Neurogenic hyperalgesia: the search for the primary cutaneous afferent fibers that contribute to capsaicin-induced pain and hyperalgesia. *J. Neurophysiol.*, 66:212–227.
2. Hardy, J. D., Wolff, H. G., and Goodell, H. (1950): Experimental evidence on the nature of cutaneous hyperalgesia. *J. Clin. Invest.*, 29:115–140.
3. LaMotte, R. H. (1988): Psychophysical and neurophysiological studies of chemically induced cutaneous pain and itch. The case of the missing nociceptor. In: *Progress in brain research*, vol. 74, edited by W. Hamann and A. Iggo, pp. 331–335. Elsevier, New York.
4. LaMotte, R. H., Shain, C. N., Simone, D. A., and Tsai, E. (1991): Neurogenic hyperalgesia: psychophysical studies of underlying mechanisms. *J. Neurophysiol.*, 66:190–211.
5. LaMotte, R. H., Torebjörk, H. E., and Lundberg, L. Pain, hyperalgesia and activity in nociceptive afferent C fibres in humans after intradermal injection of capsaicin. *J. Physiol. (Lond.) (in press)*.
6. Lewis, T. (1936): Experiments relating to cutaneous hyperalgesia and its spread through somatic nerves. *Clin. Sci.*, 2:373–421.
7. Simone, D. A., Baumann, T. K., and LaMotte, R. H. (1989): Dose-dependent pain and mechanical hyperalgesia in humans after intradermal injection of capsaicin. *Pain*, 38:99–107.
8. Simone, D. A., Oh, U., Sorkin, L. S., et al. (1991): Neurogenic hyperalgesia: central neural correlates in responses of spinothalamic tract neurons. *J. Neurophysiol.*, 66:228–246.
9. Torebjörk, H. E., Lundberg, L. E. R., and LaMotte, R. H. Central changes in processing of mechanoreceptive input in capsaicin-induced secondary hyperalgesia. *J. Physiol. (Lond.) (in press)*.

Hyperalgesia and Allodynia,
edited by W. D. Willis, Jr.
Raven Press, Ltd., New York © 1992.

17

Evidence for a Central Contribution to Secondary Hyperalgesia

Gisèle Guilbaud, Valérie Kayser, Nadine Attal, and Jean-Michel Benoist

*Unité de Physiopharmacologie du Système Nerveux, U161, INSERM,
75014 Paris, France*

Most studies on secondary hyperalgesia have been concerned with hyperalgesia close to the initial injury or within the same segment (see references in ref. 31; Campbell et al., Chapter 12; LaMotte, Chapter 16), as initially described (17,23,24) and in which the central nervous system is not necessarily responsible, as already discussed by Lewis (24) and suggested in a recent study (18). This is extensively discussed in several chapters of this book (Campbell et al., LaMotte, Woolf). Here, we report data on secondary hyperalgesia distant to the initial injury and located on a remote part of the body: symmetrically on the opposite limb and/or on heterosegmental areas. Thus, in this case, there is no doubt that the central nervous system participates.

These phenomena were first observed when we started studies with carrageenan-injected rats (4,14,20) in order to produce a unilateral localized inflammatory pain in contrast to the polyarthritic rats that we had previously extensively investigated (see references in ref. 6). Surprisingly, after carrageenan injection in a plantar hindpaw, we noted that modifications of pain-related behavior (vocalization threshold to paw pressure) and of some neuronal responses [in the ventrobasal (VB) thalamic complex] could be obtained by stimulating not only the injected but also the noninjected paws. Similar phenomena were later observed in a model of noninflammatory pain in rats rendered mononeuropathic by four loose ligatures around the sciatic nerve (1,2). These phenomena have been observed in both behavioral approaches based on the measure of nociceptive test thresholds and in electrophysiological recordings at the supraspinal level, mainly in the thalamus but also in the primary somatosensory cortex (SM1). The efficacy of several neuropharmacological treatments on the changes in nociceptive behaviors and on neuronal responses elicited by the injury has been also investigated.

BEHAVIORAL OBSERVATIONS

Mechanical Stimuli

To gauge the abnormal pain-related behavior to mechanical stimuli we used the measure of the vocalization threshold to paw pressure as in several previous studies (20,21,27). As seen in Fig. 17.1 the carrageenan injection in the right plantar hindpaw

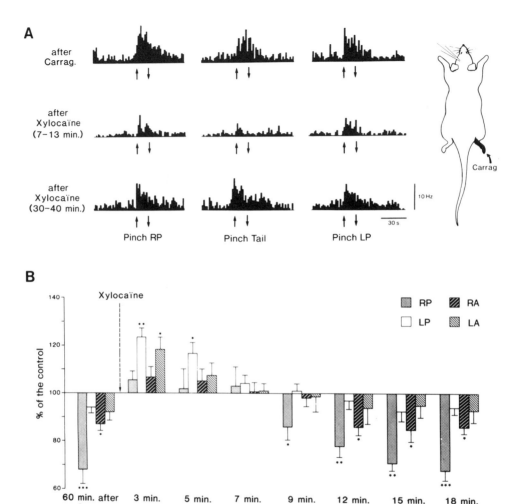

FIG. 17.1. A: Neuronal responses in the left VB thalamic complex induced by pinch applied to the carrageenan-injected or the noninjected paw (the right and left, respectively) as well as to the tail: over 1 hr after carrageenan injection in the right plantar paw (*first line*), 7 to 13 min (*second line*), and 30 to 40 min (*third line*) after lidocaine (xylocaine). (Pinch of 15-sec duration indicated between two arrows, number of spikes in 2-sec epochs in ordinates, time in abscissa). **B:** For each limb, evolution of the mean vocalization threshold to paw pressure expressed as percentages of the precarrageenan values, before and after local lidocaine in the carrageenan-injected paw. Note the threshold decrease due to carrageenan and the antinociceptive effect of xylocaine for the four paws (the decrease has been found more significant for the opposite hindpaw in several further studies). (RP, LP, right or left posterior paw; RA, LA, right and left anterior paw; Carrag., carrageenan.)

induced a decrease in the threshold from this paw, but also from the opposite hindlimb and even from the two forepaws. This was seen during the first hours following the beginning of the inflammation and was still clear 24 hr later (Figs. 17.1 and 17.2). At this time there was a significant relation between the level of hyperalgesia noted for each hindpaw; the more hyperalgesic the injected limb, the lower the vocalization threshold obtained from the opposite hindpaw (Fig. 17.3).

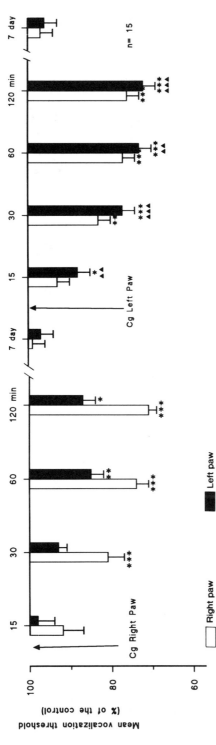

FIG. 17.2. As in Fig. 17.1, but for the two hindpaws only, evolution of the mean vocalization threshold to paw pressure expressed as percentages of the precarrageenan values, followed until a complete recovery after a first injection in the right plantar hindpaw, then after an injection in the left plantar hindpaw 7 days later.

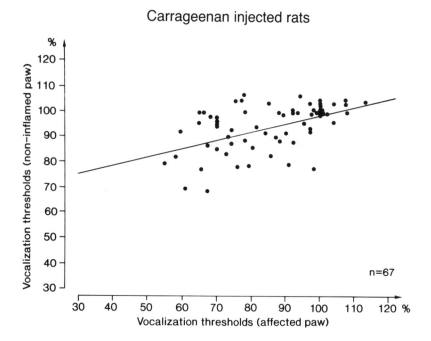

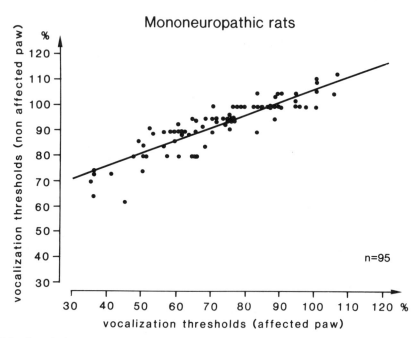

FIG. 17.3. Correlation between the vocalization threshold to paw pressure obtained from the lesioned and nonlesioned paw in the two models. **Top**, 24 hr carrageenan-injected rats; **bottom**, rats with loose ligatures around the right sciatic nerve for 2 weeks.

A comparable phenomenon was seen with a model of noninflammatory pain in rats rendered mononeuropathic by placing four loose ligatures around the common sciatic nerve (1,2). In these rats the maximal pain-related behaviors are seen 2 weeks after the ligatures have been placed. At this time it was evident that a decrease in the vocalization threshold by pressing the opposite hindpaw could be observed and that the thresholds from the two paws were significantly correlated (Fig. 17.3).

Thermal Stimuli

To gauge abnormal reaction to a thermal stimulus, we measured the struggle latency to paw immersion in successive water baths with a cutoff at 15 sec: the struggle reaction appeared with a latency below 15 sec, and this temperature was taken as the threshold to the nociceptive reaction to heat. In normal animals, it was around 44° to 45°C and remarkably stable over several successive studies (1,11) (Table 17.1). In carrageenan-injected rats, the struggle threshold was decreased by about 4°C in the first hour following the carrageenan injection; this decrease was similar but could be more pronounced at 24 hr. The threshold from the noninjected paw was still normal at 1 hr but also clearly reduced 1 day later (Table 17.1). In neuropathic rats, the mean struggle threshold to heat stimulus from the paw with the ligated nerve is usually profoundly decreased by at least 4°C, 2 weeks after surgery (1,2). In the first study performed with this rat model, a threshold decrease in the opposite paw was observed for some rats, mainly for rats with a very marked sensitivity to heat from their "lesioned" paw. However, the mean threshold obtained with 71 rats was not significantly different from the mean presurgery values. This was not the case in more recent experimental series (27; *unpublished data*) in which a significant abnormal reaction to heat either from the "lesioned" or the "nonlesioned" paw was found. In the neuropathic rats, which exhibit a marked abnormal sensitivity to cold, when

TABLE 17.1. *Struggle threshold measured by plunging a paw in successive hot water baths of graded temperature for 9 to 10 sec*

	Struggle	VB group 2 response
Normal paw	44.3 ± 1.0°C $n = 15$	44.0 ± 0.6°C $n = 10$[a]
Normal tail		44.5 ± 0.6°C $n = 11$[b]
Noninjected paw, 1hr	43.9 ± 0.9°C $n = 5$	45.3 ± 0.8°C $n = 7$[a]
Injected paw, 1 hr	40.6 ± 1.2°C $n = 10$	40.3 ± 1.4°C $n = 10$[a]
Noninjected paw, 24 hr	40.9 ± 1.4°C $n = 10$	40.2 ± 0.8°C $n = 6$[c]
Injected paw, 24 hr	39.0 ± 1.6°C $n = 10$	38.0 ± 0.6°C $n = 12$[c]

[a]Same neurons.
[b]From ref. 28a.
[c]Same neurons.

the "lesioned" paw is immersed in a 10°C water bath (1), an abnormal reaction could also be observed from the opposite side. For instance, in one of these more recent studies (unpublished), the struggle latency, normally at least 15 sec, was decreased by about 4.5 and 2.5 sec for the "lesioned" and the "nonlesioned" paws, respectively. Thus, from these various studies it clearly appears that distant hyperalgesia and allodynia to mechanical and even to thermal stimuli can be observed from parts of the body remote to the lesioned area in both inflammatory and noninflammatory pain models.

In more recent investigations, we considered whether the changes described here after a first carrageenan injection in one paw could influence the changes elicited by a further injection either in the same or the opposite paw, after a total recovery 7 days later. It was found that in the two conditions the hyperalgesia due to this second injection was more potent than after the first carrageenan injection, not only for the newly injected paw, but also, and even more marked, for the noninjected limbs. This is well illustrated in Fig. 17.2, in which the second carrageenan injection in the left paw (not previously injected) induced a dramatic threshold decrease from the right hindpaw (and the two forelimbs).

ELECTROPHYSIOLOGICAL OBSERVATIONS

Extensive studies have shown that the VB complex of the thalamus has a major role in the transmission and integration of nociceptive messages in normal and poly-arthritic rats (see references in refs. 11–14). In particular, numerous neurons in this structure are exclusively and repeatedly excited by noxious mechanical and thermal stimuli. Although these neurons were recorded under a moderate state of anesthesia ($O_2 + N_2O + 0.5-0.6\%$ halothane), their activation thresholds to both stimulus modalities fit well with those of the nociceptive reactions observed in freely moving animals when comparable stimuli are applied (11). In addition, their responses are highly sensitive to analgesic agents. Thus, investigating the putative changes in the VB neuronal responses during the settling of a hyperalgesia appears to be a suitable model to study neuronal mechanisms of hyperalgesia.

Responses to Mechanical Stimuli

Responses of a particular VB neuron to a noxious mechanical stimulus such as a pinch applied to the posterior paw were followed after carrageenan injection in the plantar area [included in the receptive field (RF) of the neuron]. It was clear that the total number of spikes in the pinch responses elicited from the injected paw increased progressively (Figs. 17.1 and 17.4); the maximum increase [about 100% by comparison with the mean initial control value as shown in several experimental series (14)] was roughly reached between the first and second hour following the carrageenan injection.

Because half of the "noxious" rat VB neurons have RFs extending to the other hindpaw and/or the tail, neurons with these characteristics were preferentially studied in order to compare responses obtained from the noninflamed part of the RF. In most cases [17 of 23 in the first systematic study (14)], there was also an increase in the response from the noninjected limb and or the tail (Fig. 17.1). In addition, ex-

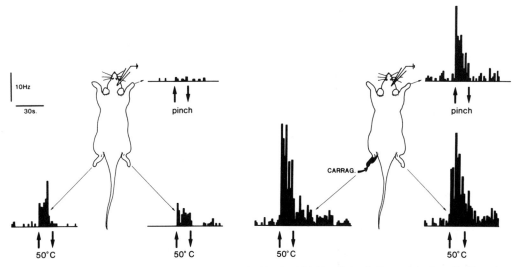

FIG. 17.4. As in Fig. 17.1, responses recorded in the VB (the right thalamus) before **(left)** and after **(right)** carrageenan injection in the left posterior paw. Note the increases of responses to a 50°C waterbath for the two hindpaws and the occurence of response from the right anterior paw.

pansion of the RFs was also observed, since stimulation of areas remote from the injected paw and not included in the RF prior to the inflammation could elicit responses to pinch after the carrageenan injection (Fig. 17.4). This was seen in eight of the 10 cases in which the opposite paw was not included in the RF prior to carrageenan injection. It was particularly striking for the forelimbs, which, in normal conditions, are extremely rarely included in RFs of VB neurons responding to pinch of the posterior part of the body: 14 of the 23 neurons of the initial study, nonresponsive at first to stimulation of either forepaw, could respond to one or even to both forepaws over the first hour following the beginning of the inflammation.

At the cortical level, the SM1 is known to be involved in transmission and integration of noxious messages in the monkey and the rat (see references in ref. 7). Using the same experimental design as for VB neuron studies, we analyzed the time course of neuronal cortical responses induced by noxious pinch, after induction of a carrageenan inflammation *(unpublished data)*. At the cortical level most of the "noxious" neurons have a unilateral contralateral RF in the normal state; thus, although the number of cells analyzed so far is limited, it is all the more surprising and significant to observe response increases not only from the injected but also the noninjected paw, ipsilateral to the recording site.

Responses to Thermal Stimuli

The increase or occurrence of responses to noxious heat (immersion into a 50°C water bath) from parts of the body distant to the carrageenan-injected paw was also a reliable phenomenon during the first hour following the beginning of the inflammation (Fig. 17.4).

However, although there was a constant decrease of the thermal activation threshold from the inflamed paw in the first stage of inflammation (decreased by about 4°C in several experimental series), there was no change for the activation threshold from the opposite paw. By contrast, in rats recorded 1 day after the carrageenan injection, the thermal threshold of VB neurons driven by pinch was found to be especially low for each hindpaw (around 38°C and 40°C for the injected and noninjected paws, respectively (Table 17.1). However, this decrease in the VB neuron activation threshold from the "nonlesioned" paw was not observed in neuropathic rats recorded 2 to 3 weeks after the nerve ligature (13), likely due to the fact that we preferentially selected rats with a clear asymmetry in the nociceptive thresholds obtained from each hindpaw.

NEUROPHARMACOLOGICAL OBSERVATIONS

On the basis of the forementioned behavioral and electrophysiological data, the question was addressed as to whether the central mechanisms responsible for the changes remote to the injured limb were resistant to the treatment of the initial injury. This was gauged using local anesthetic blocks in the two models with a unilateral injury, as reported above, as well as in a model of a more diffuse and more prolonged hyperalgesia, i.e., in rats with Freund's adjuvant-induced arthritis. In the carrageenan-injected rats we also tested whether an early treatment with antagonists of the inflammatory substances, acting only at the periphery, could prevent and/or suppress the distant secondary hyperalgesia.

Local Anesthetic Blockade

This was tested with lidocaine hydrochloride (0.05 ml of a 2% solution) or lidocaine–epinephrine hydrochloride (0.05 ml of a 1% and 0.00025%, respectively, solution) injected in the lesioned paw on behavioral and electrophysiological VB responses in the carrageenan-injected rats and with the behavioral approaches in the neuropathic animals.

Over the first stage of the carrageenan inflammation at least (i.e., 1 hr after its beginning), the local anesthetic blockade of the inflamed paw also induced a hypoalgesic effect from the parts of the body that were distant to the injected paw and originally exhibiting hyperalgesia (Fig. 17.1). This block was also able to suppress the distant hyperalgesia following a carrageenan-reinjection (Fig. 17.2) 1 week after the first inflammation.

The effect of such a block on the distant modifications due to an inflammatory process over several days has not been tested so far with the carrageenan model, but has been studied with polyarthritic rats, 3 to 4 weeks after the adjuvant inoculation. It was clear in these rats that a unilateral lidocaine blockade induced a hypoalgesic effect in the two hindpaws and that VB neuronal responses elicited by mild stimulation of each ankle were similarly depressed (Fig. 17.5). From preliminary studies it appears that in neuropathic rats, a local injection of lidocaine–epinephrine in the "lesioned" paw can also suppress the hyperalgesia seen on the "nonlesioned" limb 2 weeks after the nerve ligatures.

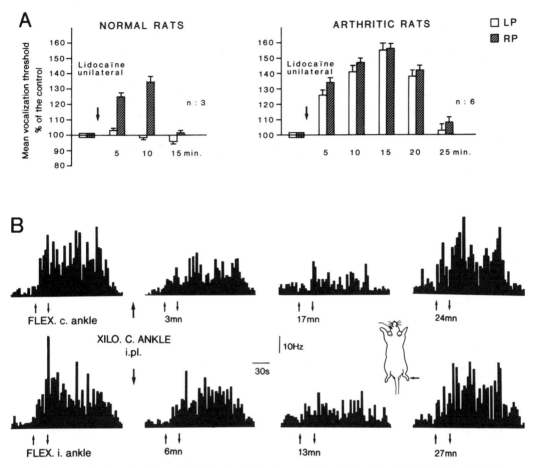

FIG. 17.5. A: In arthritic rats, bilateral effect of a unilateral injection of lidocaine on mean vocalization thresholds to paw pressure on each side. Note on the left, the unilateral effect of lidocaine when injected in normal rats. **B:** Bilateral effect of a unilateral injection of lidocaine on responses recorded in the VB of polyarthritic rats and induced by flexion of each ankle. LP, left paw; RP, right paw. (Figure designed as Fig. 17.1.)

Local Antagonists of Inflammatory Substances Released in the Exudate

In the early 1980s, when we started the use of intraplantar carrageenan as a model of localized inflammatory pain, most mechanistic studies of anti-inflammatory drugs had focused on the factors behind edema development, and the timing of production of inflammatory mediators in acute carrageenan edema was well-known (see references in ref. 15). Far fewer studies had focused on hyperalgesia per se. We attempted to determine to what extent some of the inflammatory mediators, such as histamine and serotonin, released early in the exudate (from 1 to 60 min) and known to activate and/or sensitize nociceptors by close intra-arterial injection (see references in ref. 15) could participate pathophysiologically in the first stage of carrageenan hyperalgesia and consequently in the distant hyperalgesia that we observed.

Antagonists acting at the peripheral level were used in both behavioral and electrophysiological approaches, i.e., for studies based on changes of the vocalization threshold to paw pressure, on the one hand, and the neuronal VB thalamic responses on the other. A quarternary antihistamine, thiazinamium, which does not cross the blood–brain barrier, and (3-α-tropanyl)-1H-indole-3-carboxylic ester (ICS 205-930), a potent specific antagonist of the peripheral neural serotonergic 5-HT₃ receptors (see references in ref. 15), were used for these studies, with different treatment protocols. We took into account the sequence of release of the inflammatory mediators: the antihistamine was injected 10 min prior to or 20 min after carrageenan; ICS was injected simultaneously with, prior to, or 20 to 60 min after carrageenan.

In the behavioral studies it appeared that both agents were able to prevent and/or to suppress the carrageenan hyperalgesia obtained from the injected paw, according

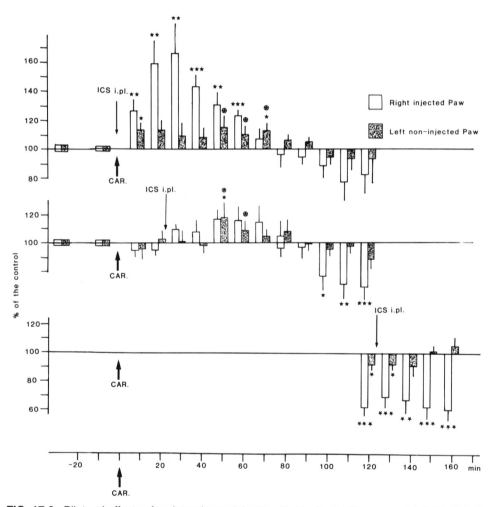

FIG. 17.6. Bilateral effects of an intraplantar injection (i.pl.) of a 5-HT₃ antagonist (ICS) (10⁻¹¹ mol/kg, i.e., 3.2 ng/kg) simultaneously with, or 20 min or 2 hr after carrageenan into the same paw on the mean vocalization thresholds to paw pressure. (Carrageenan [CAR.] in the right plantar hindpaw.) ★, *p*<0.05; ★★, *p*<0.01; ★★★, *p*<0.001. ⊛, *p*<0.05 values obtained in CAR.-treated rats. (From ref. 10a.)

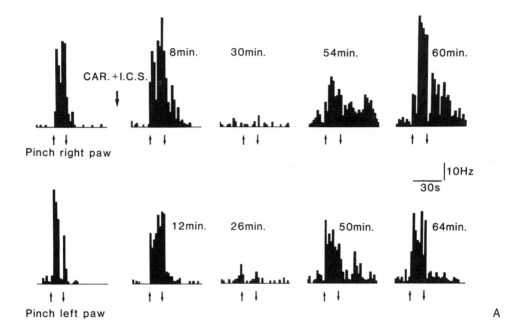

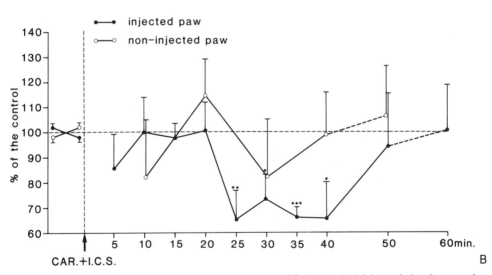

FIG. 17.7. A: Illustration of the bilateral effect of local ICS (3.2 ng/kg) injected simultaneously with carrageenan (CAR) in the right plantar paw on neuronal VB responses to pinch. Note the lack of carrageenan sensitization and, to the contrary, the depression of the response elicited by pinch applied alternately to each hindpaw. **B:** Mean curves obtained with the same protocol, illustrating the mean total number of spikes counted in each response expressed as a percentage of the mean control value (mean ± SEM). For the right injected paw, $n = 7$ until 50 min following injections, and 5 after this time (*dotted line*); for the noninjected paw, $n = 6$ until 40 min, then 4 (*dotted line*). *, $p < 0.1$; **, $p < 0.01$; ***, $p < 0.001$. (From ref. 15.)

to the time of their administration. ICS injected prior to or simultaneously with carrageenan was even able to induce an antinociceptive effect (Fig. 17.6). When injected after carrageenan (20 and 60 min for thiazinamium and ICS, respectively), they did not influence the initial hyperalgesia (Fig. 17.6). Interestingly the prevention or the suppression of the hyperalgesia from the inflamed paw was also seen for the opposite hindpaw (Fig. 17.6) with a striking parallelism throughout all the successive experimental series.

Similar observations were obtained with the electrophysiological recordings (15): the increase in VB neuronal responses to pinch from the two paws was prevented, halted, or even reduced after administration of antagonists. The time course of their efficacy was comparable to that observed with the nociceptive behavioral test (Fig. 17.7). Thus, again it was possible to prevent the secondary distant hyperalgesia with these drugs akin to the effects of the local anesthetic blockade.

DISCUSSION AND CONCLUSIONS

The various studies summarized here clearly emphasize that a unilateral limb injury may induce hyperalgesia and allodynia, not only from the injured limb but also from the other limbs. This can be observed in the case of inflammation in carrageenan-injected rats and also in neuropathic rats with loose ligatures around the sciatic nerve. These observations relate to those of several authors who observed a bilateral decrease in the foot withdrawal latency after a unilateral heat injury (9) or repeated injections of saline (22), and facilitation of the contralateral flexion reflex after a local injury on one hindlimb in decerebrate animals (33,34). They are also reminiscent of some clinical descriptions after prolonged thermal irradiation by Hardy et al. (17) in which "pain could be experienced on the side opposite the site of noxious stimulation." The electrophysiological observations at the VB level reported here and in several investigations (4,14,15), then subsequently for spinal dorsal horn neurons (28,30) and observed recently in the SM1 (Christian et al., *unpublished observations*) after carrageenan inflammation, could account for our behavioral observations. Several basic mechanisms described in the past and most recently could account for these phenomena: (a) the increased excitability of dorsal horn neurons, motoneurons, and interneuronal circuits after repetitive noxious stimulations or localized injury monitored by electrophysiological studies at the spinal level (10,17,28,30,31; references in Woolf, Chapter 19); (b) the massive, widespread, and persistent presence of immunoreactive neurokinin A in ipsi- and contralateral primary afferents in the spinal cord of cat with a kaolin–carrageenan-injected knee (19; elsewhere in this volume), (c) the large proportion of afferent fibers and propriospinal axons in the rat dorsal and dorsolateral funiculus (8,32), which could be an anatomical substrate for the heterosegmental modifications. Along these lines, it has also been demonstrated that a unilateral cervical dorsal rhizotomy could increase nociceptive thresholds in the three other innervated limbs, suggesting that the deafferentation of one limb could influence the tonic level of activity present in the other segments of the spinal cord (21). Although there are several arguments supporting the concept of cross-talk between the two sides and between different segments of the spinal cord, there is no evidence to discard similar phenomena at supraspinal levels.

The fact that after an initial inflammation followed by recovery, a new injection of carrageenan reinforced the distant hyperalgesia, whereas the second edema was comparable to the first, is surely of interest and suggests that after an initial injury that has recovered, there is a kind of trace in the nervous system that makes a further injury more painful, not only locally but also in the territories not lesioned initially. This might relate, among several putative causes, to the dramatic changes in the various neuropeptides including endogenous opioids and the activation of onco-genes, described in various types of inflammation and after lesions of the nervous system (3,25,26,29; elsewhere in this volume). However, the time course of all these changes is not yet known and further experiments are required. Another point in the successive experimental series summarized here is that it was possible to prevent and/or to suppress the distant hyperalgesia by agents acting locally on the peripheral injury itself. It is clear from several aspects that the various agents used in the various experiments were really acting at the periphery.

The question of a systemic diffusion of lidocaine, particularly in inflammatory states and therefore a putative central effect of the drug, has been hypothesized but can be ruled out (see references in ref. 20) by: (a) epinephrine limiting the possible systemic diffusion of lidocaine, (b) the time course of the different observed effects was in the range of the reduced compound action potential of peripheral axons after a local anesthetic block, whereas effects described after a systemic injection of li-docaine have a longer latency and duration, (c) at nontoxic doses systemic lidocaine seems not to be analgesic and does not depress VB responses to pinch, and finally (d) comparable data have been obtained in inflammatory and noninflammatory models as well.

Such a relief of a remote hyperalgesia by a lidocaine blockade has also been re-ported in animal and human investigations (17,22; references in ref. 20); the lack of effect reported by Woolf (33,34) might be explained by the different experimental conditions in that study: spinal reflexes in decerebrate animals, tested more than 10 min after the anesthetic injection, a time at which the anesthetic action is likely to have declined.

Although claimed to have a specific peripheral action (see references in ref. 15), a possible central action of the histamine and serotonin antagonists can also be con-sidered but is unlikely since (a) these substances have no depressive action on the neuronal VB responses when injected alone and even systematically and (b) their respective action fit well with that of their release in the exudate, and they were ineffective when injected late after the carrageenan injection.

Thus, it appears that it is possible to block the central mechanisms triggered by the peripheral process. That can be done early in the process, and later (2 weeks at least after the hyperalgesia has started), as shown in polyarthritic and in mononeu-ropathic rats. It is also important to stress that this antinociceptive action can be observed even after a newly reproduced hyperalgesia, as shown with experiments using a reinjection of carrageenan after recovery.

It is not clear whether and to what extent the sympathetic nervous system partic-ipates in the occurrence of the distant hyperalgesia; on the basis of preliminary data it does not seem to have a major role. However, different roles in the various noci-ceptive tests used to gauge hyperalgesia mean that further experiments are neces-sary.

Finally, although it seems well established that the presence of one localized hy-peralgesic lesion seems to increase the level of excitation of the neuronal pools cor-responding to distant parts of the body, it does not rule out the inverse phenomena, i.e., that "pain can inhibit pain." On the basis of a few observations we suggest that a further increase in the initial hyperalgesia at the injury level could subsequently trigger the various inhibitory controls, whether segmental, heterosegmental, or diffuse (see references in ref. 5).

ACKNOWLEDGMENTS

The authors wish to thank Dr. A. H. Dickenson for English revision, Mrs. M. Gautron for technical assistance, and Mr. E. Dehausse for illustrations.

REFERENCES

1. Attal, N., Kayser, V., Jazat, F., and Guilbaud, G. (1990): Further evidence for 'pain-related' behaviors in a model of unilateral peripheral mononeuropathy. *Pain*, 41:235–251.
2. Bennett, G. J., and Xie, Y. K. (1988): A peripheral mononeuropathy in rat that produces abnormal pain sensation like those seen in man. *Pain*, 33:87–107.
3. Bennett, G. J., Kajander, K. C., Sahara, Y., Iadarola, M. J., and Sugimoto, T. (1989): Neurochemical and anatomical changes in the dorsal horn of rats with an experimental painful peripheral neuropathy. In: *Processing of sensory information in the superficial dorsal horn of the spinal cord,* edited by F. Cervero, et al. pp. 463–472. Plenum, New York.
4. Benoist, J. M., Kayser, V., Gautron, M., and Guilbaud, G. (1984): Inflammation aigue et hyperalgie: leurs conséquences sur les résponses de certains neurones du complexe ventrobasal du thalamus chez le rat. *C.R. Acad. Sci.*, 299:401–404.
5. Besson, J. M., and Chaouch, H. (1987): Peripheral and spinal mechanisms in nociception. *Physiol. Rev.*, 67:67–186.
6. Besson, J. M., and Guilbaud, G. (1988): *The arthritic rat as a model of clinical pain?* Excerpta Medica, Amsterdam.
7. Chudler, E. H., Anton, F., Dubner, R., and Kenshalo, D. R., Jr. (1990): Responses of nociceptive SI neurons in monkeys and pain sensation in humans elicited by noxious thermal stimulation: effect of interstimulus interval. *J. Neurophysiol.*, 63:559–569.
8. Chung, K., Langford, L. A., and Coggeshall, R. E. (1987): Primary afferent and propriospinal fibers in the rat dorsal and dorsolateral funiculi. *J. Comp. Neurol.*, 263:68–75.
9. Coderre, T. J., and Melzack, R. (1985): Increased pain sensitivity following heat injury involves a central mechanism. *Behav. Brain Res.*, 15:259–262.
10. Dickenson, A. H., and Sullivan, A. F. (1987): Subcutaneous formalin-induced activity of dorsal horn neurones in the rat: differential response to an intrathecal opiate administered pre or post formalin. *Pain*, 30:349–360.
10a. Eschalier, A., Kayser, V., and Guilbaud, G. (1989): Influence of a specific 5-HT$_3$ antagonist on carrageenan-induced hyperalgesia in rats. *Pain*, 36:149–155.
11. Guilbaud, G. (1987): Responses of ventrobasal thalamic neurons to carrageenin-induced inflammation in the rat. In: *Fine afferent fibers and pain,* edited by R. F. Schmidt, H. G. Schaible, C. Vahle-Hinz, pp. 411–426. VCH, Weinheim.
12. Guilbaud, G. (1988): Peripheral and central electrophysiological mechanisms of joint and muscle pain. In: *Proceedings of the Vth World Congress on Pain,* edited by R. Dubner, G. F. Gebhart, and M. R. Bond, pp. 201–215. Elsevier, Amsterdam.
13. Guilbaud, G., Benoist, J. M., Jazat, F., and Gautron, M. (1990): Neuronal responsiveness in the ventrobasal thalamic complex of rats with an experimental peripheral mononeuropathy. *J. Neurophysiol.*, 64:1537–1554.
14. Guilbaud, G., Benoist, J. M., Kayser, V., and Gautron, M. (1986): Modifications in the responsiveness of rat ventrobasal thalamic neurons at different stages of carrageenin-produced inflammation. *Brain Res.*, 385:86–98.
15. Guilbaud, G., Benoist, J. M., Eschalier, A., Gautron, M., and Kayser, V. (1989): Evidence for peripheral serotonergic mechanisms in the early sensitization after carrageenin-induced inflammation: electrophysiological studies in the ventrobasal complex of the rat thalamus using a potent specific antagonist of peripheral 5-HT receptors. *Brain Res.*, 502:187–197.
16. Guilbaud, G., Benoist, J. M., Eschalier, A., Kayser, V., Gautron, M., and Attal, N. (1989): Evidence for central phenomena participating in the changes of responses of ventrobasal thalamic neurons in arthritic rats. *Brain Res.*, 484:283–332.

17. Hardy, J. D., Wolff, H. G., and Goodell, H. (1967): *Pain sensations and reactions*. Hafner, New York.
18. Hoheisel, U., and Mense, S. (1989): Long-term changes in discharge behavior of cat dorsal horn neurones following noxious stimulation of deep tissues. *Pain*, 36:239–247.
19. Hope, P. J., Jarott, B., Schaible, H. G., Clarke, R. W., and Duggan, A. W. (1990): Release and spread of immunoreactive neurokinin A in the cat spinal cord in a model of acute arthritis. *Brain Res.*, 533:292–299.
20. Kayser, V., and Guilbaud, G. (1987): Local and remote modifications of nociceptive sensitivity during carrageenin-induced inflammation in the rat. *Pain*, 28:99–107.
21. Kayser, V., Basbaum, A. I., and Guilbaud, G. (1990): Deafferentation in the rat increases mechanical nociceptive threshold in the innervated limbs. *Brain Res.*, 508:329–332.
22. Levine, J. D., Dardick, S. J., Basbaum, A. I., and Scipio, E. (1985): Reflex neurogenic inflammation. I. Contribution of the peripheral nervous system to spacially remote inflammatory responses that follow injury. *J. Neurosci.*, 5:1380–1386.
23. Lewis, T. (1935): Experiments relating to cutaneous hyperalgesia and its spread through somatic nerves. *Clin. Sci.*, 2:373–423.
24. Lewis, T. (1942): *Pain*. Macmillan, London.
25. Menetrey, D., Gannon, A., Levine, J. D., and Basbaum, A. I. (1989): The expression of c-fos protein in interneurons and projection neurons of the rat spinal cord in response to noxious somatic, articular and visceral stimulation. *J. Comp. Neurol.*, 285:177–195.
26. Millan, M. J., Czlonkowski, A., Morris, B., et al. (1988): Inflammation of the hind limb as a model of unilateral, localized pain: influence on multiple opioid systems in the spinal cord of the rat. *Pain*, 35:299–312.
27. Neil, A., Attal, N., and Guilbaud, G. (1991): Effects of adrenergic depletion with guanethidine before and after the induction of a peripheral neuropathy subsequent mechanical, heat and cold sensitivities in rats. In: *Pain research and clinical management, Proceedings of the VIth World Congress on Pain*, edited by M. Bond, et al. Elsevier, Amsterdam.
28. Neugebauer, V., and Schaible, H. G. (1990): Evidence for a central component in the sensitization of spinal neurons with joint input during development of acute arthritis in cat's knee. *J. Neurophysiol.*, 64:299–311.
28a.Pechanski, M., Guilbaud, G., Gautron, M., and Besson, J.-M. (1980): Noxious heat messages in neurons of the ventrobasal thalamic complex in the rat. *Brain Res.*, 197:401–413.
29. Ruda, M. A., Iadarola, M. J., Cohen, L. V., and Young III, W. S. (1988): In situ hybridization histochemistry and immunocytochemistry reveal an increase in spinal dynorphin biosynthesis in a rat model of peripheral inflammation and hyperalgesia. *Proc. Natl. Acad. Sci. USA*, 85:622–626.
30. Schaible, H. G., Schmidt, R. F., and Willis, W. D. (1987): Enhancement of the responses of ascending tract cells in the cat spinal cord by acute inflammation of knee joint. *Exp. Brain Res.*, 66:489–499.
31. Simone, D. A., Baumann, T. K., Collins, J. G., and LaMotte, R. H. (1989): Sensitization of cat dorsal horn neurons to innocuous mechanical stimulation after intradermal injection of capsaicin. *Brain Res.*, 486:185–189.
32. Verburgh, C. A., Voogd, J., Kuypers, H. G. J. M., and Stevens, H. P. J. D. (1990): Propriospinal neurons with ascending collaterals to the dorsal medulla, the thalamus and the tectum: a retrograde fluorescent double-labeling study of the cervical cord of the rat. *Exp. Brain Res.*, 80:577–590.
33. Woolf, C. J. (1983): Evidence for a central component of post-injury pain hypersensitivity. *Nature*, 306:686–688.
34. Woolf, C. J. (1984): Long term alteration in the excitability of the flexion reflex produced by peripheral tissue injury in the chronic decerebrate rat. *Pain*, 18:325–343.

Hyperalgesia and Allodynia,
edited by W. D. Willis, Jr.
Raven Press, Ltd., New York © 1992.

18

Nociceptive Processes in the Spinal Cord Evoked by Acute Arthritis

Hans-Georg Schaible

Institute of Physiology, University of Würzburg, D-8700 Würzburg, Germany

During development of an acute arthritis in the cat's knee joint, spinal neurons with articular input are rendered hyperexcitable. Since this inflammation-evoked hyperexcitability occurs in ascending as well as in nonascending neurons, it may account for the pain sensations in the arthritic joint and the impairment of motor functions associated with an inflammation in the joint (23,41,49). In order to get a better understanding of the spinal nociceptive processes associated with inflammation, detailed studies were carried out to determine the features of this hyperexcitability and the mechanisms involved.

This chapter summarizes some of our studies on the spinal mechanisms of articular nociception with special reference to inflammatory lesions in the joint. The experiments were performed in chloralose-anesthetized cats, most of which were spinalized at the thoracolumbar junction (see below). As a model of arthritis, an acute joint inflammation was used that was induced by the intraarticular injections of kaolin and carrageenan into the knee joint. These compounds evoke an inflammation that develops within 1 to 3 hr. In the awake cat this inflammatory lesion leads to hyperalgesia, which is obvious from limping and quick removal of the leg when the inflamed knee is pressed. The inflammation has a duration of at least 24 hr (45,46).

SPINAL NEURONS WITH INPUT FROM THE KNEE JOINT

A study using the transganglionic transport of horseradish peroxidase showed that afferent fibers of the medial articular and posterior articular nerves (MAN and PAN) projected mainly to the segments L5 to L7. Within these segments projection fields of articular afferents were identified in the cap of lamina I, in laminae V–VI, and in the dorsal part of lamina VII. There was no evidence for a projection into laminae II, III, and IV. A sparse projection was found caudally as far as S2 and rostrally up to L1, with a dense projection of the PAN into the medial portion of Clarke's column (8).

In electrophysiological experiments neurons driven by pressure applied to the knee joint were located in the superficial and deep dorsal horn and also in the ventral horn. They showed either convergent input from the knee and the adjacent deep structures (muscles) or convergent input from the joint, muscles, and the skin (47,48). In the intact spinal cord the neurons usually had receptive fields that were confined to the ipsilateral hindlimb, whereas neurons in the spinalized cord often had an additional receptive field in the contralateral leg (41,44).

Following a commonly used classification (2,13,55), the neurons with articular input were categorized after their response thresholds into nociceptive-specific and wide dynamic range neurons. Neurons with articular input were classified as nociceptive specific if they responded only to noxious compression of the joint and other structures of the hindlimb(s) and to noxious movements of the knee or if they responded mainly to noxious stimuli and showed only a few impulses to some innocuous stimulation (see below). Wide dynamic range neurons had substantial responses to innocuous pressure and movements within the working range of the knee and more pronounced responses to noxious stimulus intensities (41,48). Many nociceptive-specific neurons were located in laminae VII and VIII, and some of them were ascending tract cells. Wide dynamic range neurons were more often found in the deep dorsal horn (41,48). In the cat only a few neurons were recorded in the superficial dorsal horn. A recent study in the rat, however, showed that of superficially located neurons with ankle joint input, about 20% were nociceptive specific, whereas 80% were wide dynamic neurons (Grubb et al., *unpublished observations*).

The borderline between nociceptive-specific and wide dynamic range neurons is not entirely strict since a proportion of the neurons responded strongly to noxious stimuli but showed a few action potentials to innocuous stimuli (see above). A weak response to innocuous stimuli could be evoked, during reversible spinalization, in 10 of 15 neurons in the deep dorsal and ventral horn that responded in the intact spinal cord exclusively to noxious stimulus intensities (44). This suggests that the actual response thresholds of these spinal neurons are controlled by the afferent input as well as by supra- and intraspinal mechanisms. Tonic descending inhibition of spinal neurons with knee input has been demonstrated recently (5,44). In addition to changes in mechanical threshold, the size of the total receptive fields is controlled by supraspinal influences since the excitatory receptive fields expanded to the ipsilateral paw when the cord was cold-blocked in nine of 17 neurons tested (44).

SPINAL NEURONS IN ARTHRITIS

Development of Inflammation-Evoked Hyperexcitability in the Spinalized Cat

Long-term recordings from identified spinal neurons with knee input showed the spectrum of alterations in the discharges evoked by the development of an acute arthritis in the knee (41). Changes in responses were found for stimuli applied to the injected knee, for mechanical stimuli applied to noninflamed regions of the hindlimb(s) adjacent to and remote from the injected knee, and for electrical stimuli applied to peripheral nerves and descending axons in the spinal cord. Examples of two neurons in two experiments are shown in Fig. 18.1. The nociceptive-specific neuron in Fig. 18.1A developed a considerable response to flexion of the injected knee, whereas no responses to flexion of the contralateral normal knee were observed. In parallel the responses to electrical stimuli applied with a constant amplitude to the ipsi- and contralateral sural nerves and descending axons in the spinal cord increased during the development of the inflammation. Similar changes were observed in the wide dynamic range neuron displayed in Fig. 18.1B. In this neuron, however, the

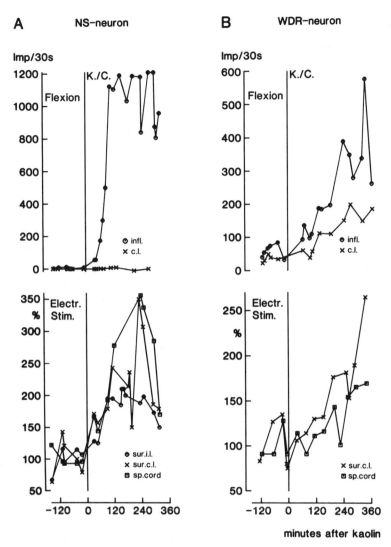

FIG. 18.1. Induction of hyperexcitability in a spinal nociceptive specific neuron (**A**) and in a wide dynamic range neuron (**B**) with knee input during developing inflammation of the knee joint. Both neurons were recorded from for several hours. The top graphs show the responses of these neurons to flexion of the ipsilateral (i.l.) and the contralateral (c.l.) knee. At the time point 0 min the inflammatory compounds kaolin and carrageenan (K./C.) were injected into the ipsilateral knee. The bottom graphs show the responses of these neurons to electrical stimulation of the sural nerve(s) and descending axons in the spinal cord. For electrical stimulation the responses in the control period were averaged and the mean was set to 100%. All values in the control and inflammatory periods were then expressed as percentage of the control mean. The cord was stimulated with impulses of 5 (A) and 3 V (B) (duration 0.2 msec). Stimulation of the sural nerves was sufficient to evoke "A responses" in the spinal neurons (latencies between 10 and 25 msec). Selected voltages were kept constant throughout the experiments. (From ref. 41.)

TABLE 18.1. *Spinal neurons with knee input in the spinalized cord: changes of responsiveness during developing inflammation in the knee*

Altered responsiveness for stimuli applied	Number of neurons
Injected knee only	1/23
Injected knee and adjacent thigh/lower leg	2/23
Injected knee, adjacent thigh/lower leg, and ipsilateral paw	2/23
Injected knee, adjacent thigh/lower leg, ipsilateral paw, and contralateral leg	18/23

responses to flexion of the contralateral normal knee also increased after injection of the ipsilateral joint.

These observations and those made in another 21 neurons with knee input are summarized in Table 18.1. All neurons were located in laminae VI, VII, and VIII, and 15 of 23 neurons had an ascending axon. Nine neurons were classified as nociceptive-specific neurons, 12 cells had a wide dynamic range responsive profile, and two neurons were activated by stimuli applied to the knee, but they were inhibited by most stimuli applied to regions remote from the knee. During the development of inflammation all of these neurons exhibited alterations of the responsiveness to mechanical stimuli applied to the injected knee. In 20 of 23 neurons the responses were also altered for mechanical stimuli applied to regions remote from the inflamed knee. In parallel to the changes in the responsiveness to mechanical peripheral stimuli, increased responses were found for electrical stimuli applied to the sural nerve(s) and descending fibers (tested in four experiments), and in addition ongoing discharges appeared or started to increase in many of the neurons (41).

The spectrum of changes suggests that spinal neurons with joint input are rendered hyperexcitable. These changes are probably induced by afferent discharges from the inflamed joint since a high percentage of myelinated and unmyelinated afferent fibers show a sensitization for mechanical stimulation of the joint, and many of them are becoming spontaneously active (12,17,45,46). The significance of the afferent input is supported by the observation that four neurons without knee input did not change responsiveness to mechanical (and electrical) stimuli during development of inflammation in the knee. Presumably the changes of excitability are not only due to the reception of the afferent barrage but may also result from intraspinal mechanisms. The contribution of central mechanisms to postinjury discharges was recently proposed after the observation that brief stimulation of afferent C fibers may cause changes of excitability in motor reflexes and an expansion of receptive fields in dorsal horn neurons that outlast the actual stimulus (7,58). Expanded receptive fields were also described for lamina I cells in a chronic model of inflammation (28).

Alterations of Descending Inhibition During Development of Inflammation

It is well established that at least under experimental conditions many spinal neurons are under tonic descending inhibitory influences that reduce the spinal nociceptive processing efficiently (for reviews, see refs. 2,16,55,56). This tonic descending inhibition may also determine the size of the receptive fields of the spinal neurons and/or the excitation thresholds (see first paragraph).

From the present knowledge it should be expected that descending inhibitory pathways also inhibit the spinal nociceptive processes evoked by inflammation. It had not been investigated, however, whether tonic descending inhibition is changing during acute inflammation. In order to investigate this matter, the occurrence of hyperexcitability was studied in cats with intact spinal cords, and the effect of descending inhibition was assessed by applying cold blocks at the thoracolumbar junction, which reversibly eliminated the descending influences (44).

Figure 18.2 displays a typical experiment. It shows a nociceptive-specific neuron located in lamina VI that was monitored for several hours during the preinflammatory control period and some hours after the injection of the inflammatory compounds. Within the control period and during the developing inflammation, the cord was reversibly blocked several times. Cooling the cord in the control period led to a disinhibition that was quantitatively reproducible. When the conduction in descending pathways was blocked, the neuron showed resting discharges (Fig. 18.2A) and responses to light pressure applied to normal joint (Fig. 18.2B). The responses to strong pressure were increased (Fig. 18.2B). During developing inflammation the neuron showed some resting discharges, an induction of a response to light compression of the knee, and an increase of the responses to noxious pressure applied to the injected knee. Cooling in the period of developing inflammation revealed a progressive enhancement in the amount of disinhibition: although the activity in the intact state showed some increase per se (as a result of inflammation), the differences between the responses and/or the resting discharges in the intact and spinalized state were augmented as well.

Table 18.2 summarizes the results obtained in 14 neurons in 14 experiments. These neurons were located in laminae IV through VIII; 10 were nociceptive specific and four had a wide dynamic range character. The majority of the neurons tested showed results similar to those the neuron displayed in Fig. 18.2. It was concluded from these experiments that the hyperexcitability evoked by arthritis is counteracted by an increase of the effectiveness of the tonic descending inhibition. It is not known at the moment whether this increase in the effectiveness is due to an increased inflow from supraspinal structures or whether the spinal neurons develop an increased sensitivity for the inhibitory input simultaneously with an increase of sensitivity for the excitatory drive from the periphery.

STUDIES OF MECHANISMS POSSIBLY INVOLVED IN THE HYPEREXCITABILITY OF SPINAL NEURONS

An analysis of the relevant processes is far from complete due to the complex nature of this matter. It is unlikely that these changes in excitability are "unspecific" processes due to changes in the extracellular ion concentration. In a recent study the extracellular concentration of $[K^+]_0$ was measured in the spinal cord using ion-sensitive microelectrodes (24). Rises in $[K^+]_0$ in the spinal gray matter were observed during innocuous stimulation such as brushing of the skin or flexion of the knee joint. Noxious stimuli produced somewhat larger increases in $[K^+]_0$, but this additional component was relatively small: electrical stimulation of the PAN sufficient to excite the unmyelinated axons was only slightly more effective in raising

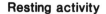

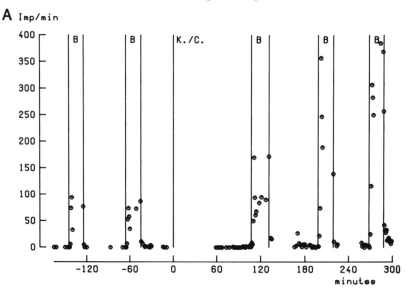

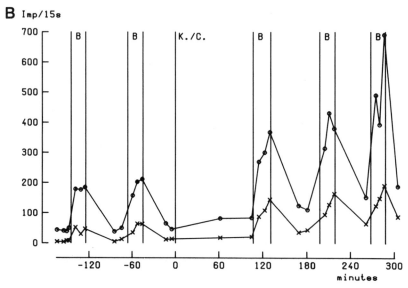

FIG. 18.2. Changes in the tonic descending inhibition of a spinal neuron with knee input during developing inflammation of the knee. The cell was nociceptive specific and located in lamina VI. The recordings were performed prior to the induction of inflammation and postinjection of the inflammatory compounds (K./C.). During the periods indicated by B the spinal cord was cooled at the thoracolumbar junction. In the intervals between, the conduction was not blocked. **A:** Resting discharges counted in impulses per minute (Imp/min). **B:** Responses to light (x) and noxious (o) pressure applied to the knee. The duration of each stimulus was 15 sec. From the total activity during application of the stimulus the resting discharges of the preceding 30 sec were subtracted.

TABLE 18.2. *Changes of responses and ongoing activity in neurons with knee input during developing inflammation in the intact and spinalized state*

	Induction or increase of activity in intact cord (neurons)	Induction or increase of activity in cold blocked state (neurons)	Increase of differences (neurons)
Resting discharges	9/14	12/14	11/14
Responses to flexion of the injected knee	12/14	9/14	8/14
Responses to light compression of the injected knee	12/14	13/14	12/14
Responses to noxious compression of the injected knee	12/14	12/14	12/14

$[K^+]_0$ above the levels reached during electrical stimulation of myelinated group II and III afferents. During development of an acute arthritis (induced by kaolin and carrageenan) stimulus-evoked increases in $[K^+]_0$ became larger by about 25%. The study revealed that the absolute $[K^+]_0$ level reached depended more on the site and type of stimulation than on the actual stimulus intensity itself.

Another argument against a major role of unspecific factors is the observation that neurons without joint input did not change their responsiveness within the first hours of the developing inflammation (41). An unspecific process would probably also affect neurons without knee input. In order to identify mechanisms responsible for the arthritis-induced excitability changes, experiments were performed that examined the involvement of N-methyl-D-aspartate (NMDA) receptors in the activity of hyperexcitable cells. Other experiments started to examine the intraspinal release of neuropeptides during arthritis.

Effects of NMDA Antagonists on the Spinal Discharges Evoked by Acute Inflammation

Involvement of NMDA receptors in the processing of nociceptive information was discussed recently (cf. ref. 1). Although the "normal processing" of afferent impulses in the spinal cord is effectively blocked by non-NMDA antagonists, a contribution of NMDA receptors has been ascribed to the "windup" phenomenon, which may occur after repetitive stimulation of C fibers (10,11,52). With noxious mechanical stimulation, suppression of neuronal responses was reported in the ventral but not in the dorsal horn (22). In other studies there was no involvement of NMDA receptors in the processing of noxious information in the dorsal horn under "normal circumstances," but a contribution of NMDA mechanisms to nociception-associated discharges was observed after formalin injection into the paw (20) and after occlusion of the femoral artery (50). These observations suggest that particular conditions may be required for an involvement of NMDA receptors in the nociceptive processing in the spinal cord. Specific requirements for the activation of NMDA channels have been demonstrated in biophysical studies (34,39).

In a series of experiments we tested whether the activity in neurons with input from an inflamed knee could be suppressed by the application of NMDA antagonists that were applied intravenously and/or ionophoretically. We chose D-2-amino-5-phosphonovalerate (APV) as a competitive antagonist and ketamine as a noncompetitive one. As in our previous studies the neurons were located in the deep dorsal and ventral horn. Some cells were ascending tract neurons (40; Schaible et al., *unpublished observations*).

NMDA antagonists had suppressive effects on about 70% of the neurons tested. These effects consisted of a reduction in either the ongoing discharges or the responses to mechanical stimulation of the knee such as flexion. Table 18.3 gives a summary of the results of this study. Most effective was the intravenous injection of ketamine. Less effective was the focal ionophoretic application of this compound. This may be due to technical reasons (NMDA receptors not reached by the antagonist), but it could also indicate that some neurons had no NMDA receptors. Ionophoretically applied APV, however, reduced the activity in most neurons tested with this compound.

In some neurons specificity of the compounds for NMDA receptors was assessed by testing them against ionophoretically applied NMDA and quisqualate. The doses of ketamine used in these experiments were specific for NMDA receptors, and the same was found for APV except for the observation that it reduced responses to quisqualate in some cases when high ejection currents (>50 nA) were used.

These results show that an NMDA–receptor-associated component is active in hyperexcitable cells. They do not exclude a contribution of NMDA receptors to the activity in these neurons under normal conditions, although an effect of NMDA receptor antagonists on responses to innocuous stimuli has not been reported. In order to show a contribution of the NMDA receptors in the generation of the arthritis-evoked hyperexcitability, some neurons were recorded from during the development of the arthritis, and NMDA antagonists were applied thereafter to assess their effect on these inflammation-induced discharges. An example is shown in Fig. 18.3. This neuron was located in lamina VIII, had an ascending axon and was nociceptive spe-

TABLE 18.3. *Effects of NMDA antagonists on the activity of spinal neurons with afferent input from the inflamed knee joint*

	Intravenous ketamine (neurons)	Ionophoretic ketamine (neurons)	Ionophoretic APV (neurons)
Reduction of ongoing activity and responses to flexion	18/26	2/21	6/24
Reduction of ongoing activity; no change of flexion response	5/26	5/21	4/24
Reduction of flexion response; no change of ongoing discharges	1/26	4/21	2/24
Reduction of ongoing discharges; flexion not tested	1/26	0/21	5/24
No effect on ongoing activity and no effect on responses to flexion	1/26	10/21	7/24

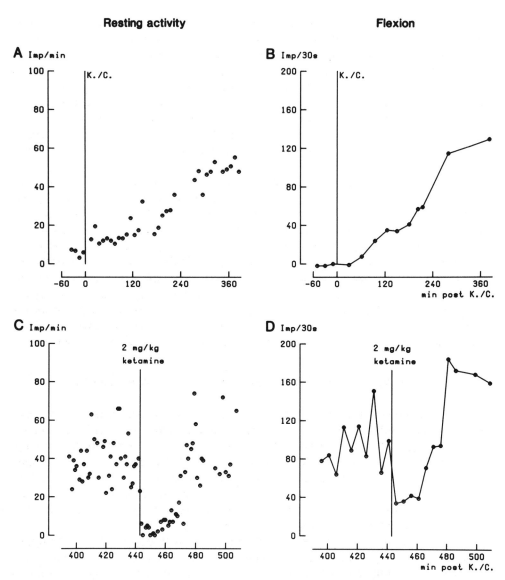

FIG. 18.3. Effects of intravenous ketamine on the inflammation-evoked discharges in an ascending nociceptive-specific neuron located in lamina VIII. **A:** Increase of the resting discharges during developing inflammation. The graph shows the mean values in periods of 10 min prior to inflammation and postinjection of the inflammatory compounds (K./C.). **B:** Increase of flexion-evoked responses after injection of the inflammatory compounds. The duration of each flexion was 30 sec. **C:** Reduction of the inflammation-evoked resting discharges by intravenous ketamine. Each value corresponds to 1 min. **D:** Effect of ketamine on the inflammation-evoked flexion responses.

cific with receptive fields in the deep tissue of both hindlimbs. During developing inflammation responses were induced to flexion of the injected knee, but a smaller response was also induced to flexion of the contralateral normal knee. In addition the neuron showed an expansion of its excitatory receptive field during inflammation. The inflammation-evoked resting discharges are displayed in Fig. 18.3A, and the induction of the responses to flexion of the injected knee is shown in Fig. 18.3B. Intravenous ketamine in an NMDA–receptor-specific dose (2 mg/kg) reduced the inflammation-evoked resting discharges (Fig. 18.3C) and the responses to flexion (Fig. 18.3D). The suppression was maximal within a few minutes and then the activity recovered.

Since the NMDA antagonists suppressed activity within minutes after or during their application, they must have interfered with ongoing events, most likely by reducing a tonic synaptic activation of NMDA receptors. This suggests that hyperexcitability of spinal neurons in arthritis is, at least in part, a process that is dependent on continuous synaptic activation of NMDA receptors. Since NMDA receptors allow the inflow of calcium into the neurons (32,33,57), the activation of NMDA receptors may be important for the state of neuronal excitability by regulation of the intracellular calcium content. The effects of the NMDA antagonists on the hyperexcitable neurons during arthritis could thus result either from a direct contribution of NMDA receptors to the depolarization of the neurons or from a reduction of the calcium influx, which may reduce excitability of the neurons by intracellular events.

Intraspinal Release of Tachykinins Evoked by an Acute Arthritis

Using antibody-bearing microprobes (15,25), the intraspinal release of immunoreactive substance P (ir-SP) and immunoreactive neurokinin A (ir-NKA) was investigated during development of an acute arthritis in the knee (27,43). Both neuropeptides were found in afferent fibers of the knee joint (21; Hanesch et al., *unpublished observations*). The antibody microprobe technique allows a spatial resolution of the release and presence of a neuropeptide in defined areas and depths of the spinal cord (15,25). Due to their relatively atraumatic nature, microprobes are suitable to identify the stimulus conditions under which neuropeptides are released.

For the recognition of SP three different antisera were used for coating the probes: (a) a rabbit polyclonal antiserum directed against the C terminus of SP, (b) a rabbit polyclonal antiserum directed against the N terminus of SP, (c) a rat monoclonal antibody directed against the C terminus of SP. For detection of NKA a polyclonal antibody was used for coating. This antibody had, however, a 100% crossreactivity with neuropeptide K (an N terminal extended form of NKA).

Release of Immunoreactive Substance P

In 10 cats 115 antibody-bearing microprobes were inserted to a depth of 4 mm in the segments L5–L7. With the normal joint there was no evidence for intraspinal release of ir-SP neither during periods of "no stimulation" nor periods in which the joint was repeatedly flexed and extended or pressed with innocuous intensity. With joint inflammation different results were obtained. In seven of 10 cats release of ir-SP was found on probes that were inserted following induction of joint inflammation. The time point for the first SP release varied from 2 to 10 hr with a mean time of 6.5 hr after injection of the knee.

Figure 18.4 shows the averaged images of two groups of microprobes bearing N–terminus-directed antibodies to SP. All these probes were from "posttransitional" periods, i.e., they were in the cord after ir-SP had been detected for the first time in the experiment, at various times after injection of the inflammatory compounds (see last paragraph). Figure 18.4A shows the averaged image of probes present in the cord during periods of no stimulation, Fig. 18.4B displays the image of probes of periods in which the inflamed joint was flexed, and Fig. 18.4C shows the differences between these groups and the statistical analysis. Probes present in the cord during flexion of the knee showed a marked inhibition of binding of radioactive [^{125}I]SP from the surface of the cord to about 1.5 mm (corresponding to lamina V), which indicates binding of ir-SP in the spinal cord. Probes present in the cord during periods of "no joint movement" also showed some inhibition, but this was only seen at the surface of the cord. The statistical analysis shows a significant difference between the "no joint movement" and the "joint flexion" group, from the surface to a depth of about 1.5 mm with a peak at about 0.8 mm, which corresponds to lamina I in the cat. This pattern indicates flexion-evoked release of ir-SP mainly in the superficial dorsal horn.

Microprobes bearing C–terminus-directed antibodies showed a similar result. The presence of ir-SP at the cord surface was even more pronounced. During joint inflammation release of SP was also evoked by pressure applied to the knee and twisting the joint. The pattern was similar to that evoked by flexion, i.e., significant presence was found in the superficial dorsal horn and in the region up to the surface. Individual probes, however, showed release in the deep dorsal horn as well.

Release of Immunoreactive Neurokinin A

There was some basal release of ir-NKA, which was detected by probes present in the cord during periods of "no stimulation." Flexion of the normal joint did not cause additional release of ir-NKA. The pattern was different when the joint was inflamed. In this situation ir-NKA was detected by the whole length of the probe, i.e., from the surface of the spinal cord to the ventral horn, suggesting diffuse presence of the peptide in several laminae. Figure 18.5 shows averaged images of probes present in the spinal cord during periods of "no stimulation." Compared to the baseline in the preinjection period (Fig. 18.5A), there was a marked inhibition of binding of [^{125}I]NKA on probes that had been in the cord for 30 min during the indicated times postinjection of the inflammatory compounds (Fig. 18.5B and C).

In later stages this pattern was almost identical, whether the inflamed joint was stimulated mechanically or left unstimulated, i.e., there was no obvious dependency of the release of ir-NKA on the presence of peripheral mechanical stimulation. This diffuse presence of ir-NKA was found after a transitory period following injection of the inflammatory compounds in which ir-NKA was mainly detected focally in the superficial dorsal horn and at the surface of the spinal cord. This suggests that ir-NKA was diffusing within the gray and white matter.

The main differences between the release of ir-SP and ir-NKA are displayed in Table 18.4. At first sight it is difficult to explain why ir-NKA and ir-SP should be

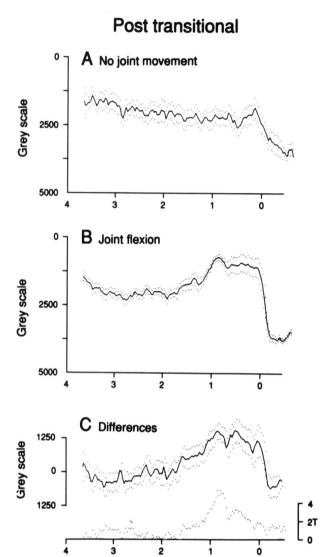

FIG. 18.4. Detection of ir-SP in the spinal cord during arthritis in the knee. The graphs display averaged images of microprobes bearing N–terminus-directed antibodies to SP that had been inserted in the spinal cord and then incubated in a solution with [^{125}I]SP overnight. Each graph shows the mean gray density (*solid line*) ± S.E.M. (*dots*) of the radioactive images along the length of the probes that had been inserted in the spinal cord to a depth of 4 mm (see x-axis, the surface of the cord corresponds to 0 mm). Inhibition of binding of radioactive peptide (reduction of the gray density) is equated with previous binding of peptide released in the cord. All probes were present in the spinal cord for periods of 30 min in the "posttransitional" period (see text). **A:** Probes ($n = 9$) inserted in periods of "no joint movement." These probes show an image that is similar to that of probes that have bound [^{125}I]SP without preincubation in the nonradioactive ligand. **B:** Probes ($n = 6$) present in the spinal cord while the inflamed joint was flexed and extended. These probes show inhibition of binding of radioactive peptide (reduced gray density) in the superficial part of the spinal cord indicating previous binding of SP in the cord. **C:** Differences between the images in A and B and statistical analysis of intervals of 30 μm. 2T and 4T correspond to the 5% and 1% level in Student's *t*-test. (From ref. 43.)

Developing arthritis & no movement

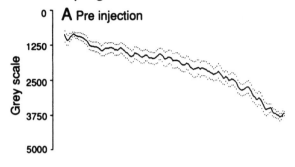

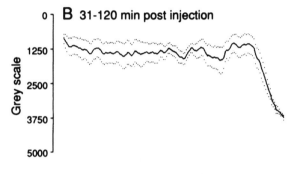

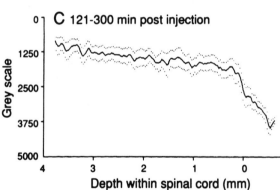

FIG. 18.5. Detection of ir-NKA in the spinal cord during joint inflammation. The graphs show averaged images of microprobes bearing antibodies to NKA. All probes were in the spinal cord with the tip at a depth of 4 mm for periods of 30 min and then incubated in [^{125}I]NKA, which produced the autoradiographic images of the probes. The principles of the analysis and the display are the same as in Fig. 18.4. While these probes were in the cord, no mechanical stimulation was performed, but the knee joint was either normal (seven probes in A) or inflamed (10 probes in B and eight in C). Compared to the probes in A, the probes in B and C show a broad zone of inhibition of binding of the radioactive NKA, indicating previous binding of endogenous ir-NKA in the cord. (From ref. 27.)

released at different times postinjection of the inflammatory compounds since both tachykinins are coexistent in primary afferents (9). There is the possibility that ir-NKA was better detected by higher sensitivity of the antibody to NKA, whereas ir-SP escaped detection in the early stage. An alternative explanation is that SP is released and rapidly degraded, whereas NKA is more resistant to degradation. In fact this has been shown for SP and NKA in plasma where the latter is resistant to peptidases and the former is rapidly degraded (51). This difference in the degradation rate may also account for the different pattern of these peptides in the spinal cord. NKA may diffuse widely, whereas SP is degraded and prevented from diffusion, at least in the time range covered by these experiments.

The present results indicate that ir-SP was predominantly released from high-threshold afferents. There was no detectable stimulus-evoked release during innoc-

TABLE 18.4. *Intraspinal release of tachykinins in arthritis*

Conditions of release	Substance P	Neurokinin A
Normal knee joint		
Basal release	0	+
Release evoked by flexion of the knee	0	0
Inflamed knee joint		
Basal release	0	+
Release evoked by flexion of the knee	+	?
Presence of neuropeptide		
First appearance	2–10 hr postinjection, (mean: 6.5 hr)	0–30 min postinjection
Location in the cord		
Surface of the cord	+	+
Dorsal columns	+	+
Superficial dorsal horn	+	+
Deep dorsal horn	Some probes	+
Ventral horn	Some probes	+

0, no release; +, release; ?, not known.

uous stimulation of the normal joint (flexion), but release was achieved by these stimuli when the joint was inflamed. During joint inflammation high-threshold afferents and initially mechanically insensitive afferents are sensitized and respond now to innocuous mechanical stimuli such as flexion (45,46). Since SP was mainly released in a stimulus-dependent mode, it may have a role in the stimulus-related processing of nociceptive discharges from the inflamed joint. It is unlikely, however, that SP is critical in the early stages of the inflammation-evoked hyperexcitability, since it was detected at the earliest in stages in which the spinal neurons are already hyperexcitable (see Fig. 18.1). SP may play a dominant role in chronic stages of inflammation. In the polyarthritic rat the content of SP is enhanced in peripheral nerves and dorsal root ganglia (6,31) and in the spinal cord (38). During chronic polyarthritis SP is released in the spinal cord by stimuli that normally do not cause release of this peptide (42). These observations suggest a tonic activation of tachykininergic neurons in polyarthritis. The distribution of ir-NKA within the spinal cord shows that peripheral stimulation may lead to release of compounds that persist in the cord beyond the period of stimulation (see also ref. 14). The function of NKA is not known, but presumably it may have a tonic modulatory rather than a stimulus-related effect.

CONCLUDING REMARKS

These studies suggest that different mechanisms may contribute to the hyperexcitability of spinal neurons during developing arthritis. The experimental evidence is insufficiently complete to provide a profound understanding of the possible interactions between the different consequences of an acute inflammation. The present data show, however, that afferent, spinal, and supraspinal components are changing in a synchronized way with a balance of excitatory and inhibitory mechanisms. Of special significance could be the presence of neuropeptides that may be released from afferent fibers and persist in the spinal cord for minutes and up to hours after release.

In the long-term range of days and weeks these changes may become more pronounced and further modified. In the chronic polyarthritic and monoarthritic rat there is a sensitization of joint afferents over weeks (18,19) and excitatory and inhibitory changes have been described in the dorsal horn of the spinal cord in the polyarthritic rat (3,4,35). In addition to electrophysiological alterations neurochemical changes have been reported that may provide the base for these long-term changes under chronic conditions. In addition to higher contents of SP (see last paragraph) dorsal roots of polyarthritic rats contain higher amounts of calcitonin gene-related peptide (30), and pronounced alterations have also been described in these animals for endogenous opioid peptides in the spinal cord (26,29,36,37,53,54). The functional role of these neurochemical changes has still to be determined.

REFERENCES

1. Aanonsen, L. M., Lei, S., and Wilcox, G. L. (1990): Excitatory amino acid receptors and nociceptive neurotransmission in rat spinal cord. *Pain*, 41:309–321.
2. Besson, J.-M., and Chaouch, A. (1987): Peripheral and spinal mechanisms of nociception. *Physiol. Rev.*, 67:67–186.
3. Calvino, B., Villanueva, L., and LeBars, D. (1987): Dorsal horn (convergent) neurons in the intact anaesthetized arthritic rat. I. Segmental excitatory influences. *Pain*, 28:81–98.
4. Calvino, B., Villanueva, L., and LeBars, D. (1987): Dorsal horn (convergent) neurones in the intact anaesthetized arthritic rat. II. Heterotopic inhibitory influences. *Pain*, 31:359–379.
5. Cervero, F., Schaible, H.-G., and Schmidt, R. F. (1991): Tonic descending inhibition of spinal cord neurones driven by joint afferents in normal cats and in cats with an inflamed knee joint. *Exp. Brain Res.*, 83:675–678.
6. Colpaert, F. C., Donnerer, J., and Lembeck, F. (1983): Effects of capsaicin on inflammation and on the substance P content of nervous tissues in rats with adjuvant arthritis. *Life Sci.*, 32:1827–1834.
7. Cook, A. J., Woolf, C. J., Wall, P. D., and McMahon, S. B. (1987): Dynamic receptive field plasticity in rat spinal cord dorsal horn following C-primary afferent input. *Nature*, 325:151–153.
8. Craig, A.D., Heppelmann, B., and Schaible, H.-G. (1988): The projection of the medial and posterior articular nerves of cat's knee to the spinal cord. *J. Comp. Neurol.*, 276:279–288.
9. Dalsgaard, C.-J., Haegerstrand, A., Theodorsson-Norheim, E., Brodin, E., and Hökfelt, T. (1985): Neurokinin A-like immunoreactivity in rat primary sensory neurons: coexistence with substance P. *Histochemistry*, 83:37–40.
10. Davies, S. N., and Lodge, D. (1987): Evidence for involvement of N-methylaspartate receptors in 'wind-up' of class 2 neurones in the dorsal horn of the rat. *Brain Res.*, 424:402–406.
11. Dickenson, A. H., and Sullivan, A. F. (1990): Differential effects of excitatory amino acid antagonists on dorsal horn nociceptive neurones in the rat. *Brain Res.*, 506:31–39.
12. Dorn, T., Schaible, H.-G., and Schmidt, R. F. (1991): Response properties of thick myelinated group II afferents in the medial articular nerve of normal and inflamed knee joints of the cat. *Somatosens. Mot. Res.*, 8:127–136.
13. Dubner, R., and Bennett, G. J. (1983): Spinal and trigeminal mechanisms of nociception. *Annu. Rev. Neurosci.*, 6:381–418.
14. Duggan, A. W., Hope, P. J., Jarrott, B., Schaible, H.-G., and Fleetwood-Walker, S. M. (1990): Release, spread and persistence of immunoreactive neurokinin A in the dorsal horn of the cat following noxious cutaneous stimulation. Studies with antibody microprobes. *Neuroscience*, 35:195–202.
15. Duggan, A. W., Hendry, I. A., Green, J. L., Morton, C. R., and Hutchison, W. D. (1988): The preparation and use of antibody microprobes. *J. Neurosci. Meth.*, 23:241–247.
16. Fields, H. L., and Basbaum, A. J. (1978): Brainstem control of spinal pain transmission neurons. *Annu. Rev. Physiol.*, 40:217–248.
17. Grigg, P., Schaible, H.-G., and Schmidt, R. F. (1986): Mechanical sensitivity of group III and IV afferents from posterior articular nerve in normal and inflamed cat knee. *J. Neurophysiol.*, 55:635–643.
18. Guilbaud, G., Iggo, A., and Tegner, R. (1985): Sensory receptors in ankle joint capsules of normal and arthritic rats. *Exp. Brain Res.*, 58:29–40.
19. Grubb, B. D., Birrell, J., McQueen, D. S., and Iggo, A. (1991): The role of PG E2 in the sensitization of mechanoreceptors in normal and inflamed ankle joints of the rat. *Exp. Brain Res.*, 84:383–392.

20. Haley, J. E., Sullivan, A. F., and Dickenson, A. H. (1990): Evidence for spinal N-methyl-D-aspartate involvement in prolonged chemical nociception in the rat. *Brain Res.*, 518:218–226.
21. Hanesch, U., Heppelmann, B., and Schmidt, R. F. (1991): Substance P- and calcitonin gene-related peptide-immunoreactivity in primary afferent neurons of the cat's knee joint. *Neuroscience*, 45:185–193.
22. Headley, P. M., Parsons, C. G., and West, D. C. (1987): The role of N-methylaspartate receptors in mediating responses of rat and cat spinal neurones to defined sensory stimuli. *J. Physiol. (Lond.)*, 385:169–188.
23. He, X., Proske, U., Schaible, H.-G., and Schmidt, R. F. (1988): Acute inflammation of the knee joint in the cat alters responses of flexor motoneurones to leg movements. *J. Neurophysiol.*, 59:326–340.
24. Heinemann, U., Schaible, H.-G., and Schmidt, R. F. (1990): Changes in extracellular potassium concentration in cat spinal cord in response to innocuous and noxious stimulation of legs with healthy and inflamed knee joints. *Exp. Brain Res.*, 79:283–292.
25. Hendry, I. A., Morton, C. R., and Duggan, A. W. (1988): Analysis of antibody microprobe autoradiographs by computerized image processing. *J. Neurosci. Meth.*, 23:249–256.
26. Höllt, V., Haarmann, J., Millan, M. J., and Herz, A. (1987): Prodynorphin gene expression is enhanced in the spinal cord of chronic arthritic rats. *Neurosci. Lett.*, 73:90–94.
27. Hope, P. J., Jarrott, B., Schaible, H.-G., Clarke, R. W., and Duggan, A. W. (1990): Release and spread of immunoreactive neurokinin A in the cat spinal cord in a model of acute arthritis. *Brain Res.*, 533:292–299.
28. Hylden, J. L. K., Nahin, R., Traub, R. J., and Dubner, R. (1989): Expansion of receptive fields of spinal lamina I projection neurons in rats with unilateral adjuvant-induced inflammation; the contribution of dorsal horn mechanisms. *Pain*, 37:229–243.
29. Iadarola, M. J., Douglass, J., Civelli, O., and Naranjo, J. R. (1988): Differential activation of spinal cord dynorphin and enkephalin neurons during hyperalgesia: evidence using cDNA hybridization. *Brain Res.*, 455:205–212.
30. Kuraishi, Y., Nanayama, T., Ohno, H., Fujii, N., Otaka, A., Yajima, H., and Satoh, M. (1989): Calcitonin gene-related peptide increases in the dorsal root ganglia of adjuvant arthritic rat. *Peptides*, 10:447–452.
31. Lembeck, F., Donnerer, J., Colpaert, F. C. (1981): Increase of substance P in primary afferent nerves during chronic pain. *Neuropeptides*, 1:175–180.
32. MacDermott, A. B., Mayer, M. L., Westbrook, G. L., Smith, S. J., and Barker, J. L. (1986): NMDA-receptor activation increases cytoplasmic calcium concentration in cultured spinal cord neurons. *Nature*, 321:519–522.
33. Mayer, M. L., MacDermott, A. B., Westbrook, G. L., Smith, S. J., and Barker, J. L. (1987): Agonist- and voltage-gated calcium entry in cultured mouse spinal cord neurons under voltage clamp measured using arsenazo III. *J. Neurosci.*, 7:3230–3244.
34. Mayer, M. L., and Westbrook, G. L. (1987): The physiology of excitatory amino acids in the vertebrate central nervous system. *Prog. Neurobiol.*, 28:197–276.
35. Menetrey, D., and Besson, J.-M. (1982): Electrophysiological characteristics of dorsal horn cells in rats with cutaneous inflammation resulting from chronic arthritis. *Pain*, 13:343–364.
36. Millan, M. J., Czlongkowski, A., Pilcher, C. W. T., et al. (1987): A model of chronic pain in the rat: functional correlates of alterations in the activity of opioid systems. *J. Neurosci.*, 7:77–87.
37. Millan, M. J., Millan, M. H., Pilcher, C. W. T., Czlongkowski, A., Herz, A., and Colpaert, F. C. (1985): Spinal cord dynorphin may modulate nociception via a κ-opioid receptor in chronic arthritic rats. *Brain Res.*, 340:156–159.
38. Minami, M., Kuraishi, Y., Kuwamura, M., et al. (1989): Enhancement of preprotachykinin A gene expression by adjuvant-induced inflammation in the rat spinal cord: possible involvement of substance P-containing spinal neurons in nociception. *Neurosci. Lett.*, 98:105–110.
39. Monaghan, D. T., Bridges, R. J., and Cotman, C. W. (1989): The excitatory amino acid receptors: their classes, pharmacology and distinct properties in the function of the central nervous system. *Annu. Rev. Pharmacol. Toxicol.*, 29:365–402.
40. Neugebauer, V., and Schaible, H.-G. (1988): Ketamine depresses inflammation-induced activity in spinal neurons with articular input. *Pflugers Arch.*, 412:R62.
41. Neugebauer, V., and Schaible, H.-G. (1990): Evidence for a central component in the sensitization of spinal neurons with joint input during development of acute arthritis in cat's knee. *J. Neurophysiol.*, 64:299–311.
42. Oku, R., Satoh, M., and Tagaki, H. (1987): Release of substance P from the spinal dorsal horn is enhanced in polyarthritic rats. *Neurosci. Lett.*, 74:315–319.
43. Schaible, H.-G., Jarrott, B., Hope, P. J., and Duggan, A. W. (1990): Release of immunoreactive substance P in the cat spinal cord during development of acute arthritis in cat's knee: a study with antibody bearing microprobes. *Brain Res.*, 529:214–223.
44. Schiable, H.-G., Neugebauer, V., Cervero, F., and Schmidt, R. F. (1991): Changes in tonic de-

scending inhibition of spinal neurons with articular input during the development of acute arthritis in the cat. *J. Neurophysiol.*, 66:1021–1033.

45. Schaible, H.-G., and Schmidt, R. F. (1985): Effects of an experimental arthritis on the sensory properties of fine articular afferent units. *J. Neurophysiol.*, 54:1109–1122.

46. Schaible, H.-G., and Schmidt, R. F. (1988): Time course of mechanosensitivity changes in articular afferents during a developing experimental arthritis. *J. Neurophysiol.*, 60:2180–2195.

47. Schaible, H.-G., Schmidt, R. F., and Willis, W. D. (1986): Responses of spinal cord neurones to stimulation of articular afferent fibres in the cat. *J. Physiol. (Lond.)*, 372:575–593.

48. Schaible, H.-G., Schmidt, R. F., and Willis, W. D. (1987): Convergent inputs from articular, cutaneous and muscle receptors onto ascending tract cells in the cat spinal cord. *Exp. Brain Res.*, 66:479–488.

49. Schaible, H.-G., Schmidt, R. F., Willis, W. D. (1987): Enhancement of the responses of ascending tract cells in the cat spinal cord by acute inflammation of the knee joint. *Exp. Brain Res.*, 66:489–499.

50. Sher, G., and Mitchell, D. (1990): N-methyl-D-aspartate receptors mediate responses of rat dorsal horn neurons to hindlimb ischemia. *Brain Res.*, 522:55–62.

51. Theodorsson-Norheim, E., Hemson, A., Brodin, E., and Lundberg, J. M. (1987): Sample handling techniques when analyzing regulatory peptides. *Life Sci.*, 41:845–848.

52. Thompson, S. W. N., King, A. E., and Woolf, C. J. (1990): Activity-dependent changes in rat ventral horn neurons in vitro; summation of prolonged afferent evoked postsynaptic depolarizations produce a D-2-amino-5-phosphonovaleric acid sensitive windup. *Eur. J. Neurosci.*, 2:638–649.

53. Weihe, E., Millan, M. J., Höllt, V., Nohr, D., and Herz, A. (1989): Induction of the gene encoding prodynorphin by experimentally induced arthritis enhances staining for dynorphin in the spinal cord of rats. *Neuroscience*, 31:77–95.

54. Weihe, E., Millan, M. J., Leibold, A., Nohr, D., and Herz, A. (1988): Colocalization of proenkephalin and prodynorphin-derived opioid peptides in laminae IV/V spinal neurons revealed in arthritic rats. *Neurosci. Lett.*, 85:187–192.

55. Willis, W. D. (1985): *The pain system. The neural basis of nociceptive transmission in the mammalian nervous system.* Karger, Basel.

56. Willis, W. D. (1988): Anatomy and physiology of descending control of nociceptive responses of dorsal horn neurons: a comprehensive review. *Prog. Brain Res.*, 77:1–29.

57. Womack, M. D., MacDermott, A. B., and Jessell, T. M. (1988): Sensory transmitters regulate intracellular calcium in dorsal horn neurons. *Nature*, 334:351–353.

58. Woolf, C. J. (1983): Evidence for a central component of post-injury pain hypersensitivity. *Nature*, 306:686–688.

Hyperalgesia and Allodynia,
edited by W. D. Willis, Jr.
Raven Press, Ltd., New York © 1992.

19

Excitability Changes in Central Neurons Following Peripheral Damage

Role of Central Sensitization in the Pathogenesis of Pain

Clifford J. Woolf

*Department of Anatomy and Developmental Biology, University College London,
London WC1E 6BT, England*

One of the most disturbing features of clinical pain states is the presence of tenderness, a state of increased pain sensitivity. The production of this hypersensitivity or hyperalgesia represents a dramatic conversion of the normal situation where pain is only produced by intense, potentially damaging, or noxious stimuli to a pathological state where low intensity, or what would normally be innocuous, stimuli begin to produce pain. The contribution of changes in the transducer sensitivity of high-threshold primary afferent nociceptors, peripheral sensitization to hyperalgesia, is reviewed elsewhere in this volume. In this chapter I will review work that my colleagues and I have performed over the past 10 years that has shown that peripheral inputs, particularly those related to peripheral tissue damage and inflammation, have the capacity to modify the excitability of neurons within the spinal cord and that these changes constitute a state of central sensitization. I will show that alterations in the receptive field properties of dorsal horn neurons parallel changes in pain sensation in humans and that we are beginning to appreciate the cellular mechanisms involved in this form of activity-dependent plasticity.

BEHAVIORAL STUDIES

The 1970s were an important decade for pain research for two reasons. The first was the growing appreciation, as a direct result of the Melzack-Wall spinal gate control theory, that neurons in the spinal cord were subject to local and descending controlling influences. The second was the discovery of opiate receptors and their endogenous ligands. The combination of these two led to an intensive search for evidence for a tonic modulation by the endogenous opioid system of the reaction by the central nervous system to noxious stimuli. The major approach was to use the narcotic antagonist naloxone to see if changes in pain sensitivity occurred. The simplicity of this approach was unfortunately inadequate for unraveling the complexity of a system containing different opioid receptor subtypes, local opiate actions in the spinal cord and brain, and a complex combination of tonic and phasic control systems. As a consequence a bewildering set of contradictory results emerged with hyperalgesia, analgesia, and biphasic changes reported following naloxone (24). Our own studies using the intrathecal administration of naloxone in the rat found that a low dose of naloxone produced a small analgesia, but at higher doses a hyperalgesia occurred (15) (Fig. 19.1). At the highest doses the latency of a rat to withdraw its tail from a water bath at 49°C was reduced by over half, and these animals also exhibited an exaggerated escape response to a standard pinch stimulus. Although these results indicated that in the absence of any peripheral damage, it was possible to produce hyperalgesia, this hyperalgesia represented a reduction in nociceptive threshold, not the generation of nociceptive responses by innocuous inputs. This implied that the level of sensitivity, or gain of the nociceptive system, was controlled to some extent by endogenous opioids in the spinal cord.

An extension of this study was an investigation of the response of rats to intrathecal morphine at a wide range of doses (16). A quite unexpected finding was that at high doses, the morphine, instead of producing antinociception, produced hyperalgesia (Fig. 19.1). This hyperalgesia was not naloxone reversible and was only partially stereospecific. A similar effect could be produced by low doses of morphine-3-glucuronide. Almost identical results were later reported by Yaksh and Harty in 1988 (30). In contrast to the hyperalgesia associated with intrathecal naloxone, high-dose intrathecal morphine produced a state where innocuous stimuli, such as light touch, brush, or puffs of air elicited vigorous flexion withdrawal reflexes and coor-

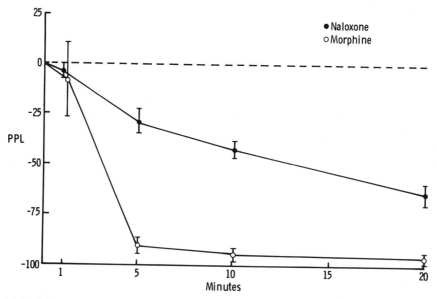

FIG. 19.1. A demonstration of the hyperalgesic effect of high-dose intrathecal naloxone (100 μg) and morphine (150 μg) on the response latency of rats to the hot water (40°C) tail immersion test. Pretrial latencies were found for each animal before the experiment. The animals were then injected intrathecally with the drug in 10 μl over 1 min and the tail latencies remeasured at 1, 5, 10, 15, and 20 min. Results are expressed as percentage changes from pretrial latencies (PPL), each animal acting as its own control. Results are mean ± SEM. (Modified from refs. 15, 16).

dinated escape responses. Similar effects were produced by heating the tail to 40°C. This was a true allodynia and was restricted to the dermatome in the vicinity of the injection cannula, lasting from 20 to 35 min after the injection. These results showed that in addition to the control of nociceptive responsiveness by local inhibitory systems, the differences between the high-intensity stimulus–pain system and the low-intensity stimulus–innocuous sensation system were not absolute. It was possible by a pharmacological manipulation to create a state where pain-like reactions could be generated by completely innocuous inputs. Such pharmacological changes have since then also been shown to be produced by gamma-aminobutyric acid and glycine antagonists (29). My work in this field since then has essentially been a search for the natural stimuli that can precipitate such centrally mediated allodynia and an attempt to discover the mechanisms involved.

The first step was to study the reaction of rats to peripheral damage and inflammation. For ethical reasons these experiments were performed in chronic decerebrate rats (18). These rats possess intact brain stem and spinal reflexes. Mild noxious cutaneous thermal and mechanical stimuli of an intensity that does not produce damage evoked transient flexion withdrawal reflexes, vocalization, and coordinated escape responses. Localized tissue damage by thermal or chemical means produced long-term (up to 6 weeks) changes in the thresholds and responsiveness of the flexion reflex ipsilateral and contralateral to the injury. Figure 19.2 shows an example of the reduction in mechanical thresholds produced, in this case by an intraplantar injection of the irritant turpentine oil. Twenty-four hours after the injection, the hindpaw was swollen and red, and the von Frey threshold for eliciting a flexion reflex had fallen both on the ipsi- and contralateral foot. The increase in sensitivity was such that

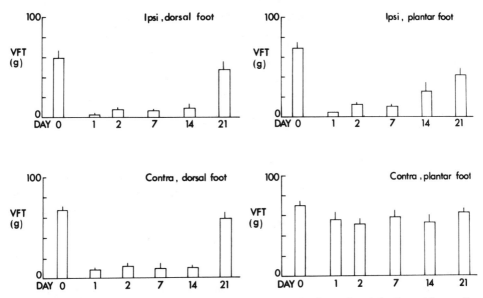

FIG. 19.2. Behavioral effects of inflammatory lesions. The effect of an injection of turpentine into a paw of five decerebrate rats to produce a focal sterile inflammatory lesion on the mechanical thresholds for eliciting flexion from the feet both ipsilateral (ipsi) and contralateral (contra) to the injection. Note the substantial and sustained change in sensitivity both ipsi- and contralateral to the lesion. (From ref. 18.)

innocuous stimuli could now evoke reflexes. These observations show that by pharmacological means and tissue injury it is possible to reproduce allodynia in experimental situations in laboratory animals.

PRIMARY AFFERENT TRIGGERS FOR THE PRODUCTION OF CENTRAL SENSITIZATION

Following the behavioral studies, electrophysiological investigations were performed to assess changes in reflex sensitivity produced by peripheral damage in terms of the response properties of single motor neurons. These studies were carried out following both acute (17) and prolonged inflammation (22). Acute thermal injury in a decerebrate-spinal rat results in an increase in the spontaneous activity of flexor motor neurons, a reduction in threshold, and an increase in responsiveness (Fig. 19.3) (17). Similar results were found when studying flexor motor neurons ipsilateral to a turpentine inflammation made days before (22). In both cases the high-threshold phasic reflex was effectively changed by the peripheral inflammatory lesion into a low-threshold tonic one. Comparable changes in primary afferents innervating the vicinity of the peripheral injury were not found (22).

It was naturally important to see how and where these changes were operating. One approach to answer this was to attempt to duplicate the effects of acute peripheral tissue damage by brief electrical stimulation of a peripheral nerve. Using the flexor reflex, Dr. Wall and I showed that, provided the stimulus strength was sufficient to activate the unmyelinated C afferents, a brief (20 sec), low-frequency (1 Hz) stimulus applied to a nerve produced a large increase in the excitability of the reflex (13). Of particular interest was the finding that the duration of the reflex excitability changes differed if a cutaneous or muscle nerve was stimulated (Fig. 19.4). This afferent-induced facilitation could be detected both when natural stimuli were used as a test input (Fig. 19.4) or when electrical stimuli were used (Fig. 19.5).

The electrophysiological studies also demonstrated that acute injury, apart from altering the threshold for eliciting the flexion reflex and increasing its responsiveness, also changed the receptive fields of single flexor motor neurons (Fig. 19.6) (17). Under normal circumstances most biceps femoris/semitendinosus flexor motor neurons have cutaneous mechanoreceptive fields restricted to the distal part of the ipsilateral hindlimb. Following an acute thermal injury, the receptive field spread to the contralateral foot.

The next issue addressed was whether the changes in the reflex excitability produced by peripheral tissue damage required an ongoing input for their maintenance. The strategy adopted to answer this was to induce a facilitation of the reflex by either tissue or nerve damage and then block subsequent activity with local anesthetics. This type of experiment was performed following acute thermal injury (Figs. 19.6 and 19.7) (17), following the intra-articular injection of the irritant chemical mustard oil (Fig. 19.8) (25) and following peripheral nerve section (Fig. 19.9) (13). In each case the manipulation in the absence of any local anesthetic produced prolonged facilitations of the flexor reflex. Blockade of sensory input from the site of the peripheral conditioning stimulus by subcutaneous local anesthetic (Figs. 19.6 and 19.7), intra-articular local anesthetic (Fig. 19.8), or application of local anesthetic to the cut end of a sectioned nerve (Fig. 19.9) failed to significantly reduce the duration of the facilitation.

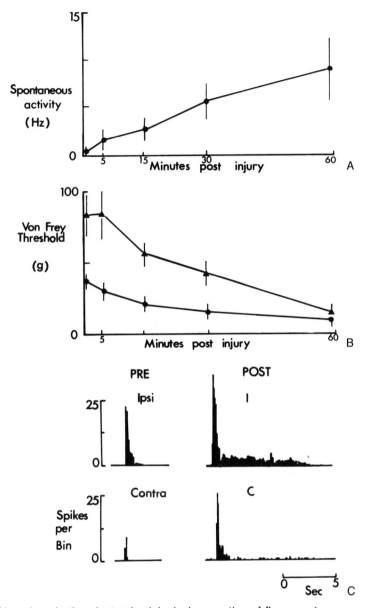

FIG. 19.3. Alterations in the electrophysiological properties of flexor motor neurons accompanying tissue damage. **A:** Time course of the increase in the spontaneous activity of biceps femoris alpha motor neuron efferents ($n = 25$) after thermal injury to the ipsilateral foot at time 0. **B:** Mechanical thresholds required to elicit responses from the plantar surface of the ipsilateral (▲) ($n = 25$) and contralateral (●) ($n = 13$) foot determined by testing with von Frey hairs. The ipsilateral tests were performed adjacent to but not on the site of the injury. **C:** Examples of responses produced in a single biceps femoris efferent by a standard pinch (150 g mm^{-2}) to the plantar surface of the ipsilateral and contralateral second toe, before a thermal injury (PRE) to the lateral side of the foot and 30 min after the injury (POST). Bin width was 500 msec. Note the bilateral increase in response amplitude and duration. Recordings of the alpha motor neurons were made from fine filaments of the hamstring nerve dissected free in the popliteal fossa in the decerebrate-spinal unanesthetized adult rat. (From ref. 17.)

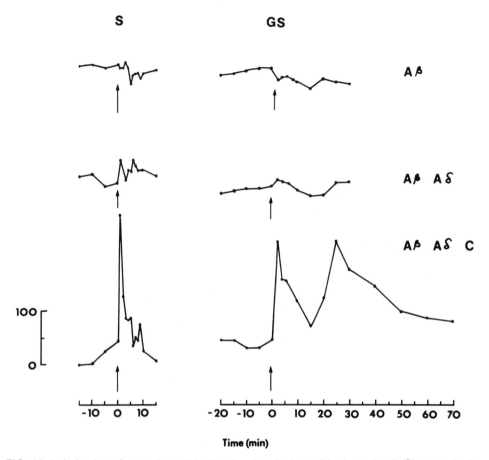

FIG. 19.4. Induction of central sensitization by electrical conditioning stimuli. Changes in the total number of action potentials elicited by an ipsilateral standard pinch in posterior biceps femoris/semitendinosus motor neurons following conditioning stimuli to the sural (S) and gastrocnemius-soleus (GS) nerves at strengths sufficient to activate large myelinated afferent fibers only (Aβ), small and large myelinated afferent fibers (Aβ and Aδ), and nonmyelinated afferents (Aβ, Aδ and C). Only the latter conditioning stimulus produced a large change in the pinch-evoked responses, with a more prolonged effect from the gastrocnemius-soleus nerve. (Vertical scale represents number of action potentials per pinch.) (From ref. 13.)

This indicates that the conditioning stimuli had triggered a change in the response properties of spinal neurons and that once this change had been initiated, it became independent for a period of tens of minutes at least from any further peripheral input to sustain it. Clearly from the results of the experiments using graded electrical stimuli, the trigger was likely to be related to C afferents. Natural stimuli that predominantly or exclusively activated C afferents would therefore be expected to produce central facilitations, and indeed this turned out to be the case. Mustard oil applied to the skin appears only to activate C afferents, producing a brief (several minutes duration) burst of activity (25), but this is followed by a facilitation of the flexor reflex that lasts for over an hour (25). Similarly tetanic stimulation of muscles to produce a model of claudication pain also produced a central facilitation (25). The

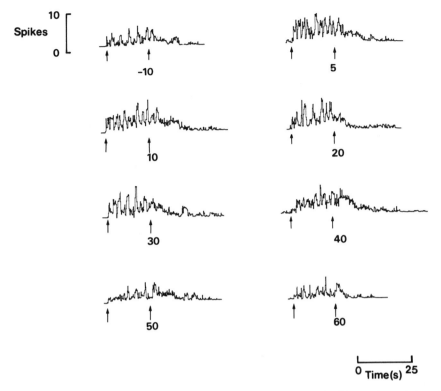

FIG. 19.5. Rate-meter recordings of the activity evoked in a posterior biceps femoris/semitendinosus motor neuron by an electrical test stimulus to the sural nerve (0.5 Hz, 20 sec, C-fiber strength) applied at the time indicated by the *arrows.* At time 0 a 20-sec, 1-Hz C-strength conditioning stimulus was applied to the gastrocnemius-soleus nerve. Note the increased test-evoked activity and the longer posttest stimulus afterdischarge that occurred for 40 min after the conditioning stimulus. (Vertical scale = number of action potentials per 200 μsec bin.) (From ref. 13.)

locus of the central change was shown by monosynaptic and antidromic excitability testing not to be located in the motor neurons themselves nor in primary afferent terminals, but in neurons somewhere between the site of termination of the conditioning input and the motor neurons in lamina IX (2).

One possible reason why C-afferent fibers and not A-beta fibers produce these prolonged changes in central excitability might be related to the differences in the chemical phenotype of these different afferents, particularly the presence of neuropeptides in small-caliber afferents (8). To test this, a study was performed in which the neuropeptide substance P and calcitonin gene-related peptide (CGRP) were administered intrathecally to see if they could mimic or modify the afferent-produced central excitability changes (27). These experiments showed that at doses that did not modify the monosynaptic reflex, substance P, CGRP, and a factor released from sural C fibers increased the excitability of the nociceptive reflex for prolonged periods in a multiplicative fashion. For example, substance P and CGRP injected together had a synergistic effect greater than either one alone, and they also facilitate the response produced by a conditioning stimulus to a peripheral nerve (Fig. 19.10).

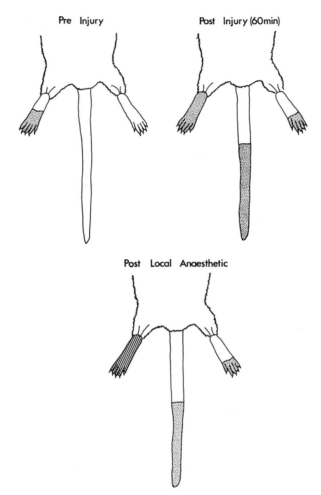

FIG. 19.6. Changes in the cutaneous receptive field of a biceps femoris flexor motor neuron following an acute thermal injury. Prior to the injury the receptive field was restricted to the ipsilateral hindpaw and toes. By 60 min after the production of the injury the receptive field had expanded to the entire ipsilateral foot, tail, and contralateral foot. The injection of local anesthetic into the site of the injury at this time failed to return the expected receptive field to its preinjury level.

These types of studies have been extended by Wiesenfeld-Hallin et al. (14), showing that a tachykinin antagonist spantide II blocks both the substance–P- and the C–fiber-evoked facilitation of the flexion reflex.

RATIONALE FOR PRE-EMPTIVE ANALGESIA

If certain types of primary afferent input have the capacity to trigger prolonged alterations in the excitability of spinal neurons, and these excitability changes modify the response properties of the neurons such that they react to normal inputs in an abnormal or exaggerated way, then it is reasonable to assume that preventing such

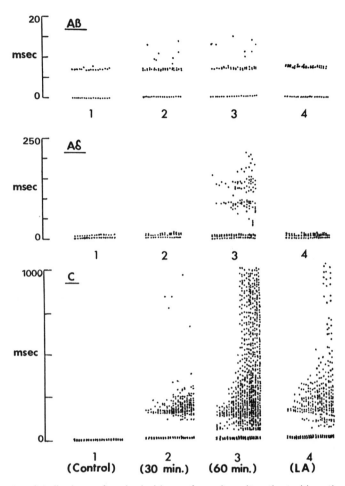

FIG. 19.7. Raster dot displays of a single biceps femoris unit activated by stimulation of the sural nerve before an ipsilateral thermal injury (control), 30 and 60 min postinjury, and 10 min after the injured foot had been completely anesthetized with lidocaine. Each dot represents an action potential. The vertical scale is the latency of the response after the sural nerve stimulus. The stimulus artefact is present at time 0, while the horizontal scale is real time (from left to right) with a new stimulus every 2 sec. The sural nerve was stimulated at strengths that only activated Aβ fibers (100 μA, 50 μsec), Aβ and Aδ fibers (250 μA, 50 μsec), and Aβ, Aδ, and C fibers (5 mA, 500 μsec). Note the different time scales used for monitoring the Aβ-, Aδ-, and C-evoked responses. In the preinjury state, only an Aβ input was evoked. Thirty minutes after the injury a C response begins to occur, while at 60 min both Aδ- and C-evoked bands of activity are present. (Note the progressive response increment or windup of the C responses). Ten minutes following the local anesthetic (administered 80 min postinjury) the sural C-evoked responses remain higher than before the injury, although not as high as immediately before the local anesthetic. (From ref. 17.)

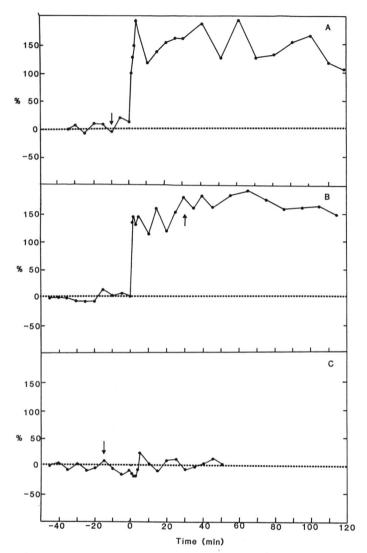

FIG. 19.8. Changes in the excitability of the flexor reflex measured as percentage deviation from baseline response to control ipsi- and contralateral test pinch evoked action potential discharges produced by intra-articular injections. **A:** *Arrow* indicates that 5 μl (0.9%) NaCl did not alter the reflex, but 5 μl mustard oil (time 0) produced increased responses to both the ipsi- and contralateral test stimuli. **B:** Mustard oil (5 μl) was injected at time 0, and then 5 μl lidocaine (2%) was also injected (*arrow*). This failed to modify the mustard–oil-induced changes. **C:** Lidocaine, 5 μl (2%) was injected (*arrow*), and then at time 0, 5 μl mustard oil was administered, which did not increase the excitability of the reflex. (From ref. 25.)

change may prevent some of the sensory problems associated with peripheral tissue injury. Stated more simply, preventing the induction of a state of central sensitization may be able to reduce hyperalgesia.

We set out to examine whether this was a possibility in a study using morphine as the analgesic (26). The first observation we made was that both the cutaneous pinch and electrical evoked response of flexor motor neurons were relatively insensitive to

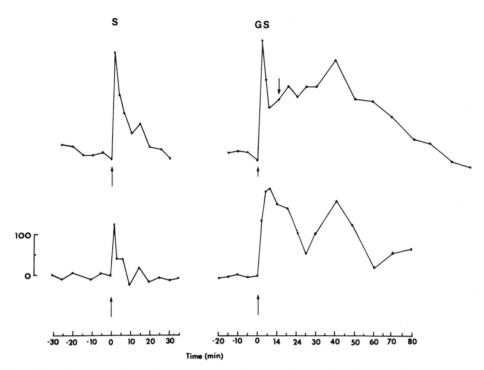

FIG. 19.9. Changes in the total number of action potentials evoked by an ipsilateral pinch in two posterior biceps femoris/semitendinosus motor neurons after section of either the sural (S) or gastrocnemius-soleus (GS) nerves at the times indicated by the *arrows*. Section of the sural nerve produced a fairly short facilitation of the reflex, whereas section of the gastrocnemius-soleus nerve caused a more prolonged increase in the reflex excitability. In the upper right trace, the *arrow* indicates the time at which the cut end of the gastrocnemius-soleus nerve was immersed in 2% xylocaine to abolish any ongoing activity. (Vertical scale represents number of action potentials per pinch.) (From ref. 13.)

morphine (Fig. 19.11). Only at 5 mg/kg^{-1} was a detectable reduction produced and the reduction only became substantial at 20 mg/kg^{-1}. Therefore morphine is a relatively poor antinociceptive agent. The second observation was that if morphine was administered at a dose that itself did not reduce the flexion reflex (0.5 mg/kg^{-1}), it could nevertheless prevent the production of a prolonged afferent-induced facilitation by stimulating a muscle nerve (Fig. 19.12). Once the effect of the morphine was antagonized by naloxone, then a repeat of the conditioning stimulus to the nerve now produced the expected prolonged changes. The reverse was not true, however; the administration of low doses of morphine (0.5 mg/kg^{-1}), once the central facilitation had been initiated, did not reduce it (Fig. 19.13). Such a reduction was only produced by the higher dose of 5 mg/kg^{-1}. These results show that a low, nonantinociceptive dose of morphine could prevent the development of central sensitization but that much higher doses were required to terminate it once it was established.

Translated into clinical practice these findings imply that the administration of analgesic before a peripheral injury would result in less pain and hyperalgesia than the administration once the pain is present. The effectiveness of pre-emptive analgesia has been tested in two clinical trials. The first used local anesthetic blocks to

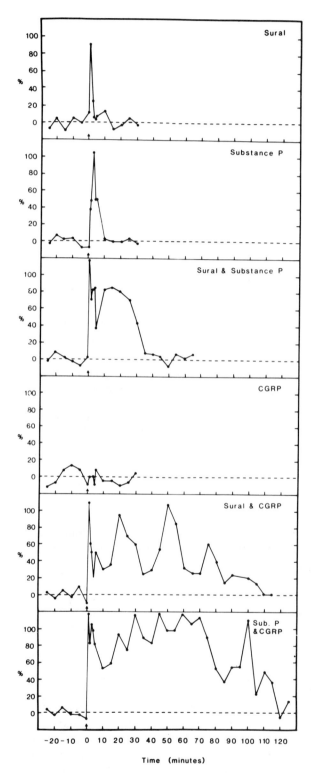

FIG. 19.10. Changes in the excitability of the flexor reflex produced by the intrathecal neuropeptides. The tracings show, from top to bottom, the effects of a sural conditioning stimulus (5 mA, 500 μsec, 1 Hz) for 20sec, 10 ng substance P, the simultaneous injection of substance P and the application of the sural conditioning stimulus, 10 ng CGRP, the simultaneous injection of CGRP (10 ng) and the application of the sural conditioning stimulus, and the simultaneous injection of 10 ng substance P and 100 ng CGRP. All injections were of 10 μl. (From ref. 27.)

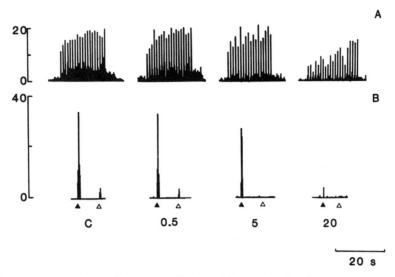

FIG. 19.11. The effect of morphine on the flexion withdrawal reflex. Rate-meter recordings of the responses evoked in a hamstring flexor alpha motor neuron by stimulation of the sural nerve at 1 Hz for 20sec at C-fiber strength (**A**) and by a standard pinch (150 g) applied to the ipsi (▲) and contralateral (△) hindpaws (**B**). The vertical scale represents the number of action potentials per 200 msec bin. Recordings were made from a control animal (C) and 10 min following the administration of 0.5, 5, or 20 mg/kg morphine. (From ref. 26.)

prevent sensory input during surgery (11) and the second administered opioids preoperatively (7). In both cases a reduction in postoperative analgesic requirement was found, and in the first trial postoperative pain and tenderness were significantly reduced compared to patients given conventional anesthetics.

MECHANISMS OF CENTRAL SENSITIZATION

That the prolonged excitability changes in the spinal cord produced by brief C-afferent inputs occurred in the dorsal horn was first demonstrated by a study of the receptive field properties of dorsal horn neurons (3). Extracellular recordings were made from 46 neurons in lamina I and laminae III to VI including 10 whose axons projected to the brain. In the absence of any disturbing stimulus in the control situation, the size and mechanical threshold of the receptive fields remained stable. Following a brief conditioning stimulus to the gastrocnemius nerve (1 Hz for 20 sec), no change was produced if only large myelinated afferents were activated; a transient change in receptive field properties was produced by stimuli that recruited A-delta afferents, whereas a prolonged (>40 min) expansion of receptive fields occurred in 60% of the cells when C-fiber strength stimuli were used. At this strength a prolonged facilitation of the flexion reflex also occurs when stimulating this nerve (see Figs. 19.4 and 19.5). In three of 10 cells that originally responded only to noxious cutaneous mechanical stimulation, the conditioning stimulus to the gastrocnemius nerve at C-fiber strength reduced the mechanical threshold of the receptive field such that low-intensity stimuli (e.g., light touch or brush) began to activate the cells (Fig.

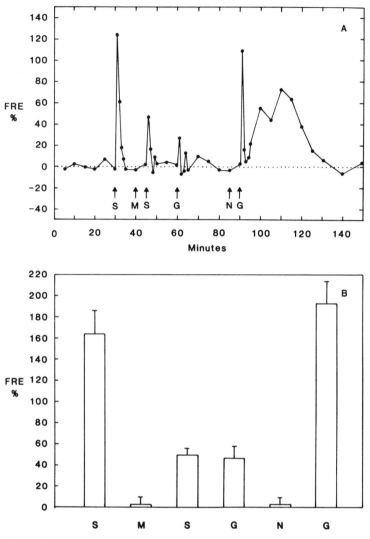

FIG. 19.12. The effect of pretreatment with morphine on afferent-induced central excitability increases. Changes in the flexor reflex excitability (FRE) expressed as a percentage of the mean baseline response to a standard pinch (150 g) applied to the middle three toes of the ipsilateral foot. **A:** Results from a single experiment. **B:** Mean values ± SEM obtained from five experiments. At 30 min after the start of the experiment a sural conditioning stimulus (S) (1 Hz, 20 sec, C-fiber strength) was applied, followed 10 min later by the injection of morphine (M) (0.5 mg/kg), and the sural conditioning stimulus was then repeated. A conditioning stimulus was applied to the gastrocnemius-soleus nerve (G) (1 Hz, 20 sec, C-fiber strength) 20 min after morphine. This was followed by the administration of 1 mg/kg naloxone (N) after which the gastrocnemius-soleus conditioning stimulus was repeated. (From ref. 26.)

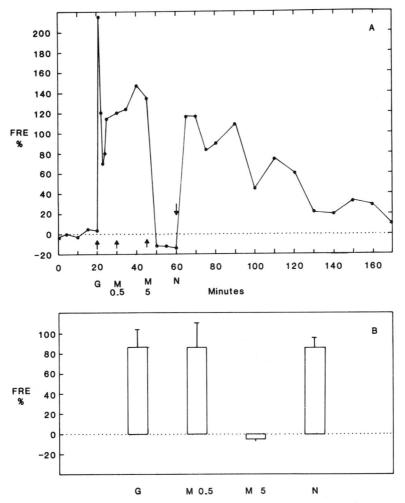

FIG. 19.13. The effect of morphine on established excitability increases. Changes in flexor reflex excitability (FRE) illustrated from one animal (**A**) and the means ± SEM in four experiments (**B**). Twenty minutes after commencement of recording a conditioning stimulus was applied to the gastrocnemius-soleus nerve (G) (1 Hz, 20 sec, C-fiber strength). Ten minutes later 0, 5 mg/kg morphine was administered (M 0.5) and 15 min after this 5 mg/kg morphine was injected (M 5). Naloxone (N) 1 mg/kg was then injected. (From ref. 26.)

19.14). Similar expansions of receptive fields occur after the activation of small-caliber afferents by the cutaneous application of mustard oil (21), the production of experimental inflammation (5), and the injection of irritant chemicals into joints (9), muscle (4), or skin (1). These findings show that the receptive fields of dorsal horn neurons are not fixed but can be modified by peripheral inputs. The nature of the changes produced are of interest; expansion of the size of receptive fields, increase in responsiveness to suprathreshold stimuli, reduction in threshold, and the recruitment of novel inputs, because these almost exactly parallel the postinjury sensory disturbances found in humans: spread of sensitivity to uninjured areas, hyperalgesia, and allodynia.

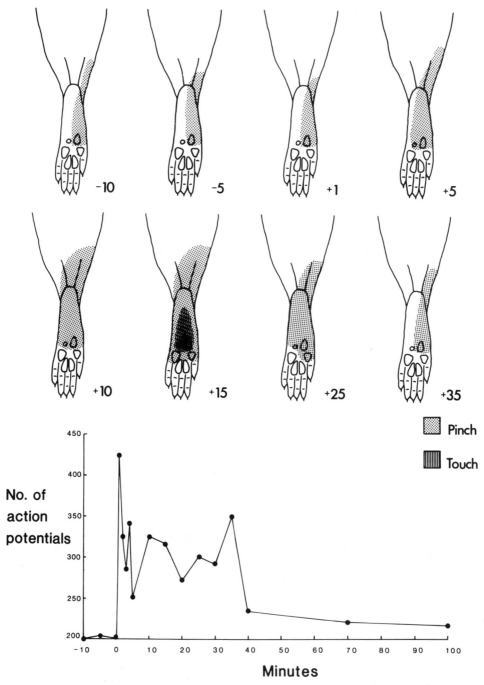

FIG. 19.14. Top: Expansion of the pinch receptive field of a dorsal horn neuron following a C–fiber-strength conditioning stimulus at time 0 to the gastrocnemius-soleus nerve (1 Hz, 20 sec). Note that 15 min after the conditioning stimulus the neuron begins to respond to a low-intensity mechanical stimulus (touch). **Bottom:** Change in the total number of action potentials in a neuron evoked by a standard pinch applied for 3 sec to the medial edge of the foot following the gastrocnemius-soleus conditioning stimulus at time 0. (From ref. 3.)

The next key questions were: how did the change in receptive field properties occur and what was responsible for the induction and maintenance of these changes. The answer to the first seems to be that the receptive field of dorsal horn neurons comprises both a suprathreshold and a subliminal component. From an intracellular analysis of action and synaptic potentials it was possible to define both components, the first constituting the firing zone of the receptive field and the second a low-probability firing fringe where subthreshold but not suprathreshold responses could be reliably evoked (20) (Fig. 19.15). What this actually means is that stimulation of some peripheral areas will evoke synaptic potentials of sufficient amplitude in a given dorsal horn to generate an action potential discharge, whereas stimulation of other areas will evoke synaptic potentials that are predominantly subthreshold. If the receptive field is defined purely in terms of its action potential discharge, then the subthreshold input to the cell is subliminal and undetected. However, if either synaptic efficacy or membrane excitability is changed, then these subliminal inputs could be recruited to the firing zone. This recruitment could be spatial, expanding the size of the receptive field, increasing the suprathreshold response in the existing firing zone, or recruiting novel inputs such as A-beta input to cells with a normal

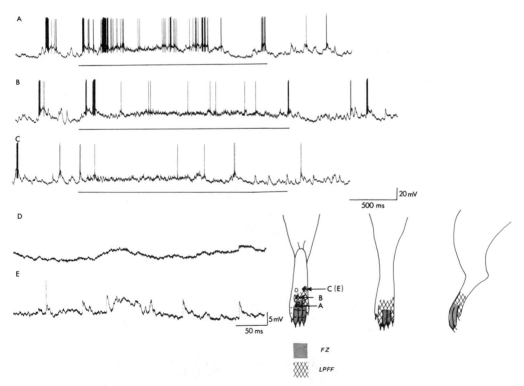

FIG. 19.15. Changes in the response evoked in a neuron by the application of a standard pinch to different areas of skin within the firing zone (FZ) and in the low-probability firing fringe (LPFF). **A–C,** and **E:** Responses evoked from locations indicated in drawing of rat hindlimb. **D** and **E:** Amplified and expanded examples of spontaneous and pinch-evoked excitatory post-synaptic potentials, respectively. (From ref. 20.)

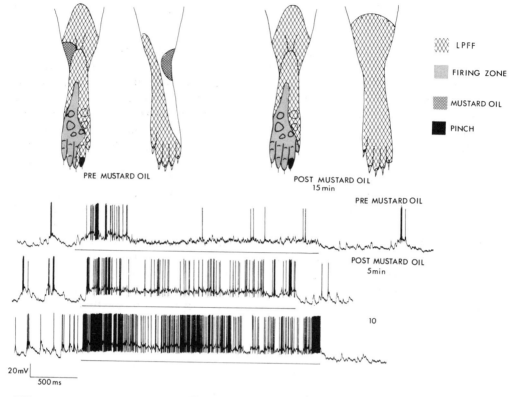

FIG. 19.16. Changes in the size and responsiveness of high-threshold (pinch) cutaneous receptive fields of a dorsal horn neuron following the application of mustard oil to the skin. The change in the size of the firing zone and the LPFF at 15 min (cell 2) after the mustard oil is illustrated. Intracellular records showing alterations of responses to a standard pinch (150 g) to toes 2 and 5 and 10 min after mustard oil. (From ref. 21.)

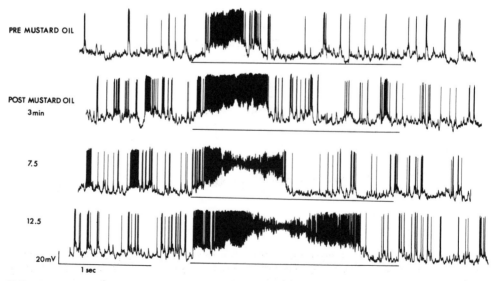

FIG. 19.17. The effect of a standard pinch (150 g) applied to the firing zone of a dorsal horn before and at various times after the cutaneous application of mustard oil, showing the increase in the depolarization elicited, which eventually resulted in spike inactivation. (From ref. 21.)

238

high-threshold receptive field. That these changes do occur has been shown by a study using the cutaneous application of mustard oil to generate prolonged receptive field changes (21). Figure 19.16 illustrates how a subliminal input can be recruited following a noxious conditioning input to the firing zone, expanding the receptive field. Increases in responsiveness also occur as a result of an increased amplitude of synaptic potentials, and this is illustrated in Fig. 19.17. What is obvious from these figures is that the changes in excitability produced by a C-fiber conditioning input are large. In these studies we also found an example of a nociceptive dorsal horn neuron, which in the control situation had a subthreshold brush input but that, after mustard oil application, became suprathreshold (21). This shows that allodynia may be due to a recruitment of normal low-threshold A-beta inputs, in addition to any reduction in peripheral thresholds of nociceptors that occurs as part of peripheral sensitization.

CELLULAR MECHANISMS OF CENTRAL EXCITABILITY INCREASES FOLLOWING PERIPHERAL DAMAGE

The sequence of cellular and molecular events, from the activation of certain classes of small-caliber afferents in the periphery to the production of a prolonged change in the excitability of dorsal horn neurons, remains inadequately understood. Exactly which classes of afferents have the capacity to produce these changes, which transmitters they release, and how these transmitters initiate persistent changes in postsynaptic cells are not fully known. However, we do have some clues. The more interesting of these relates to the role of the *N*-methyl-D-aspartic acid (NMDA) excitatory amino acid receptor. Small-caliber afferents have the capacity, unlike large-diameter myelinated afferents, to produce slow synaptic potentials when recorded in *in vitro* preparations (10,12,31). This enables a remarkable degree of spatial and particularly temporal summation to occur. For example, the temporal summation of slow synaptic potentials resulting from the repetitive activation of C afferents at low frequencies (0.5–1.0 Hz) results in the buildup of a large cumulative depolarization (10). This incrementing depolarization results in a greater action potential discharge per stimulus with repeated stimuli, the phenomenon of windup, and a persistent depolarization after the stimulus is terminated. The slow synaptic potentials, the cumulative depolarization on repeated stimulation, and windup are all reduced substantially by an NMDA antagonist D-2-amino-5-phosphonovalerate (D-APV) (10).

Although the cumulative depolarization and windup only seem to represent short-lasting–activity-dependent changes in the response properties of spinal neurons, they may in fact represent the trigger mechanism for the more longer lasting changes that mediate prolonged central excitability changes. The reason for stating this is that if windup is prevented from occurring by pretreatment with an NMDA antagonist *in vivo*, e.g., MK 801 or D-CPP, the prolonged facilitations do not occur (Fig. 19.18) (23). So far this is only an association and does not prove causality, but it is possible that the mechanisms that operate are as follows. Small-diameter afferents release both fast and slow transmitters, the former is likely to be glutamate or a similar compound and the latter a neuropeptide. The glutamate binds to the three receptor subtypes that are linked to ion channels: the alpha-amino-3-hydroxy-5-methyl-4-isoxazole-propionic acid (AMPA) receptor, the kainate receptor, and the

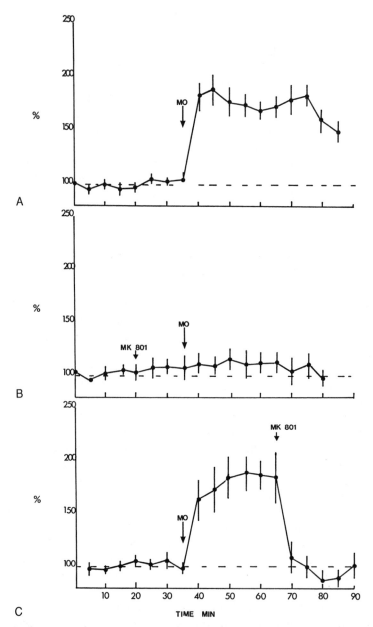

FIG. 19.18. Changes in flexor motor neuron reflex excitability produced by the cutaneous application of the chemical irritant mustard oil (MO) and its modification by the NMDA receptor antagonist MK 801. In **A** the baseline reflex (measured by counting the total number of action potentials generated in a flexor motor neuron by a standard pinch to the toes and normalized) increases by almost 200% following mustard oil application. If the mustard oil treatment is preceded by the administration of MK 801 at a dose that has no effect on its own, the mustard oil no longer produces an increase in reflex excitability (**B**). Once the excitability increase is established, treatment with MK 801 can return the reflex to the baseline level (**C**). (Modified from ref. 23.)

NMDA receptor. At normal resting membrane potentials the ion channel linked to the NMDA receptor is blocked by Mg^{2+} ions so that glutamate binding to this receptor will produce no effect (6). Binding to the AMPA receptor in particular will allow sodium ions to enter the cell and produce a short-lasting depolarization of the fast excitatory postsynaptic potentials. This depolarization lasting a few milliseconds may be slightly prolonged by the removal of Mg^{2+} ions from the NMDA receptor because of its voltage sensitivity. The neuropeptides, acting on tachykinin and other receptors, produce a long latency, long duration, but small amplitude depolarization by blocking potassium currents and increasing calcium currents. This long-lasting depolarization will produce a long-lasting removal of the magnesium blockade of the NMDA receptor linked ion channel (6). This will allow glutamate, by binding to the NMDA receptor, to produce a voltage-dependent depolarization, which will increase in amplitude with further depolarization. The source of the glutamate acting on the NMDA receptors unblocked by the peptide-induced depolarization could be from primary afferent terminals and polysynaptic interneuronal inputs to the cell. The NMDA–receptor-linked ion channel produces a depolarization by permitting the

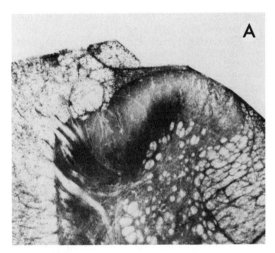

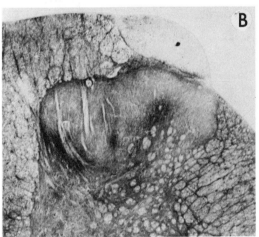

FIG. 19.19. A: The effect of the application of mustard oil to the skin of the hindlimb on the activity of the enzyme glycogen phosphorylase detected by an immunocytochemical technique (see ref. 28). Within 10 min of the application of mustard oil glycogen phosphorylase activity is increased in the ipsilateral dorsal horn. This is due to an activation of phosphorylase b kinase, which in turn is activated by calcium and cyclic AMP-dependent protein kinase. The activation of glycogen phosphorylase is an indicator therefore of second–messenger-mediated events triggered by afferent inputs. B: This shows that the intrathecal administration of D-APV 1.0 nmol (10 μl) 5 min before the mustard oil substantially reduced the glycogen phosphorylase activity increase. (Modified from ref. 19.)

entry into a cell of sodium and calcium ions. The latter may be particularly important, because it can act as a second messenger activating protein kinases (Fig. 19.19) (19) or indeed by changing gene expression via the activation of transcription factors.

Whether this scenario is correct or not can only be discovered by further experimental work. What is evident though is that peripheral stimuli, particularly those related to tissue damage and inflammation, can initiate profound and prolonged changes in the excitability of central neurons, and these changes, by recruiting subthreshold inputs, can produce sensory modifications that may underlie the clinical phenomenon of hyperalgesia.

REFERENCES

1. Chung, J. M., LaMotte, R. H., Oh, U., et al. (1989): Spinothalamic neurones and hyperalgesia; evidence from anaesthetized macaques (C). *J. Physiol. (Lond.)*, 412:13P.
2. Cook, A. J., Woolf, C. J., and Wall, P. D. (1986): Prolonged C-fibre mediated facilitation of the flexion reflex is not due to changes in afferent terminal or motoneurone excitability. *Neurosci. Lett.*, 70:91–96.
3. Cook, A. J., Woolf, C. J., Wall, P. D., and McMahon, S. B. (1987): Dynamic receptive field plasticity in the dorsal horn of the rat spinal cord following C-primary afferent input. *Nature*, 325:151–153.
4. Hoheisel, U., and Mense, S. (1989): Long-term changes in discharge behaviour of cat dorsal horn neurones following noxious stimulation of deep tissues. *Pain*, 36:239–247.
5. Hylden, J. L. K., Nahin, R. L., Traub, R. J., and Dubner, R. (1989): Expansion of receptive fields of spinal lamina 1 projection neurones in rats with unilateral adjuvant-induced inflammation: the contribution of dorsal horn mechanisms. *Pain*, 37:229–243.
6. Mayer, M. I., Westbrook, G., and Guthrie, P. B. (1984): Voltage-dependent block by Mg^{2+} of NMDA responses in spinal cord neurones. *Nature*, 309:261–263.
7. McQuay, H. J., Carroll, D., and Moore, R. A. (1988): Postoperative orthopaedic pain—the effect of opiate premedication and local anaesthetic blocks. *Pain*, 33:291–295.
8. O'Brien, C., Woolf, C. J., Fitzgerald, M., Lindsay, R., and Molander, C. (1989): Differences in chemical expression by rat primary afferent neurones which innervate skin, muscle or joint. *Neuroscience*, 32:493–502.
9. Schaible, H. G., Schmidt, R. F., and Willis, W. D. (1987): Enhancement of the responses of ascending tract cells in the cat spinal cord by acute inflammation of the knee joint. *Exp. Brain Res.*, 66:489–499.
10. Thompson, S. W. N., King, A. E., and Woolf, C. J. (1990): Activity-dependent changes in rat ventral horn neurones in vitro; summation of prolonged afferent evoked postsynaptic depolarizations produce a d-APV sensitive windup. *Eur. J. Neurosci.*, 2:638–649.
11. Tverskoy, M., Cozacov, C., Ayache, M., Bradley, E. L., and Kissin, I. (1990): Primary afferent evoked synaptic responses and slow potential generation in rat substantia gelatinosa neurons in vitro. *J. Neurophysiol.*, 62:96–108.
12. Urban, L., and Randic, M. (1984): Slow excitatory transmission in rat dorsal horn: possible mediation by peptides. *Brain Res.*, 290:336–341.
13. Wall, P. D., and Woolf, C. J. (1984): Muscle but not cutaneous C-afferent input produces prolonged increases in the excitability of the flexion reflex in the rat. *J. Physiol. (Lond.)*, 356:443–458.
14. Wiesenfeld-Hallin, Z., Xu, X-J., Haakanser, R., Feng, D. M., and Folkers, K. (1990): The specific antagonist effect of intrathecal spantide II on substance P and C-fibre conditioning stimulation-induced facilitation of the nociceptive flexor reflex in rat. *Brain Res.*, 526:284–290.
15. Woolf, C. J. (1980): Analgesia and hyperalgesia produced in the rat by intrathecal naloxone. *Brain Res.*, 189:593–597.
16. Woolf, C. J. (1981): Intrathecal high dose morphine produces hyperalgesia in the rat. *Brain Res.*, 209:491–495.
17. Woolf, C. J. (1983): Evidence for a central component of postinjury pain hypersensitivity. *Nature*, 306:686–688.
18. Woolf, C. J. (1984): Long term alterations in the excitability of the flexion reflex produced by peripheral tissue injury in the chronic decerebrate rat. *Pain*, 18:325–343.
19. Woolf, C. J. (1987): Excitatory amino acids increase glycogen phosphorylase activity in the rat spinal cord. *Neurosci. Lett.*, 73:209–214.

20. Woolf, C. J., and King, A. E. (1989): Subthreshold components of the cutaneous mechanoreceptive fields of dorsal horn neurons in the rat lumbar spinal cord. *J. Neurophysiol.*, 62:907–916.
21. Woolf, C. J., and King, A. E. (1990): Dynamic alterations in the cutaneous mechanosensitive receptive fields of dorsal horn neurons in the rat spinal cord. *J. Neurosci.*, 10:2717–2726.
22. Woolf, C. J., and McMahon, S. B. (1985): Injury-induced plasticity of the flexor reflex in chronic decerebrate rats. *Neuroscience*, 16:395–404.
23. Woolf, C. J., and Thompson, S. W. N. The induction and maintenance of central sensitization is dependent on N-methyl-D-aspartic acid receptor activation: implications for the treatment of postoperative pain. *Pain*, 44:293–301.
24. Woolf, C. J., and Wall, P. D. (1983): Endogenous opioids and pain mechanisms—a complex relationship. *Nature*, 306:739–740.
25. Woolf, C. J., and Wall, P. D. (1986): The relative effectiveness of C-primary afferent fibres of different origins in evoking a prolonged facilitation of the flexor reflex in the rat. *J. Neurosci.*, 6:1433–1442.
26. Woolf, C. J., and Wall, P. D. (1986): Morphine sensitive and morphine insensitive actions of C-fibre input on the rat spinal cord. *Neurosci. Lett.*, 64:221–225.
27. Woolf, C. J., and Wiesenfeld-Hallin, Z. (1986): Substance P and calcitonin gene related peptide synergistically modulate the gain of the nociceptor reflex in the rat. *Neurosci. Lett.*, 66:226–230.
28. Woolf, C. J., Chong, M. S., and Rashdi, T. (1985): Mapping increased glycogen phosphorylase activity in dorsal root ganglia and in the spinal cord following peripheral stimuli. *J. Comp. Neurol.*, 234:60–76.
29. Yaksh, T. L. (1989): Behavioral and autonomic correlates of tactile evoked allodynia produced by spinal glycine inhibition; effects of modulatory receptor system and excitatory amino acid antagonists. *Pain*, 37:111–123.
30. Yaksh, T. L., and Harty, G. J. (1988): Pharmacology of the allodynia in rats evoked by high dose intrathecal morphine. *J. Pharmacol. Exp. Ther.*, 264:501–507.
31. Yoshimira, M., and Jessell, T. M. (1989): Primary afferent evoked synaptic responses and slow potential generation in rat substantia neurons in vitro. *J. Neurophysiol.*, 62:96–108.

Hyperalgesia and Allodynia,
edited by W. D. Willis, Jr.
Raven Press, Ltd., New York © 1992.

20

Pharmacology of Nerve Compression-Evoked Hyperesthesia

Tony L. Yaksh, Tatsuo Yamamoto, and Robert R. Myers

*Department of Anesthesiology, University of California,
San Diego, La Jolla, California 92093*

Focal injuries to peripheral nerve that leave it in continuity are frequently associated with pronounced hyperesthesia. Several animal models have recently been developed to study this phenomenon. Bennett and Xie (2) reported that placement of loose ligatures around the sciatic nerve proximal to the popliteal fossa results in a progressive decrease in the withdrawal latency of the ligated paw to a local thermal stimulus with little change in the response latency of the contralateral, nonligated paw. This finding has also been observed by other investigators (1,21). In this chapter, we describe the light and electron microscopic findings following focal nerve compression with loose ligatures and the effect of pharmacological interventions on the thermal hyperesthesia produced by this intervention.

METHODS

Animal Model

Male Sprague-Dawley rats were anesthetized with halothane. A local incision was made over the biceps femoralis of each leg, and the muscle was bluntly dissected at mid-thigh to expose the sciatic nerves. Each nerve was then carefully mobilized, with care taken to avoid undue stretching. Four 4-0 chromic gut sutures were each tied loosely around the right sciatic nerve, as described by Bennett and Xie (2). The left sciatic nerve was only mobilized and served as sham control. Both incisions were closed in layers with 3-0 silk sutures, and the rats allowed to recover from anesthesia. The animals were maintained individually in clear plastic cages with solid floors covered with 3 to 6 cm sawdust. All animals displayed normal feeding and drinking postoperatively.

To permit intrathecal injections, groups of rats were prepared under halothane anesthesia with intrathecal catheters (PE-10) that extended from the cisterna magna to the lumbar enlargement (8 cm). Catheters were placed 2 days prior to the ligation of the sciatic nerve.

Test System

The thermal nociceptive threshold was measured with a device similar to that previously reported (8). The rats were placed in a clear plastic cage (10×20 cm) placed on an elevated floor of clear glass (2 mm thick). A radiant heat source (halogen projector lamp CXL/CXP 50W 8V, Ushio, Inc., Tokyo, Japan) was contained in a movable holder placed beneath the glass floor. The voltage to the thermal source was controlled by a constant voltage supply. The interior of the box under the animal was heated and regulated so that the underplate temperature was kept constant at 30°C. The calibration of the thermal test system was adjusted so that the average response latency in normal untreated rats, measured prior to the initiation of an experimental series, was 10 ± 0.5 sec. To initiate a test, the rat was placed in the box and allowed 5 to 10 min to accommodate. The underfloor heat source was then positioned so that it focused at the plantar surface of one hindpaw. The light was then activated, which initiated a timing circuit. The time interval between the application of the light beam and the brisk hindpaw withdrawal latency (PWL) was measured to the nearest 0.1 sec. The trial was terminated and the lamp removed in the absence of a response within 20 sec. This value was then assigned as its withdrawal latency.

Anatomical Changes

To examine the neuropathological changes in the peripheral nerve, four to six sciatic nerves were harvested at intervals after the placement of the ligatures. The nerve segments were immersed in phosphate-buffered 2.5% glutaraldehyde for 48 hr after which the ligatures were removed by fine dissection and the tissue cut into 2-mm blocks for processing for electron microscopy (EM). Following dehydration, osmium infiltration, and embedding in araldite, 1-μm thick sections were cut for light microscopy. EM thin sections were subsequently cut from selected blocks. Light microscopic sections were stained with paraphenylenediamine; EM sections were stained with uranyl acetate and lead citrate and viewed in a Siemens 101 electron microscope operating at 80 KeV.

RESULTS

Upon recovery from surgery, the animals displayed a mild weakness of the lower ligated limb. This was correlated with a reliable loss of the placing and stepping response of that paw and a tendency for the paw to display a mild eversion. The contralateral paw with a sham lesion showed no evidence of any change in function. Measurement of the thermal response threshold revealed that during the induction of the compression injury there was a progressive reduction in the thermal response latency of the paw of the lesioned nerve, with no change in the paw of the unlesioned nerve. The maximum reduction in response latency was observed by 5 to 7 days with the decreased latency being maintained for a period of up to 14 days. After that there was a progressive increase in the response latency of the lesioned paw such that by 3 weeks the lesioned paw tended to show a longer latency than the nonlesioned paw. In normal, nonsurgically treated animals, the average baseline PWL

($\pm$ S.D.) was 9.8 ± 1.7 sec ($n = 75$). The mean baseline PWL ($\pm$ S.D.) in the nonligated paw of the lesioned animal was 10.6 ± 2.0 sec, a difference that was modest but significantly different ($t = 2.714$, $df = 182$; $p = 0.007$). In the lesioned rat, the mean PWL ($\pm$ S.D.) for the ligated paw (8.2 ± 1.7 sec) was significantly less than the nonligated paw, with the average difference score ($\pm$ S.D.) being -2.5 ± 1.7 sec ($t = -15.0$, $df = 107$; $p < 0.0001$).

Anatomical Changes

In all animals examined, epineurial fibrosis was a striking feature of the tissue associated with the ligatures and could be seen in all sections. Endoneurial edema was also a prominent finding seen in experimental sections, primarily in the subperineurial and perivascular spaces but also throughout the entire interstitium in more severely injured fascicles. Fibroblasts were noted in the edematous areas within the endoneurium. Endothelial hypertrophy was a distinctive feature in the neuropathy that was observed in both epineurial and endoneurial vessels. Endothelial cells had enlarged and prominent nuclei with swollen cytoplasm that protruded into the luminal space (Fig. 20.1).

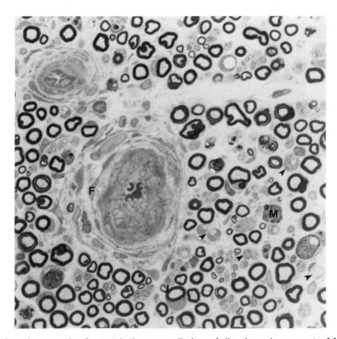

FIG. 20.1. Light micrograph of rat sciatic nerve 7 days following placement of four loose constriction ligatures. Note endoneurial edema in the perivascular space and throughout the interstitium that separates the normally tightly packed myelinated fibers. Vessel pathology is striking with hypertrophied endothelial cells nearly occluding the lumen of the two vessels in the field. Note the numerous fibroblasts (F) in the perivascular space. Macrophages (M) are present throughout the endoneurium phagocytozing myelin debris from demyelinated axons (*arrowheads*). Paraphenylenediamine. Original magnification = 200×.

   Demyelination was the principal pathological change in nerve fibers, although degenerated axons could be seen in severe lesions with concomitant wallerian degeneration. EM revealed swollen Schwann cell cytoplasm, occasionally associated with normal myelin, suggesting that Schwann cell injury was the cause of the demyelination. There was active phagocytosis of myelin debris by numerous macrophages. Although detailed morphometric analysis has not been completed, it seems clear on the basis of the present qualitative analysis that myelinated fibers were preferentially affected, with unmyelinated fibers generally appearing normal (Fig. 20.2).

   There was still ongoing nerve fiber injury 23 days following placement of the ligatures as indicated by continuing demyelination and occasional dark axons, fibrosis, and edema. Nevertheless, clear evidence of remyelination was observed, and this appeared to be the dominant process that could be seen throughout the injured fascicles.

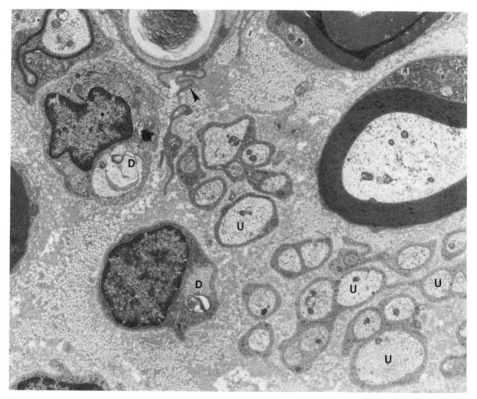

FIG. 20.2. Electron micrograph of rat sciatic nerve 7 days after loose ligature placement demonstrating Schwann cell pathology and demyelination but preservation of unmyelinated fibers. Abnormal Schwann cell cytoplasm can be seen in the large fiber in the upper right corner that has normal-appearing myelin. Completely demyelinated fibers (D) can be seen at the left. Remnant basal lamina (*arrowhead*) is associated with phagocytic Schwann cell activity. Unmyelinated fibers (U) appear normal. Uranyl acetate, lead citrate. Original magnification = 12,000×.

Pharmacological Treatment

Topical Colchicine

To determine if the changes in neural function were the results of alterations in axonal transport from the region of injury, the effects of blocking axonal transport by the topical application of colchicine (7,9) were assessed. In these studies, groups of animals were prepared with unilateral compression of the sciatic nerve as described. At the time of surgery, pledgets of gelfoam ($3 \times 3 \times 1$ mm) were placed around the nerve at a site just proximal to the ligations. In separate groups of rats, the pledgets of gelfoam were immersed in either saline, colchicine 5 mM, or colchicine 50 mM in saline. In a fourth group of rats, the pledget of gelfoam immersed in the highest concentration of colchicine was placed distal to the nerve compression. The wounds were closed.

In these experiments, placement of the pledget soaked in saline was without effect. Placement of the pledget with the highest concentration of colchicine around a normal nerve was without effect on the response latency of the left and right paw. However, placement of the pledget proximal to the compression injury resulted in a dose-dependent abolition of the hyperesthesia. Placement of the pledget soaked in 50 mM colchicine distal to the compression was without effect on the hyperesthesia (see Table 20.1).

Intrathecal Capsaicin

Capsaicin administered intrathecally will result in a loss of markers for small primary afferents [such as substance P (SP)] and an elevation in the thermal nociceptive response threshold (12,27). In the present studies, animals prepared with indwelling intrathecal catheters were then subjected to a unilateral sciatic nerve compression as described. After the compression, the animals were anesthetized with halothane and received intrathecal injection of capsaicin (75 μg/15 μl) dissolved in 20% 2-hydroxy-propyl-b-cyclodextrin or the cyclodextrin vehicle alone. The animals were tested at 7 days and were then terminally anesthetized and the spinal cords removed. The lumbar cord was divided into dorsal and ventral portions and extracted and the

TABLE 20.1. *Effects of topical colchicine on hyperesthesia following unilateral compression injury*

Treatment	Response latency (sec)		
	Control paw	Lesioned paw	Difference score (sec)[d]
Saline[a]	10.5 ± 0.6	7.5 ± 0.6	-3.0 ± 0.3
Colchicine 5 mM[a]	9.0 ± 0.4	7.8 ± 0.4^c	-1.2 ± 0.2
Colchicine 50 mM[a]	10.1 ± 0.2	10.0 ± 0.4	-0.1 ± 0.3
Colchicine 50 mM[b]	11.1 ± 0.7	8.0 ± 6^c	-3.1 ± 0.4

[a]Proximal pledget placement.
[b]Distal pledget placement.
[c]$p < 0.05$ as compared to nonligated paws.
[d]Mean $\pm$ SE; $n = 8$–10 rats.

levels of sP and calcitonin-gene related peptide (CGRP) assessed by radioimmunoassay.

In these studies, the intrathecal injection of vehicle had no effect on the response latency of the normal or lesioned paw and there was no change in difference score. Intrathecal capsaicin resulted in a significant elevation in the thermal response latency of the normal paw. In contrast, the mean response latency of the lesioned paw was not altered (see Table 20.2). Consequently, the difference scores were substantially increased.

Measurement of the CGRP levels in vehicle-treated animals revealed no difference between left and right dorsal horns, and these levels did not differ from the levels of CGRP in normal (nonlesioned) rats. In the capsaicin-treated animals, there was a significant bilateral reduction in the levels of CGRP (see Table 20.2). Comparable results were observed with sP (data not shown).

Intrathecal Strychnine

Previous work has indicated that the incidence of transsynaptic changes following peripheral nerve section or compression was enhanced by the intrathecal injection of the glycine antagonist strychnine (25). In the present studies, groups of rats were prepared with lumbar intrathecal catheters. The compression injuries were performed as described above. At the time of surgery and at 1 and 2 days after the lesion, the rats were briefly anesthetized with halothane and received intrathecal injection of either saline or strychnine (30 μg) in saline. At 7 days, the animals were tested for thermal response latency.

In these studies, the intrathecal injection of strychnine had no effect on the response latency of the normal paw. There was, however, a marked reduction in the response latency of the otherwise hyperesthetic paw (see Table 20.3).

Modulatory Pharmacology of the Hyperesthetic State

In the present series of experiments, rats were prepared with compression injuries. The modulatory effect of several spinal receptor systems on the response latencies of the lesioned and nonlesioned paws was then assessed by intrathecally administering one of several doses of different receptor-selective agents. Each animal was used twice, at 7 and 14 days, with no animal receiving two injections of the same class of agent. The drugs examined were morphine (mu opioid: 0.3–30 nmol),

TABLE 20.2. *Effects of intrathecal capsaicin on hyperesthesia and dorsal horn CGRP levels following unilateral compression injury*

Treatment	Response latency (sec)			Dorsal horn CGRP (ng/g)	
	Normal paw	Lesioned paw	Diff. score[a]	Normal	Lesioned
Capsaicin (n = 10)	16.9 ± 0.9[b]	11.2 ± 1.2	−5.7 ± 1.3[b]	2,000 ± 210[b]	1,900 ± 200[b]
Vehicle (n = 10)	10.5 ± 0.6	7.5 ± 0.5	−3.7 ± 0.4	700 ± 170	610 ± 107

[a]Mean ± SE.
[b]$p < 0.05$ as compared to saline.

TABLE 20.3. *Effects of intrathecal strychnine on hyperesthesia and dorsal horn CGRP levels following unilateral compression injury*

	Response latency (sec)		
Treatment	Normal paw	Lesioned paw	Diff. score[a]
Vehicle (n = 6)	10.5 ± 0.1	7.7 ± 0.4	−2.8 ± 0.5
Strychnine (n = 9)	11.3 ± 0.4	6.8 ± 0.3	−4.5 ± 0.3[b]

[a]Response latency of lesioned paw − response latency of normal paw; mean ± SE.
[b]$p < 0.05$ as compared to saline.

DPDPE (delta opioid: 15–150 nmol), U50488 (kappa agonist: 20–200 nmol), ST-91 (alpha-2: 0.05–150 mol), NECA (adenosine: 0.01–1.0 nmol) baclofen (GABA-B: 0.05–5 nmol), muscimol (GABA-A: 2–30 nmol), MK801 (NMDA antagonist: 1–60 nmol), 2-amino-5-phosphonovalerate (AP-5, NMDA antagonist: 5–50 nmol), ketamine (NMDA antagonist: 40–800 nmol), kynurenic acid (non-NMDA antagonist: 20–60 nmol); g-D-glutamylaminomethyl sulfonate (GAMS, non-NMDA glutamate antagonist: 5–50 nmol), zomepirac sodium (cyclooxygenase inhibitor: 100 nmol) and CP96345 (NK-1 antagonist: 1,600 nmol).

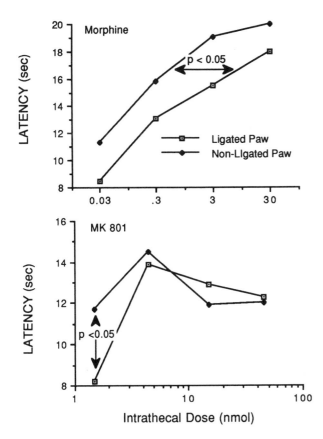

FIG. 20.3. Dose–response curves for the paw withdrawal latency in the normal (nonligated) and lesioned (ligated) paw after intrathecal morphine (**top**) or intrathecal MK 801 (**bottom**). Each point represents the mean of six to eight rats. $p < 0.05$ (top) indicates the significant right shift as indicated by ANOVA. $p < 0.05$ (bottom) indicates difference by Newman Keuls.

In these studies, mu, delta, and alpha-2 agonists resulted in a clear dose-dependent increase in the response latency of the nonligated paw. GABA-A and B and adenosine agonists also exerted a mild antinociceptive effect. NMDA and non-NMDA antagonists had no effect on paw latency until evidence of a motor dysfunction was noted. Figure 20.3 presents the dose–response curves for intrathecal morphine and intrathecal MK801 as representative of the dose–response curves for the active and inactive agents. The ED_{50} values are presented in Table 20.4. In separate experiments, intrathecal dose–response curves for these agents in unlesioned animals were obtained and the ED_{50} values were not different from those reported in Table 20.4 (data not shown).

Examination of the dose–response curves for the lesioned paw revealed opioid and alpha-2 agonists also resulted in a monotonic dose-dependent increase in the thermal response latency. As indicated in Fig. 20.3 and Table 20.4, the dose–response curves for the hyperesthetic paw are parallel to and shifted to the right of the curves for the nonlesioned paw. Of particular interest, examination of the dose–response relationship for other agents, notably the GABA-B and adenosine agonists and the NMDA antagonists, revealed that at low doses, which had no detectable effect on motor function, the agents had a highly selective effect on the hyperesthesia of the lesioned paw. At higher doses there were no further changes in response latencies until dose-related motor dysfunction was also observed.

TABLE 20.4. *Summary of dose–response analysis showing the ED 15 sec (dose required to raise the response latency to 15 sec) with 95% confidence interval (CI) for intrathecally administered receptor-preferring agonists in the paws of normal rats and in the normal and hyperesthetic paws of rats with unilateral partial ligation of the sciatic nerve and the minimum intrathecal dose that selectively blocked the hyperesthesia*

| | | Dose summary | | |
| | | Ligated paw | Nonligated paw | |
Drug	Receptor	ED 15 sec (95% CI)	ED 15 sec (95% CI)	Hyperesthesia blocking dose[a]
Morphine	Mu (agonist)	2.0 nmol (0.9–4.7)	0.2 nmol[b] (0.07–0.9)	
U50488	Kappa	>200 nmol[c]	>200 nmol	
DPDPE	Delta (agonist)	43.0 nmol (25.2–73.5)	23.7 nmol (13.8–40.9)	
ST 91	Alpha-2 (agonist)	>100 nmol	0.6 nmol (0.2–2.3)	
Baclofen	GABA-B (agonist)	0.3 nmol (0.1–0.6)	0.1 nmol (0.06–0.2)	
Muscimol	GABA-A (agonist)	11.6 nmol (5.0–26.7)	4.7 nmol[d] (2.6–8.6)	
NECA	Adenosine (agonist)		0.06 nmol (0.02–0.2)	
MK 801	NMDA (antagonist)	>60 nmol	>60 nmol	4.5 nmol
AP-5	NMDA (antagonist)	>60 nmol	>60 nmol	15 nmol
Ketamine	NMDA (antagonist)	>800 nmol	>800 nmol	370 nmol
Kynurenic acid	non-NMDA (antagonist)	>50 nmol	>50 nmol	>50 nmol
GAMS	non-NMDA (antagonist)	>40 nmol	>40 nmol	>40 nmol

[a]Minimum intrathecal dose at which the response latency of the hyperesthetic paw is not different from the nonlesioned saline response latency.
[b]Significantly different from the ligated paw ($p < 0.005$).
[c]Inactive at this dose. Upper dose limitation was typically the result of developing motor dysfunction.
[d]Significantly different from the ligated paw ($p < 0.05$).

DISCUSSION

Peripheral nerve injuries in humans can give rise to spontaneous reports of pain as well as marked changes in the reported intensity of a given stimulus. The observation that chronic compression of the sciatic nerve results in a thermal hyperesthesia thus represents a model that provides some parallels to these injury-induced disorders of sensation. Although the animal appears to favor the lesioned limb, it is difficult to determine that this represents a source of "spontaneous and ongoing discomfort." The animals appeared to thrive over the experimental period, although this was not systematically quantified. Thus, while we cannot exclude the presence of an ongoing spontaneous event, these data, although indirect, suggest that the lesion did not result in an ongoing stress from which the animal could not gain relief. On the other hand, there seems little question that the unconditioned response to the thermal stimulus reflects an exaggeration of the processing of the high-intensity thermal input, i.e., a hyperesthesia.

The time of onset and the failure to see concurrent changes in the response latency of the contralateral paw argue for a progressive change in the functioning of the afferent processing system. The fact that these changes can be modified by treatments directed at the spinal cord, as well as the nerve, argues that the observed alterations in behavior are mediated by local changes in afferent processing.

Anatomical Changes

The compression injury itself results in profound changes in the nerve in the vicinity of the ligation. The most prominent changes are Schwann cell injury and the associated loss of myelin and the phagocytic activity of macrophages. At the EM level it is clear that, in spite of the progressive loss of myelinated afferents, there is preservation of unmyelinated, small-diameter fibers, a finding previously reported (6,15). These results are consistent with the finding in the present studies that the levels of sP and CGRP in the lumbar dorsal horns ipsi- and contralateral to the compressed nerve failed to reveal any differences.

Of equal significance to the changes in the fiber degeneration are the neuropathologic changes that proceed the injury to the nerve fibers. At the light level, by 4 days, all ligated nerves displayed prominent increases in: (a) edema and endoneurial space, (b) endoneurial fibroblasts, and (c) a highly significant endothelial hypertrophy. These observations are consistent with increased endoneurial fluid pressure, decreased local nerve blood flow, and blockade of axonal transport. Previous work with other rodent models of focal nerve injury share this common picture, and it has been posited that the commonality is the development of a biomechanically induced ischemic state (17). In this regard, it is interesting to note that femoral artery occlusion and/or the local stripping of the surface vessels of the nerve have also produced evidence suggestive of hyperesthesia in rats (Myers, Yamamoto, and Yaksh, *unpublished observations*).

Mechanisms

An important question relates to the substrate over which the afferent message is transmitted following the induction of the compression injury. Capsaicin will selectively destroy spinal C-fiber terminals (19). Intrathecal treatment with the C-fiber neurotoxin capsaicin will result in a depletion of markers for small unmyelinated primary afferents, notably sP and CGRP (12,27; Yaksh et al., *present work*). The intrathecal dose given in the present study resulted in a prominent bilateral depletion of both peptides. The smaller depletion of sP suggests that a fraction of the peptide being contained in bulbospinal pathways is insensitive to this toxin. As anticipated, the normal, unlesioned paw displayed an elevation in the thermal response latency consistent with previous studies showing increases in hot plate and tail flick response latency. Of particular interest was the observation that in the same animal the response latency of the hyperesthetic paw was unaltered. These observations were entirely unexpected, given the preservation of unmyelinated profiles and the significant loss of myelinated nerve fibers. However, other groups have recently suggested that the hyperesthetic state may be mediated by A-fiber afferents (6,21). Regardless of the precise substrate, the present capsaicin results emphasize that the afferent populations that support the thermal nociceptive event in the lesioned paw differ substantially from those that support thermal nociception in the normal paw. It is important to note that in the present studies, the levels of sP and CGRP in the lumbar dorsal horns ipsilateral and contralateral to the compression injury did not differ at 7 days. The fact that the capsaicin treatment served to lower both dorsal horn levels of these peptides, but only served to elevate the response latency of the nonlesioned paw, suggests a dissociation between those peptide-containing terminals and the observed effect. These data, in fact, raise the likelihood that changes in the thermal response latency in the *normal* paw induced by capsaicin are mediated by spinal systems that do not employ afferents that contain or release sP or CGRP, although they are capsaicin sensitive. For example, it is known that FRAP-sensitive neurons are capsaicin sensitive, but to our knowledge the transmitter content of these FRAP neurons has not been identified.

Significantly, neither the response latency of the normal paw nor the hyperesthetic state with thermal stimuli is blocked by the intrathecal administration of the potent NK-1 sP antagonist CP96345.

The compression injury itself results in several changes in tropic axon function, one of which is the blockade of axon transport. While colchicine treatment (7,9) does not affect the long-term viability of the axon (11), we considered the likelihood that the block of transport might alone result in a hyperesthesia. This did not occur. Rather, the treatment with colchicine prevented the development of the hyperesthetic state. The observation that in the normal paw there is an accumulation of sP and CGRP with the colchicine treatment emphasizes that the dosing was adequate. That this effect of topical colchicine was not due to a systemic action is demonstrated by the fact that placement of the pledget peripheral to the compression did not alter the development of the hyperesthesia. This observation also suggests the hypothesis that the ligation initiates the hyperesthetic state by the transport of factors from the site of compression to the spinal cord and not by a transport of some factor to the nerve ending. In this regard, the prominent activity of macrophages in this neuropathy may play a role. It is known that the recruitment of hematogenous macrophages is an important step in the digestion of myelin debris, Schwann cell division, and Schwann cell release of nerve growth factor that is transported retrogradely to the first-order sensory neuron (3,23). Additionally, nonresident macrophages are potent sources of cytokines with varied biological effects. For example, macrophage-liberated tumor necrosis factor has been shown to induce distinct patterns of endothelial activation (16) that might have been associated with the pathologic changes in the endothelium that we report. Spontaneous activity arising from ectopic foci has also been shown to be blocked by blockade of axon transport (4). It is interesting to note that Kajander and colleagues (14) have observed increases in the firing of dorsal horn cells in these compression neuropathies.

Pharmacology of the Compression-Evoked Mononeuropathy

The present results indicate that the decreased response latency of the lesioned nerve may be elevated in a dose-dependent fashion by opioids and alpha-2 agonists. Comparison of the dose–response curves obtained with the contralateral paw and the activity in nonlesioned animals indicated that there was a parallel right shift in the dose–response curve. Whereas this right shift may be interpreted as a diminished sensitivity of the lesioned system to modulators of dorsal horn pain processing, the parallel shift and the ability to achieve a maximum blockade seem to reflect a system that is not fundamentally different from the normal paw with regard to its sensitivity to these modulatory agents, but might be modeled by an apparent increase in the magnitude of the sensory message. In other words, by modestly increasing the stimulus intensity, one would induce a right shift in the intrathecal dose–response curves for these agents (20a,26b).

In contrast, the hyperesthetic component of this compression model appears to represent a component that has a distinct pharmacology. Thus, NMDA antagonists at doses that did not elevate the normal response threshold resulted in a selective attenuation of the hyperesthesia otherwise produced in this mononeuropathy. These agents have little effect on normal thermal nociceptive thresholds at doses that do not influence motor function, a finding consistent with previous studies (26a). In previous studies, it has been shown that the intrathecal administration of strychnine will produce a transient, tactile-evoked allodynia. This syndrome is modestly sensitive to opioids but is blocked in a dose-dependent fashion by NMDA antagonists and adenosine agonists (22a,26a). NMDA antagonists have been shown to block polysynaptic excitation in the dorsal horn without altering monosynaptic excitation by primary afferents (3a). This class of agents has also been shown to have prominent effects on the facilitated activity evoked by C-fiber stimulation [windup (5)].

Although adenosine has been shown to induce a mild antinociceptive effect and may have postsynaptic actions in the dorsal horn, unlike the opiates these agents have no apparent effect on release of transmitters from C afferents (22a). Of interest in the present context, this family of agents has been shown to block glutamate release (5a,5b). As such, adenosine agonists may serve to block actions mediated by glutamate receptor systems by preventing the release of the appropriate neurotransmitter.

Central Changes Following Peripheral Nerve Injury

Peripheral nerve lesion may induce *central* changes in the organization of the systems that process afferent input. While there are no direct data, it should be emphasized that in this peripheral mononeuropathy, transsynaptic changes in the dorsal horn have been noted. Thus, "dark-staining" neurons have been reported to increase following both section and compression of the peripheral nerve in the rat (2,25).

While the identity of these dark-staining neurons is not known, it should be emphasized that many neurons in the dorsal horn are thought to be GABAergic and glycinergic (26). Strychnine binding is elevated in that region (29). Sugimoto and colleagues (25) reported that the incidence of dark-staining neurons in the dorsal horn was elevated by the administration of strychnine. In the present study, the treatment of the spinal cord twice during the period following the lesion resulted in a marked exaggeration of the hyperesthetic state at 7 days, with no change in the response latency of the contralateral paw. This correlation between these dorsal horn changes and the observed hyperesthetic state may be of pathogenetic significance.

The evidence outlined above correlating the modulatory pharmacology and the covariance of the magnitude of the hyperesthesia with treatments known to augment transsynaptic changes argues that the loss of an intrinsic modulation (perhaps glycinergic) might remove control over a facilitatory linkage (mediated in part by the release of glutamate, which acts subsequently on an NMDA receptor). This facilitation might thus be responsible in part for the observed hyperesthesia. It will be of particular interest to determine if the colchicine treatment alters the appearance of the dark-staining neurons in a manner that covaries with hyperesthesia. Additional information is clearly required as to the nature of the substrate that transmits the sensory information.

CONCLUDING HYPOTHESES

Based on the above discussions, there are several hypotheses that may be advanced regarding the time-dependent hyperesthesia induced by focal compression injury of the nerve.

1. The hyperesthetic state results from an increased activity in peripheral axons, leading to a central facilitation (akin to windup). This phenomenon would be sensitive to spinal agents such as opioids and alpha-2 agonists. The facilitation component would also be sensitive to NMDA and adenosine agonists.

2. The central facilitation could reflect a normal central processing in the face of an exaggerated afferent input and/or an alteration in the central processing systems leading to an exaggerated outflow from the dorsal horn.

3. Exaggerated outflow from the peripheral nerve could arise as a result of one or more of the following:

a. An increase in spontaneous neural activity could arise from the vicinity of the compression, and this could be locally antagonized by as yet undetermined effects of colchicine.

b. The exaggerated activity might arise from changes in the activity of dorsal root ganglion cells as a result of products transported from the compressed region such as cytokines liberated from hematogenous macrophages.

c. Secondary biomechanical effects of increased endoneurial fluid pressure. In preliminary studies we have observed that such peripheral lesions can also give rise to significant increases in endoneurial fluid pressure at the level of the rat dorsal root ganglion (18). Dorsal root ganglion cells have been shown to be sensitive to mechanical distortion such as might be caused by increased endoneurial fluid pressure, giving rise to trains of spontaneous discharges (10).

d. Alteration in the substrate activated by the afferent stimulus due to a change in transduction characteristics secondary to the injury.

4. Alterations in central processing result in a loss of central glycinergic and/or GABAergic neurons that exert a modulatory influence over the activity of interneuronal systems that release glutamate and facilitate dorsal horn outflow through a facilitatory event mediated by the NMDA receptor. The above considerations represent hypotheses that may be addressed to define the complex events leading to the compression-evoked hyperesthesia. Interestingly, it appears that a variety of nerve insults including those that are secondary to toxic events, trauma, and ischemia may share common mechanisms of hyperesthesia.

5. Finally, these observations suggest potential directions in the development of novel therapies directed at managing the hyperesthetic state. Of particular interest is the blockade of axon transport as an alternative to nerve sectioning where a peripheral nerve injury is associated with allodynia and the potential use of NMDA antagonists. Because the presumed mechanism of NMDA action reflects an effect within the spinal dorsal horn for a number of these syndromes, this should be the theoretical target site for the administration of such agents to increase their therapeutic ratio, toxicology studies permitting.

ACKNOWLEDGMENTS

We would like to thank Ms. Kristin Hagaman for carrying out the measurement of peptides and Ms. Laura Breen and Ms. Heidi Heckman for assisting with the animal studies and histology.

REFERENCES

1. Attal, N., Jazat, F., Kayser, V., and Guilbaud, G. (1990): Further evidence for 'pain-related' behaviours in a model of unilateral peripheral mononeuropathy. *Pain*, 41:235–251.
2. Bennett, G. J., and Xie, Y. K. (1988): A peripheral mononeuropathy in rat that produces disorders of pain sensation like those seen in man. *Pain*, 33:87–107.
3. Brown, M. C., Perry, V. H., Lunn, E. R., Gordon, S., and Heumann, R. (1989): Macrophage dependence of peripheral sensory nerve regeneration: possible involvement of nerve growth factor. *Neurology*, 6:359–370.
3a. Davies, S. N., and Lodge, D. (1987): Evidence for involvement of N-methylaspartate receptors in 'wind-up' of class 2 neurones in the dorsal horn of the rat. *Brain Res.*, 424:402–406.
4. Devor, M., and Govrin-Lippmann, R. (1983): Axoplasmic transport block reduces ectopic impulse generation in injured peripheral nerves. *Pain*, 16:73–85.
5. Dickenson, A. H., and Sullivan, A. F. (1990): Differential effects of excitatory amino acid antagonists on dorsal horn nociceptive neurones in the rat. *Brain Res.*, 506:31–39.
5a. Dolphin, A. C., and Prestwich, S. A. (1985): Pertussis toxin reverses adenosine inhibition of neuronal glutamate release. *Nature*, 316:148–152.
5b. Fastbom, J., and Fredholm, B. B. (1985): Inhibition of [^{3}H] glutamate release from rat hippocampal slices by L-phenylisopropyladenosine. *Acta Physiol. Scand.*, 25:121–123.
6. Gautron, M., Jazat, F., Ratinahirana, H., Hauw, J. J., and Guilbaud, G. (1990): Alterations in myelinated fibres in the sciatic nerve of rats after constriction: possible relationships between the presence of abnormal small myelinated fibres and pain-related behaviour. *Neurosci. Lett.*, 111: 28–33.
7. Grafstein, B., and Forman, D. S. (1980): Intracellular transport in neurons. *Physiol. Rev.*, 60:1167–1283.
8. Hargreaves, K., Dubner, R., Brown, F., Flores, C., and Joris, J. (1988): A new and sensitive method for measuring thermal nociception in cutaneous hyperalgesia. *Pain*, 32:77–88.

9. Hinkley, R. E., and Green, L. S. (1971): Effects of halothane and colchicine on microtubules and electrical activity of rabbit vagus nerves. *J. Neurobiol.,* 2:97–105.

10. Howe, J. F., Loeser, J. D., and Calvin, W. H. (1977): Mechanosensitivity of dorsal root ganglia and chronically injured axons: a physiological basis for the radicular pain of nerve root compression. *Pain,* 3:25–41.

11. Jackson, P., and Diamond, J. (1977): Colchicine block of cholinesterase transport in rabbit sensory nerves without interference with the long-term viability of the axons. *Brain Res.,* 130: 579–584.

12. Jhamandas, K., Yaksh, T. L., Harty, G., Szolcsanyi, J., and Go, V. L. W. (1984): Action of intrathecal capsaicin and its structural analogues in the content and release of spinal substance P: selectivity of action and relationship to analgesia. *Brain Res.,* 306:215–225.

13. Kajander, K. C., and Bennett, G. J. (1988): Analysis of the activity of primary afferent neurons in a model of neuropathic pain in the rat. *Soc. Neurosci. Abstr.,* 14:912.

14. Kajander, K. C., Wakisaka, S., and Bennett, G. J. (1989): Early ectopic discharges are generated at the dorsal root ganglion in rats with a painful peripheral neuropathy. *Soc. Neurosci. Abstr.,* 15:816.

15. Munger, B. L., and Bennett, G. J. (1990): The peripheral axonal pathology in the constrictive model of peripheral neuropathy. *Anat. Rec.,* 226:70A.

16. Munro, J. M., Pober, J. S., and Cotran, R. S. (1989): Tumor necrosis factor and interferon gamma induced distinct patterns of endothelial activation and associated leukocyte accumulation in skin of papio anubis. *Am. J. Pathol.,* 135:121–133.

17. Myers, R. R., Heckman, H. M., Galbraith, J. A., and Powell, H. C. (1991): Subperineurial demyelination associated with reduced nerve blood flow and oxygen tension after epineurial vascular stripping. *Lab. Invest.,* 65:41–50.

18. Myers, R. R., Rydevik, B. L., Heckman, H. M., and Powell, H. C. (1988): Proximodistal gradient in endoneurial fluid pressure. *Exp. Neurol.,* 102:368–370.

19. Palermo, N. N., Brown, H. K., and Smith, D. L. (1991): Selective neurotoxic action of capsaicin on glomerular C-type terminals in rat substantia gelatinosa. *Brain Res.,* 208:506–510.

20. Rydevik, B. L., Myers, R. R., and Powell, H. C. (1989): Pressure increase in the dorsal root ganglion following mechanical compression: closed compartment syndrome in nerve roots. *Spine,* 14:574–576.

20a. Saeki, S., and Yaksh, T. L. Suppression by spinal alpha-2 agonists of motor and autonomic responses evoked by low and high intensity thermal stimuli. *J.P.E.T. (in press).*

21. Shir, Y., and Seltzer, Z. (1990): A-fibers mediate mechanical hyperesthesia and allodynia and C-fibers mediate thermal hyperalgesia in a new model of causalgiform pain disorders in rats. *Neurosci. Lett.,* 115:62–67.

22. Snider, R. M., Constantine, J. W., Lowe III, J. A., et al. (1991): A potent nonpeptidic antagonist of the substance P (NK$_1$) receptor. *Science,* 252:435–437.

22a. Sosnowski, M., and Yaksh, T. L. (1989): Role of spinal adenosine receptors in modulating the hyperesthesia produced by spinal glycine receptor antagonism. *Anesth. Analg.,* 69:587–592.

23. Stoll, G., Griffin, J. W., and Trapp, B. D. (1989): Wallerian degeneration in the peripheral nervous system: participation of both Schwann cells and macrophages in myelin degradation. *J. Neurocytol.,* 18:671–683.

24. Sugimoto, T., Takemura, M., Sakai, A., and Ishimaru, M. (1986): Topical application of colchicine, vinblastine and vincristine prevents strychnine-enhanced transsynaptic degeneration in the medullary dorsal horn following transection of the inferior alveolar nerve in adult rats. *Pain,* 27:91–100.

25. Sugimoto, T., Bennett, G. J., and Kajander, K. C. (1990): Transsynaptic degeneration in the superficial dorsal horn after sciatic nerve injury: effects of chronic constriction injury, transection and strychnine. *Pain,* 42:205–213.

26. Todd, A. J., and Sullivan, A. C. (1990): Light microscopic study of the coexistence of GABA-like and glycine-like immunoreactivities in the spinal cord of the rat. *J. Comp. Neurol.,* 296:496–505.

26a. Yaksh, T. L. (1988): Behavioral and autonomic correlates of the tactile evoked allodynia produced by spinal glycine inhibition: effects of modulatory receptor systems and excitatory amino acid antagonists. *Pain,* 37:111–123.

26b. Yaksh, T. L. (1990): The analgesic pharmacology of spinally administered mu opioid agonists. *Eur. J. Pain,* 11:66–71.

27. Yaksh, T. L., Farb, D. H., Leeman, S. E., and Jessell, T. M. (1979): Intrathecal capsaicin depletes substance P in the rat spinal cord and produces prolonged thermal analgesia. *Science,* 206: 481–483.

28. Yamamoto, T., and Yaksh, T. L. (1991): Stereospecific effects of a nonpeptidergic NK-1 selective antagonist, CP 96–345: antinociception in the absence of motor dysfunction. *Life Sci.,* 49:1955–1963.

29. Zarbin, M. A., Wamsley, J. K., and Kuhar, M. J. (1981): Glycine receptor: light microscopic autoradiographic localization with [3H]-strychnine. *Neuroscience,* 1:532–547.

Hyperalgesia and Allodynia,
edited by W. D. Willis, Jr.
Raven Press, Ltd., New York © 1992.

21

Role of Central Changes in Secondary Hyperalgesia

Discussion

Howard L. Fields, Moderator

Dr. Fields: I'd like to ask Dr. Yaksh a question. How do you draw your circuit diagram in the dorsal horn to permit a strychnine hyperesthesia to escape opioid inhibition? How could opioids not have an inhibitory effect on that behavior?

Dr. Yaksh: Well, the answer is that they do. Opioids have an inhibitory effect; the dose–response curve data which I didn't show indicate a mild effect.

Dr. Fields: I thought you said the hyperesthesia was resistant to opioids.

Dr. Yaksh: The effect was pretty minimal.

Dr. Fields: Almost nonexistent?

Dr. Yaksh: No, the data we published show that there is definitely some responsiveness.

Dr. Fields: Statistically significant?

Dr. Yaksh: The important thing is that, if you look at the degree of suppression, which is clearly dependent on how we measure hyperesthesia, the phenomenon that you can get with MK801 or AP5 is really significant, whereas the effect of morphine is not. The only thing I would add to that is why is that so? Simplistically, I used to think that observation simply reflects the pre- and postsynaptic effects of morphine in the dorsal horn. In the presence of strychnine with A-beta drive coming in, we know that the terminals of A-beta primary afferents are relatively insensitive to narcotics, that is to say that the presynaptic binding is on capsaicin-sensitive primary afferents (probably C fibers) and not on noncapsaicin-sensitive afferents and that what we observed, in effect, was the effect of morphine postsynaptically only.

Dr. Fields: Dr. Guilbaud.

Dr. Guilbaud: Thank you. I want to continue on this effect of morphine in this model because we have some comparable and some different data to compare to that of Dr. Yaksh. Indeed, we are working with intravenous, not intrathecal injection.

Dr. Fields: Intravenous injection of what?

Dr. Guilbaud: Intravenous injection of morphine.

Dr. Guilbaud: In the neuropathic rat at very low doses, 0.3 to 1 mg/kg i.v. maximum, there was a clear dose-related effect of morphine on the nociceptive threshold to paw pressure. In this case the effect was more pronounced on the paw on the lesioned than on the nonlesioned side, taking into account the modification of the initial pressure. But, when we look at the effect of the same doses of morphine on the abnormal neural activity to cold, 10°C, or to all stimuli, there was no effect of morphine in this condition. So I think we have to be careful to consider the test that is used, the dose that is used, and the route of administration before making definite conclusions.

Dr. Fields: Excellent point. Dr. Perl has a comment.

Dr. Perl: I have a comment and a couple of questions. The comment is that it's been established in the rodent, at least, that the transmitter for thin primary afferent fibers is probably a glutamate-like agent. But for the thick fibers, particularly those that are associated with tactile kinds of input, it is something else. Whatever it is, it doesn't seem to be interfered with by the usual glutamate antagonists, and that, I think, needs to be factored into any kind of model. I don't think it does any damage to Dr. Woolf's model, but it may raise some issues for some of the other models. For the two questions, one is about substance P. How do you differentiate in the various discussions of substance-P effects between what is obviously presumed to be of primary afferent origin and that which is integral in the spinal cord, that is from intraspinal elements? No one really seemed to come to grips with that in the various discussions. There are changes, increases and decreases of effects, or increases and presence of substance–P-like markers, but how do you know which is which, because both in the superficial dorsal horn and deeper, there is clearly some substance P of origin other than the primary afferent fibers?

I have another question, which is really for Dr. Woolf; it was Dr. Bennett who proposed the question. Where are the inhibitory potentials that everybody has observed who has recorded from the spinal cord intracellularly, in particular from the superficial spinal cord? Almost anybody who has put an afferent input into a multireceptive neuron in the spinal cord sees inhibitory potentials as well as excitatory potentials, and Dr. Bennett wondered, and I wonder, too, where were the inhibitory potentials?

Dr. Woolf: There are two answers to that. First, there are inhibitory potentials, although the examples I showed you didn't demonstrate them. One of the reasons we don't see large-amplitude inhibitory potentials is because we're dealing with a neonatal rat preparation. The development of inhibitory interneurons seems to lag the formation of projection neurons, as Beal has shown. The later we look, the larger the inhibitory potentials, so I make no pretenses that the neonatal rat preparation is a good model for man. It's a model for showing some kinds of interactions, but it's certainly not identical to the *in vivo* situation. I agree, when you look at an adult *in vivo,* inhibitory potentials are a prominent feature. But we do, *in vivo,* still get the summation of C-evoked potentials, windup, and prolonged depolarizations, but at the same time, the contribution of the disinhibitory phenomenon to them is something that we need to be aware of.

Dr. Ng: I'd like to make a comment and then a question. We've heard very elegant presentations for the past day and a half now. However, as a clinician I'm a little disappointed because most of the models that are being used are focused on cutaneous injuries. The afferent input coming from muscle fibers, for example, has a much more potent excitatory effect on spinal cord neurons. Why haven't other models been developed?

Dr. Fields: I think they have. Maybe you should proceed to the question.

Dr. Ng: The question is, from the work that Woolf and others have done, clinically we know that activation of the large-diameter fibers has an analgesic effect and here we're seeing data that activation of some of these fibers facilitates nociception. Would you like to comment on that?

Dr. Woolf: I think the critical observation is the fact that mechanical hyperalgesia is sensitive to compression block, which removes A-beta afferent input, so there's no question that, in man, removal of an A-beta input removes the mechanical hyperalgesia. At the same time, activation of A-beta afferents by transcutaneous nerve stimulation can reduce pain. How does that happen? Well, I think that relates to the previous comment that Dr. Perl made. I think that there are enormous inhibitory postsynaptic potentials generated by A-beta afferents, and if you stimulate these fibers at sufficiently high frequencies, the kind of frequencies used clinically, I think you may get a summation of those inhibitory synaptic potentials which may, in fact, shut down the NMDA-mediated phenomena. So I think the two are not incompatible.

Dr. Fields: Yes, would you identify yourself, please?

Dr. Lebedev of Leningrad: In Russia, machine guns are very popular, but I think that Dr. Yaksh fires faster. I have two questions for Dr. Yaksh. The first: you described a painful behavior and this behavior was elicited by radiant heating. Is it really painful behavior, or is it only a spinal cord motor escape reflex, because we know the tail flick can be elicited in spinal animals? And for the other question, I want you to return to yesterday's discussion about regeneration of fibers. You have the same data that Dr. Perl had in his presentation. What is your point of view when there is a restoration of hypersensitivity in 15 or 20 days—is this regeneration, or what happened with the fibers?

Dr. Yaksh: With regard to the issue of the spinal reflex, I agree with you, that's a major question. In the case of this flick model, we think that's not an issue because, for one thing, although you can generate a flick reflex in the transected animal after it's lost spinal shock, you can get a flexion withdrawal. These animals show what is a very clear behavioral component. The jerk is very limited and very motorically appropriate.

Dr. Guilbaud: When we consider another, more integrated reaction, which is a struggling reaction after immersing the paw in hot water, there is also a kind of allodynia and hyperalgesia to thermal stimulation. Concerning nerve damage, I do not understand Dr. Yaksh when he says that all the mechanisms are located at the spinal level and there is nothing to do with peripheral fibers, which are very, very dramatically damaged. So, I think that although there are surely some changes at the spinal level and maybe upstream, the peripheral fiber damage is involved initially in the various pain-related behaviors to a significant degree. With this lesion there are maximum signs of degeneration at 2 weeks, but there are already consistent signs of regeneration. So, based on our extensive studies of the anatomical damage of this nerve, we think that a great part of these pain-related behaviors is due to the localized damage, maybe to ephapses or some abnormal contact between fibers. So I don't agree with Dr. Yaksh totally concerning the origin of this disease.

Dr. Yaksh: The data that are required are the characteristics of the C fibers and A-beta and A-delta fibers proximal to the compression with the stimulus applied to the old receptive field. When those data appear and we see that in fact that there is an augmented transduction of the thermal stimulus and the stimulus response curves for the C fibers are all shifted to the left, then we'll know, but I think that at this moment in time, we were impressed by the fact that the allodynia went away with the colchicine treatment.

Dr. Wilcox: This is a question for Dr. Woolf. Many of the windup experiments you've shown, I believe, are on ventral horn neurons in the neonatal cord. How often do you see it in dorsal horn neurons?

Dr. Woolf: The reason for going for the ventral horn initially was because it was much easier to record from those cells, but in fact we see exactly the same phenomenon in dorsal horn neurons. The only caveat to that is that we went for flexor motor neurons because we knew that *in vivo* they showed similar windup. When we go for the dorsal horn neurons, we see many cells that don't have slow synaptic potentials and don't show windup, so when we do see cells with slow synaptic potentials, they do wind up and they respond to APV and in fact they do everything, sometimes in a much more dramatic sense, but it is not as easy and there are not as many cells.

Dr. Abrams: We've heard of several models of mechanical hyperalgesia. Are any of these models associated with cold allodynia as well? We see this often in our so-called RSD patients, and this is of particular interest to those of us that practice in northern climates.

Dr. Guilbaud: Yes, I can say that with the mononeuropathic rats of Dr. Bennett, there is a clear cold allodynia. Usually when the normal paw is immersed in a 10° water bath, the latency for the struggling reaction is around 15 sec. In neuropathic rats the latency is strongly decreased to 9 sec, so there is a clear abnormal cold reactivity in these rats. These abnormal reactivities to cold are sensitive to guanethidine pretreatment or treatment and also to sympathectomy. So I think this model exhibits clear signs which make it appropriate to the clinical condition of RSD.

Dr. Fields: Dr. Ronald Dubner.

Dr. Dubner: I have a question both for Dr. Guilbaud and for Dr. Schaible. It relates to the subject of central changes, central hyperexcitability. One of the questions that might be of interest mechanistically is whether the changes that one sees are changes occurring at that level, or a reflection of changes that have occurred at a previous level within the nervous system. So, for example, in Dr. Guilbaud's experiments, do we know whether the changes one is seeing in the thalamus represent changes that might have occurred at the periphery as well as in the spinal cord, or are they actually changes in excitability of the neurons in the thalamus? One way that might be addressed is what one does in looking in the spinal cord; you bypass the receptor and electrically stimulate afferents the way Dr. Schaible did to see whether there is still an increase in excitability in the spinal cord. Similarly, you could do the same thing by stimulating the projection pathways, such as the spinothalamic pathway, that ascend from the spinal cord to the thalamus. Now, the same thing applies to Dr. Schaible's issue of whether the descending effects represent an action in the spinal cord or a change in descending systems occurring at higher levels. That could also be addressed by looking at changes in spinal cord excitability by electrically stimulating descending pathways. So I ask both of you the question, have you done those experiments?

Dr. Guilbaud: No, but I have never said that the modifications that we have described were occurring only at the thalamic level. For me, what we are recording is mainly a reflection of what happens at lower levels. In any case, the thing that I wanted to show is that the peripheral process triggers some central phenomena, since the hyperalgesia seen on the opposite side cannot be explained without something which is arriving at least at the spinal cord level. Your suggestion to stimulate electrically is very good. We have not performed such electrical stimulation so far.

Dr. Schaible: We have not done the experiments you ask for, but I would like to say if we have these compounds hanging around in the spinal cord, it might be difficult to interpret the results of electrical stimulation. For example, neurokinin, whose effect we don't know in the spinal cord, is released and hangs around for hours. The data of Dr. Guilbaud I could explain perfectly well with changes in the spinal cord. Of course, Dr. Schmidt could now attack me and say I can explain your data with afferent fibers, because if neurokinin, for example, should be released from afferent fibers, then it is in fact a peripheral component which is initiating all these central changes. And now I would like to go back to the question Dr. Perl asked. With the method of antibody microprobes, we cannot respond to the question of whether substance P or any other compound is released from afferent fibers or spinal cord neurons.

Dr. Fields: Dr. Donald Price.

Dr. Price: In human neuropathic pain conditions, such as trigeminal neuralgia, as Dr. Dubner has shown, and RSD, as we have shown, under certain conditions, A-beta stimulation applied at very slow rates produces a windup of allodynic pain. I was wondering, and I ask this of Dr. Woolf and of Dr. Yaksh, is there anything you've seen in your animal models that suggests windup of responses to A-beta stimulation? If so, is it related to the NMDA receptor; that is, is it antagonizable by such things as MK801 or AP5?

Dr. Woolf: For the intracellular recordings we haven't seen anything like that. The only time I've seen it is in a pharmacological manipulation which Dr. Yaksh has subsequently also done. When you give intrathecally a high dose of morphine, you get a very bizarre state which seems to resemble the strychnine and bicuculline model. In that situation puffing of the skin repetitively does produce a buildup; now I don't know whether you've tested NMDA on that or not.

Dr. Yaksh: Not on the high-dose morphine, but of course on the strychnine-evoked allodynia. The morphine effect, of course, is probably due to the metabolite, morphine-3 glucuronide, and the effects of this on the blood pressure. We've not done anything quite so elegant as single-unit recording, obviously, but the effects on the augmented blood pressure response generated following strychnine are completely blocked by MK801 and AP5. The tactile-evoked hyperesthesia is produced merely by gently rubbing the skin. The response is a very florid phenomenon. It is not unlike that to substance P intrathecally. The animals are incredibly aggressive. You literally can't handle the animals. MK801 at doses that do not produce any effect on motor function that we can detect, at doses less than 30 µg completely abolishes this. It's extremely striking, and yet at that dose the animal has normal thermal nociception.

If you want to see the effects of endogenous modulation, I would say one extreme is morphine for its effect on C fibers; the other effect is on this low-threshold input.

Dr. Woolf: If I could just add a brief comment on something I think hasn't really been addressed. We've all spoken about mechanical allodynia, but clearly clinically it's allodynia to rapidly adapting stimuli, not to sustained stimuli. I have no satisfactory explanation for why, if you have a sustained innocuous input, you do not have the same kind of sensitivity. I don't know if Dr. LaMotte has any comment on that with your model.

Dr. LaMotte: That's true. It seems to require a movement of the stimulus. However, at times when we have injected deeper underneath the skin, you get a kind of aching hyperalgesia. Dr. Simone is doing some work on that by injecting capsaicin into the muscle. Then a blunt stimulus can produce some hyperalgesia. I was wondering if you have applied mustard oil to your own skin. If so, what is the time course of primary and secondary hyperalgesia, or is there any secondary hyperalgesia? Is there ongoing pain, and what's the time course in relation to the effects you've observed?

Dr. Woolf: Right. Firstly, if you applied mustard oil to the skin accidentally, that's something I don't advise people to do, it doesn't produce an effect because it doesn't seem to penetrate the skin. But if you have a small abrasion and you'd rapidly find out if you do, because if it contacts it, it produces the same kind of effect that you describe following capsaicin: intense burning, literally tears in the eye type of pain, with mechanical sensitivity. We haven't done anything like your sophisticated analyses.

Dr. LaMotte: Is there any secondary hyperalgesia?

Dr. Woolf: Yes, there is.

Dr. Fields: Dr. Jeftinija.

Dr. Jeftinija: Question to Dr. LaMotte. Did you try to block nerves in any other way than local anesthetic in the experiments in which you blocked the effects of capsaicin?

Dr. LaMotte: No. We, of course, anesthetized the skin by cooling, but other than that we didn't try different types of blocks.

Dr. Jeftinija: Did cooling work?

Dr. LaMotte: That was just cooling the site of injury.

Dr. Jeftinija: And not proximal to the area?

Dr. LaMotte: No. A long time ago Bickford produced a cold block. You mean by blocking a whole nerve by cooling, for example?

Dr. Jeftinija: Yes.

Dr. LaMotte: That's kind of risky because you can produce some damage if you're not careful. We haven't done that.

Dr. Fields: Two more questions. First, Dr. Boivie.

Dr. Boivie. A clinical background. I had a sad case, a woman about 50 years of age who had a small crush injury on the outer part of the left little finger. This produced ongoing pain, irritating her so much that after 5 years she asked to have the tip of the finger removed. At that time she was tender; she had allodynia or hyperalgesia, if you wish. After the amputation, the allodynia spread, as we have seen, and she was unsatisfied and went to another surgeon who removed the rest of the finger. There spread through the whole hand a very severe hypersensitivity to all stimuli of the skin. This spread up the arm, and when she came to us, she asked to have the arm removed, which we didn't do, of course. So an irritation starts this process and then you cut the nerve in two steps and you increase these reactions. Have you experimentally looked at anything similar to that?

Dr. Fields: Dr. Guilbaud?

Dr. Guilbaud: No, I have no explanation at all. We have looked at the damage which is induced by a loose ligature around the nerve. It is apparently a very modest lesion and when you see all the damage that is induced by this small lesion from the anatomical point of view, you can imagine that even a small lesion of the tip of the digit can also induce a lot of fiber degeneration, then regeneration and so on. I know that is not an answer, but I think that the study of this model was also interesting from the point of view of showing that even a small lesion of the nerve, but a persistent lesion, which I think is really important. By contrast, with a crush, we have not this kind of pain-related behavior in the following week. This very small persistent lesion can induce a very marked change of the fibers, so maybe when you cut the digit, you also have all these regenerating fibers which are forming some new endings.

Dr. Fields: Dr. José Ochoa.

Dr. Ochoa: A quick comment which was spurred on by the comment that Dr. Woolf just made concerning the clinical meaning of mechanical hyperalgesia. In patients with chronic pain and hyperalgesia there are two kinds of behavioral mechanical hyperalgesia. One is the one that most people call allodynia, in which gentle repetitive stroking causes a very unpleasant sensation, which is not painful. It is a weird sensation; it's more akin to tickling than it is to pain. That dynamic mechanical hyperalgesia disappears with an A-fiber block. But there's a very distinct mechanical hyperalgesia which does not disappear with an A-fiber block and which is triggered by sustained pressure at normally nonpainful intensity. Clearly these two kinds of mechanical hyperalgesia are served by different kinds of afferent input and must have different central mechanisms—one is peripheral, the other one is central. Now the remarkable clinical observation is that the area in skin for dynamic and static mechanical hyperalgesia when it coexists in patients is exactly the same and that turns out to be a very challenging observation because if one is postulating different mechanisms, somehow the idea of a behavioral expression of the hyperalgesia is exactly the same and somebody should investigate this.

Hyperalgesia and Allodynia,
edited by W. D. Willis, Jr.
Raven Press, Ltd., New York © 1992.

22

Mechanisms of Central Changes Produced by Peripheral Damage

Overview

G. F. Gebhart

*Department of Pharmacology, University of Iowa College of Medicine,
Iowa City, Iowa 52242-1109*

Following sensitization of nociceptive primary afferents or injury of afferent nerves, a variety of changes in the CNS have been noted. The chapters in this section address the mechanisms by which some of these central changes may occur.

Building on earlier observations that primary afferent terminals in the dorsal horn contain both substance P (sP) and glutamate, Rustioni and Weinberg report that sP and glutamate are contained in different compartments in these terminals. Glutamate is contained in clear vesicles, whereas sP is contained in dense core vesicles, raising the possibility that their release may be independently regulated. Dorsal root ganglion cells, primarily of the small type, also contain glutamate (and glutaminase) as well as aspartate and about 25% also contain sP. Interestingly, the amino acid neurotransmitters glutamate and aspartate are cocontained in primary afferent terminal profiles in the substantia gelatinosa and Rustioni and Weinberg speculate on their independent regulation. Complementing this neuroanatomy, Haley and Wilcox describe the cellular events associated with release of these neurotransmitter substances as sequentially involving activation by an excitatory amino acid of an alpha-amino-3-hydroxy-5-methyl-4-isoxazole-propionic acid (AMPA) receptor that "primes" an N-methyl-D-aspartate (NMDA) receptor, leading to a rapid depolarization of the postsynaptic element. sP, acting at NK-1 receptors on the same postsynaptic element, initiates a slower and longer lasting depolarization. Although excitatory amino acids are believed to contribute to "windup" in the dorsal horn, longer term changes (e.g., induction of early immediate genes) may require a combination of excitatory messages mediated by amino acids and peptide neurotransmitters and their second messenger systems.

This anatomy and physiology in the spinal dorsal horn are significantly altered when peripheral nerves are injured. When such injury occurs, multiple excitatory messages are generated and both immediate and long-term changes in the spinal cord are produced. After experimental peripheral nerve injury, Rustioni and Weinberg describe a fusion of dense core, peptide-containing vesicles to terminal membranes in the dorsal horn. Most interestingly, wheat germ agglutinin-horseradish peroxidase (WGA-HRP) reaction product was present in the extracellular space, raising the provocative possibility that neuroactive peptides released upon injury and excluded from the synapse contribute to a variety of CNS changes.

Other experimental approaches and different changes in the CNS are reported by Bennett and Laird, Basbaum et al., and Ruda and Dubner. Following experimental constriction of the sciatic nerve, which produces a neuropathic hyperalgesia, Bennett and Laird describe transsynaptic degeneration and the appearance of "dark neurons" in the superficial dorsal horn. The transsynaptic degeneration is believed to occur primarily in inhibitory interneurons in the spinal dorsal horn. They hypothesize that peripheral nerve injury leads to a reduction in presynaptic inhibitory mechanisms in the dorsal horn (i.e., disinhibition) and that this transsynaptic process, mediated by excitatory amino acids, leads to central hyperexcitability. Bennett and Laird speculate that excitatory amino acid receptor antagonists would be efficacious against neuropathic hyperalgesia and also prevent transsynaptic degeneration/central hyperexcitability following nerve injury.

Consistent with longer term changes in the spinal cord following nerve injury, Basbaum et al. transected the sciatic nerve and observed persistent expression of the c-fos proto-oncogene for up to 1 month after surgery. The expression of Fos protein oscillated in some areas of the dorsal horn, but was strikingly stable in other areas of the spinal cord. Fos protein is presumed to result from excitation of neurons, and it was hypothesized that activity within the sciatic nerve neuroma contributes to expression of the Fos protein. In support of such an interpretation, local anesthesia of the nerve reduced the number of labeled cells in some areas of the spinal cord, but failed to do so at all times tested and influenced Fos expression in different patterns when tested at different times. Thus, whereas long-term central changes in this putative "third messenger" clearly result following peripheral nerve injury, and likely contribute to hyperalgesia, the temporal picture of changes in Fos protein after sciatic nerve injury suggest that mechanisms not yet understood contribute to neuropathic pain.

Ruda and Dubner employed a third model of nerve injury. When tested 6 to 8 weeks after capsaicin treatment as neonates, peripheral inflammation and hyperalgesia produced by an intraplantar injection of complete Freund's adjuvant were not different than those seen in vehicle-treated rats. Capsaicin treatment did, however, significantly decrease the numbers of sP-containing primary afferent terminal profiles, Fos-labeled nuclear profiles, and preprodynorphin-containing neuronal profiles in the spinal dorsal horn. Ruda and Dubner suggest thus that Fos protein and dynorphin gene expression require input from capsaicin-sensitive primary afferents and that these and other protein products are associated with central changes in response to peripheral tissue injury.

The studies reported in this section document the wide range of central changes that occur in association with a variety of peripheral nerve injuries. It is clear that we have probably underestimated how commonplace such changes are as well as their variety and magnitude. Excitotoxic events in the spinal dorsal horn, mediated by excitatory amino acid receptors that increase Ca^{2+} permeability, may be a common consequence of peripheral nerve damage and lead to persistent central alterations and pain. Mechanisms proposed and examined to date suggest that antagonists at excitatory amino acid receptors and perhaps kappa opioid receptors may be efficacious against hyperalgesic and sensitization phenomena.

Hyperalgesia and Allodynia,
edited by W. D. Willis, Jr.
Raven Press, Ltd., New York © 1992.

23

Neurotransmission in Primary Afferents to Superficial Laminae of the Dorsal Horn

A. Rustioni and R. J. Weinberg

Department of Cell Biology and Anatomy, University of North Carolina,
Chapel Hill, North Carolina 27599

Over the past decade, work in our laboratory has been aimed at the identification of neuromediators that may be released by dorsal root ganglion (DRG) neurons. Our focus has been on the immunocytochemical demonstration of amino acid neurotransmitters in DRG neurons and their terminals in the dorsal horn of the spinal cord. The immunocytochemical evidence for glutamate as neurotransmitter in DRG neurons and its coexistence with substance P (SP) in some of these neurons, as originally reported in work from our laboratory, is here summarized very briefly (for a review on this topic, see ref. 36). The rest of the work presented in this chapter deals with: (A) further immunocytochemical evidence for amino acid neurotransmitters in DRG neurons, (B) colocalization of amino acid neurotransmitters in the same primary afferent terminal, and (C) some considerations on the possible modulation of spinal cord activity by extrasynaptic neural communication.

The production of an antiglutamate antibody was a prerequisite for our investigation of amino acid neurotransmitters in DRG neurons. This antibody was raised in rabbits against glutamate conjugated with glutaraldehyde to the invertebrate carrier protein hemocyanin (14). Characterization of the antibody on sections from fixed brains and by immunoblot analysis revealed no significant cross-reactivity with conjugates of compounds structurally similar to glutamate. A similarly prepared antibody against SP was characterized and shown to have very low (<0.1%) cross-reactivity with neurokinins A and B (6).

In a quantitative survey of cervical DRGs in rats it was found that up to 70% of somata of DRG neurons are immunoreactive for glutamate (3). Glutamate-positive DRG neurons are mainly of the small type, or type B of Andres (2). The majority of the small DRG neurons immunopositive for glutamate are also immunopositive for glutaminase, an enzyme that converts glutamine into glutamate; about 25% of DRG neurons immunopositive for glutamate, all of small size, are also immunopositive for SP.

Immunopositivity for glutamate has also been observed, with pre-embedding electron microscopical immunocytochemistry, in dorsal root fibers (47) and, with both pre- and postembedding methods, in dorsal root afferent terminals in the superficial laminae (I and II) of the dorsal horn (9,26,44). Both type 1 and 2 terminals, as described by Ribeiro-Da-Silva and Coimbra (33), are immunopositive for glutamate. Many type 1 terminals—believed to be associated with unmyelinated primary affer-

ent fibers—can be double-stained for glutamate and SP (9) (Fig. 23.1). SP immunocytochemistry in these terminals is largely confined to large dense core vesicles (9).
Double-staining immunocytochemistry combined with anterograde tracing demonstrated that both type 1 and 2 glutamate immunopositive terminals are indeed from
primary afferents (9). The immunopositivity for glutamate in terminals of presumed
unmyelinated endings also containing SP established an anatomical basis for the proposal that release of glutamate is involved in the mediation of nociceptive input to
the dorsal horn of the spinal cord (1,37–39,51).

A. Following publication of the work reviewed above, immunopositivity for glutamate in primary afferents to the dorsal horn was demonstrated in cats (24) with
the antibody of Storm-Mathisen et al. (40) and confirmed in rats (25) with the antibody of Hepler et al. (14). Although neither of these papers attempted to establish
the origin of stained endings, in both cases glutamate immunoreactivity was observed in endings typical of dorsal root afferents. In cats, glutamate-stained terminals in superficial laminae presumed to originate from DRG neurons included the
dark sinuous type terminals containing large dense core vesicles (LDCVs) and "regular" synaptic terminals. The first two types may be homologous to type 1, and the
regular terminals are similar to the type 2 terminals of Ribeiro-Da-Silva and Coimbra
(33). Dense glutamate staining was present in dark sinuous terminals (in dorsal regions of lamina II) and in regular terminals (in ventral II and in lamina III). Weaker
glutamate staining was observed in LDCV terminals in lamina I and dorsal II (24).
These data indirectly confirm the coexistence of glutamate and peptides (in LDCV
terminals) and the likelihood of glutamate as neurotransmitter in unmyelinated fi-

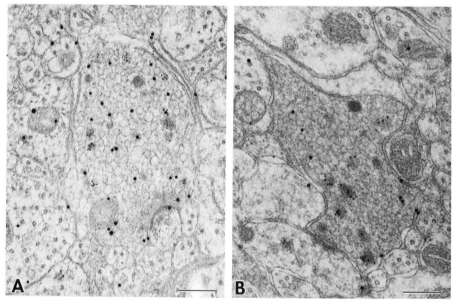

FIG. 23.1. A and **B:** Two examples of type 1 terminals (as determined by the irregular size of
vesicles and relative absence of mitochondria) in lamina II double-stained for glutamate (large
dots) and for SP (small dots). Staining for SP is clustered over large dense core vesicles.
Calibration: 0.25 μm. (Courtesy of Dr. S. De Biasi.)

bers. Colocalization of glutamate and SP was confirmed in the double-staining study of Merighi et al. (25), who also showed the coexistence of these two mediators with calcitonin gene-related peptide (CGRP). Both peptides are associated with LDCVs, most of the stained vesicles containing both SP and CGRP; however, not all LDCVs are stained for either peptide (see also ref. 31).

We have recently used an antibody for aspartate produced and characterized in the same way as our glutamate antibody (14). Once it was determined with blocking experiments that the two antibodies did not cross-react, serial sections were prepared from cervical DRGs. Aspartate immunopositivity was virtually exclusively in small (type B) DRG neurons and the majority of these neurons were stained (41). Using consecutive thin sections, it was found that all aspartate immunoreactive DRG neurons were also immunopositive for glutamate (41) (Fig. 23.2). With both pre- and postembedding immunocytochemistry for electron microscopy, it was also found that many type 1 and 2 terminals stain with the aspartate antibody (41).

Aspartate immunopositivity in DRGs has not been studied by other investigators.

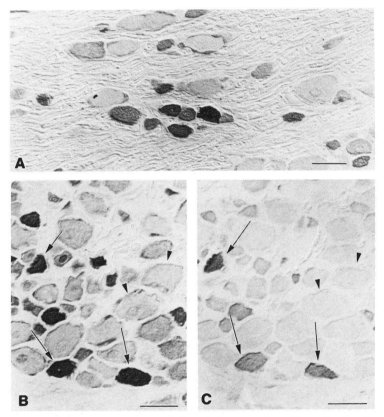

FIG. 23.2. Immunostaining in sections of dorsal root ganglia with antibodies for aspartate and glutamate. **A:** Cryostat section showing aspartate-stained cell bodies. **B** and **C:** Colocalization in adjacent cryostat sections stained for aspartate (B) and for glutamate (C). Corresponding stained neurons are indicated by *arrows* and corresponding unstained neurons are indicated by *arrowheads*. Neurons stained by the antiaspartate antibody are also stained by the antiglutamate antibody, but not with equal intensity. Calibration: 50 μm. (From ref. 41.)

Two groups who have looked for aspartate staining in the superficial laminae of the dorsal horn report either sparsely stained terminals (25) or no staining above background (24). However, Westlund et al. (48) observed aspartate immunoreactive fibers in dorsal roots. Although these fibers appeared to be more numerous than glutamate immunopositive ones (47), in both cases the percentage of stained unmyelinated afferent fibers was higher than myelinated ones. Whereas a fair degree of agreement exists in the immunocytochemical observations on staining for amino acids in DRG neurons and their terminals in superficial laminae of the dorsal horn, discrepancies exist when comparing staining of cell bodies with that of terminals in other regions. For instance, most terminals of primary afferents in the dorsal column nuclei stain for glutamate (10), whereas the large cells in the DRGs that give origin to this projection (13) are, for the most part, unstained (3). This might be related to the patterns of central arborization: Unmyelinated primary afferents may terminate more locally than large afferents; somatic concentrations of amino acid transmitters (synthesized at terminals) may be elevated only for neurons with shorter central processes.

B. To verify whether primary afferent terminals in superficial laminae are stained for both glutamate and aspartate, we injected wheat germ agglutinin-horseradish peroxidase (WGA-HRP) as transganglionic tracer in the sciatic nerve and employed postembedding immunocytochemistry using gold particles of two different sizes. Of the various immunocytochemical protocols tested, we found the following to give the best results for our postembedding colloidal gold staining (30). Wash mesh grids for 5 min in 0.05 M Tris, pH 7.6, with 0.9% NaCl and 0.1% Triton X-100 (TBST 7.6), dry and incubate in primary antiglutamate antibody (up to 1:500,000, preabsorbed for 4 hr with 1 mM aspartate) overnight in a moist chamber. This was followed by two changes of TBST 7.6 (5 and 30 min) and one change of TBST 8.2 (0.05 M Tris, pH 8.2 with 0.9% NaCl and 0.1% Triton X-100) for 5 min. Grids were subsequently incubated in secondary antibody conjugated to 20 nm (or 10 nm) gold particles diluted (1:25) in TBST 8.2 for 1 hr in a moist chamber. After two washes in TBST 7.6 for 5 min each, grids were rinsed in deionized water and then allowed to dry. For double-staining immunocytochemistry, grids were then exposed to paraformaldehyde vapors at 80°C for 1 hr, washed in TBST 7.6 for 5 min and incubated in the second primary antibody (antiaspartate, 1:10,000, preabsorbed with 1 mM glutamate for 4 hr) in TBST 7.6 overnight in a moist chamber. Subsequent steps were as described above, using secondary antibody conjugated to 10 nm (or 20 nm) gold.

Most anterogradely labeled terminals in lamina II, both type 1 and 2, were double-stained for glutamate and aspartate (Fig. 23.3). They were identified as primary afferents by the crystals of reaction product and as double-stained by the presence of above background gold particles of two sizes (Fig. 23.4). Particles were distributed rather homogeneously between or over synaptic vesicles.

The coexistence of glutamate and aspartate in primary afferent terminals in the substantia gelatinosa is consistent with previous studies of the coexistence of these two amino acids in DRG somata (41), supporting the possibility that aspartate may be a neurotransmitter in small DRG neurons. Preliminary results from our lab suggest that a large fraction of primary afferent terminals in deeper laminae also stain above background for glutamate and aspartate; thus, these amino acids may not be specific markers for nociceptive afferents. The evidence for aspartate as neurotransmitter in primary afferents is inconclusive (5,11,15,17,19,20,28,32,38,39), and the

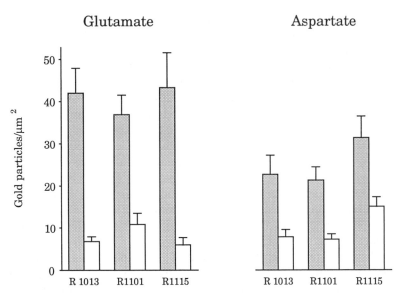

FIG. 23.3. Histogram showing the density of gold particles over primary afferent terminals in lamina II compared with that over random profiles excluding synaptic terminals. The counts are from 30 terminals from three different rats (R1013, R1101, R1115). Terminal labeling was significantly above background for both antigens. Whereas the background level for the two antigens is comparable, the number of aspartate-coding particles over terminals is lower than that of glutamate.

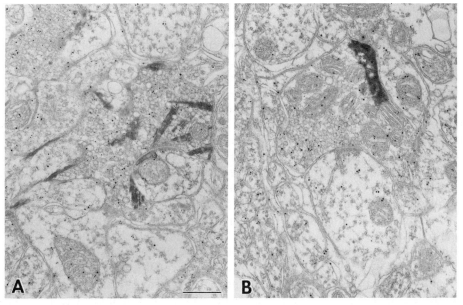

FIG. 23.4. Two examples of anterogradely labeled, double-stained primary afferent terminals, one of type 1 (**A**) and one of type 2 (**B**). Density of glutamate staining (small beads) and aspartate staining (large beads) were $56/\mu m^2$ and $12/\mu m^2$, respectively, for A (background staining $12/\mu m^2$ and $6/\mu m^2$) and $36/\mu m^2$ and $12/\mu m^2$ (background staining $14/\mu m^2$ and $6/\mu m^2$) for B. Calibration: 0.25 μm.

validity of the present results is complicated by the question of whether immuno-cytochemically detected amino acids represent neurotransmitters or merely chemi-cals of metabolic significance. Against this latter possibility are (a) terminals en-riched in gamma-aminobutyric acid (GABA) do not immunostain for glutamate or aspartate and (b) in terminals cut to include portions of the preterminal axon, glu-tamate and aspartate immunoreactivity are selectively elevated over the vesicle-rich portion; moreover, a variety of biochemical and pharmacologic evidence also sup-ports that these terminals may use an excitatory amino acid transmitter.

Taking these results at face value, what might be the functional significance of releasing glutamate and aspartate from the same terminal? Since aspartate may be a relatively specific ligand for the *N*-methyl-D-aspartate (NMDA) receptor (7,29), it is conceivable that this amino acid plays a specific role in spinal processing. NMDA receptors (present at high densities in the substantia gelatinosa) mediate windup [the increased responsiveness of spinal neurons to afferent stimulation after several vol-leys at C-fiber strength (8)]; chronic pain may involve NMDA-mediated synaptic changes at the spinal level (50). It seems at first glance puzzling that NMDA-related effects might be selectively mediated by aspartate: What biological advantage could be conferred by providing two agents to mediate actions that could be achieved by glutamate alone? By independently regulating aspartate and glutamate concentra-tions, the balance of brief [alpha-amino-3-hydroxy-5-methyl-4-isoxazole propionic acid- (AMPA) mediated] versus more sustained (NMDA-mediated) effects of activity could be modulated. It is also conceivable that aspartate and glutamate are contained in distinct vesicles having different exocytotic characteristics, but there is at present no evidence to support this possibility.

C. Several lines of evidence suggest that distinct functions may be performed by amino acids and peptides released by primary afferents in the superficial laminae of the dorsal horn. Small clear vesicles (containing amino acids) and LDCVs (contain-ing peptides) may be released under different circumstances, and exocytosis of LDCVs is preferentially away from the active zone. The evidence in the literature raises the possibility that these peptides may normally be released only during sus-tained high-frequency stimuli or secondary to injury (43,49,52).

In experiments designed to determine suitable tracing parameters to use in con-junction with double-staining immunocytochemistry, we observed some features of anterograde labeling that suggest an interpretation of the significance of coexistence of amino acids and peptides in the same DRG fiber. To establish optimal parameters for labeling fine afferent fibers, two different tracers were tested: either 0.25 to 2.5 µl of 5% to 10% WGA-HRP in dimethyl sulfoxide (DMSO) or 1.0 to 1.5 µl of 1% to 2% cholera toxin B subunit conjugated to HRP (CTB-HRP) in DMSO was injected in the sciatic nerve. After 60 to 160 hr animals were perfused with physiological saline followed by 2.5% glutaraldehyde, 0.5% paraformaldehyde, and 0.1% picric acid in pH 7.4 phosphate buffer. Pertinent spinal cord segments (L3, L4, and L5) and their DRG were removed and cut in consecutive 50-µm thick sections with a Vibratome. These were incubated according to a modified tetramethylbenzidine pro-tocol using ammonium paratungstate as stabilizer (46). For light microscopic obser-vations, sections were mounted unstained or counterstained with 0.02% thionin and examined in bright- and dark-field illumination. Sections of spinal segments and gan-glia selected for electron microscopy were wafer-embedded in Epon. Thin sections were mounted on copper or nickel mesh grids or single-hole, formvar-coated grids and counterstained with uranyl acetate and lead citrate.

With all survival times and volumes injected, only small DRG neurons were la-

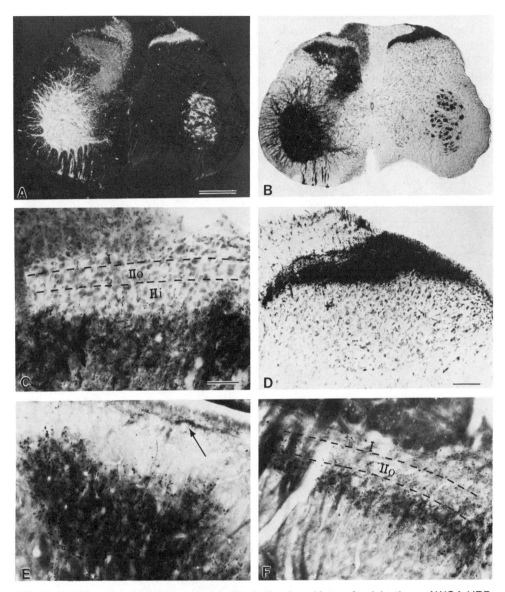

FIG. 23.5. Differences in anterograde labeling in the dorsal horn after injections of WGA-HRP or CTB-HRP in the sciatic nerve. **A** and **B** are dark- and bright-field low-power photomicrographs, respectively, of a section from L4 of a rat with injection of CTB-HRP on the left and of WGA-HRP on the right. **C** shows the sharp border between labeled and unlabeled regions on the side with CTB-HRP injection in a section counterstained to show laminar borders of the superficial dorsal horn. **D:** The reaction product in the superficial dorsal horn on the side of WGA-HRP. The ventral border of reaction product in D corresponds to the dorsal border of reaction product in C. Similar comparison is shown in **E** and **F** from plastic-embedded sections. In E the *arrow* points to CTB-HRP labeled primary afferents in lamina I. Calibration in A and B: 0.5 mm. Calibration in C pertains also to E and F and corresponds to 50 μm. Calibration in D: 100 μm.

beled after WGA-HRP injections, whereas large ones were preferentially labeled after CTB-HRP (34). This dichotomy was paralleled by the results in the spinal dorsal horn. Here WGA-HRP consistently gave very dense labeling of a band of gray matter extending up to about 110 μm from the margin of the dorsal horn encompassing laminae I and II (Fig. 23.5A and B). Labeling was densest in the inner part of lamina II (IIi) and appeared broader medially as a result of the thinning out of the lateral part of lamina II (27) (Fig. 23.5C and F). In sharp contrast with these results, CTB-HRP labeled fibers and presumed terminals throughout the spinal cord but was virtually absent from the same superficial band of gray matter heavily involved after

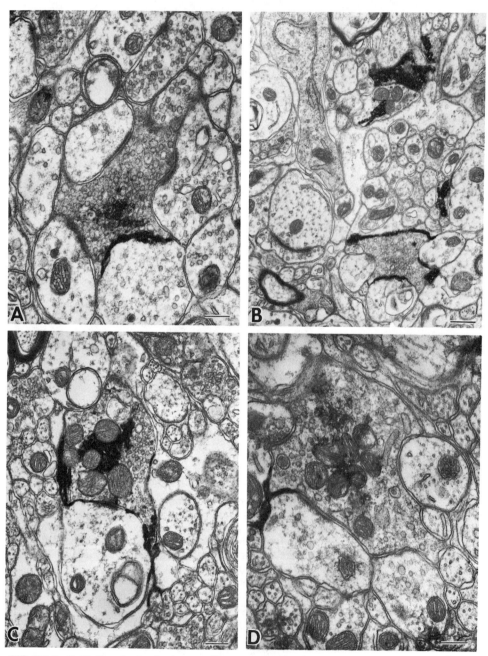

FIG. 23.6. A–D: Terminals of primary afferents in lamina II after injection of WGA-HRP in the sciatic nerve. Anterograde labeling is present inside the terminals in the form of either crystals or diffuse amorphous material. Reaction product is also present in the extracellular space surrounding the labeled terminals or its immediate vicinity. The extracellular product is never seen invading the synaptic cleft (C and D). Calibration: 0.2 μm in A, C, and D; 0.5 μm in B.

injections of WGA-HRP, except for a thin (20 μm) band immediately adjacent to the dorsal funiculus corresponding to lamina I (Fig. 23.5A–D).

Electron microscopy revealed labeled terminals of primary afferents in laminae I and II after WGA-HRP injection, whereas after CTB-HRP injection, no labeled terminals were seen in lamina II. In deeper laminae, numerous myelinated profiles and primary afferent terminals were labeled after CTB-HRP injection, whereas only sparse labeling was discernible in deep laminae after WGA-HRP. The appearance of terminal labeling with the two tracers was similar, consisting of crystals of reaction product apparently located at random, only rarely obscuring the cytological features of the terminal. Punctate reaction product was also seen, especially in areas surrounding the crystals. The discrepancy in results after injections of the two different tracers in the sciatic nerve has been reported by previous investigators (4,21,22,35). The selectivity of WGA-HRP for primary afferent fibers of small caliber reflects the membrane-bound glycoproteins specific to these neurons (42). These glycoproteins

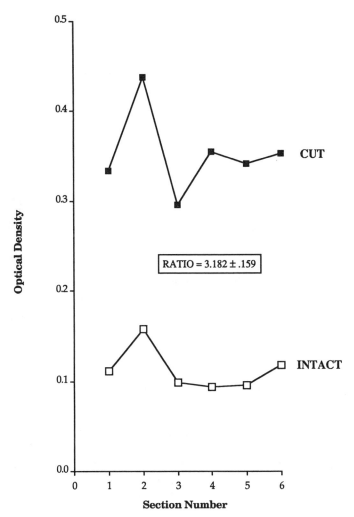

FIG. 23.7. Comparison of WGA-HRP labeling on lesioned and unlesioned sides of one representative case with sciatic nerve cut. The staining in lamina II was measured by microdensitometry in a series of 50-μm thick transverse sections.

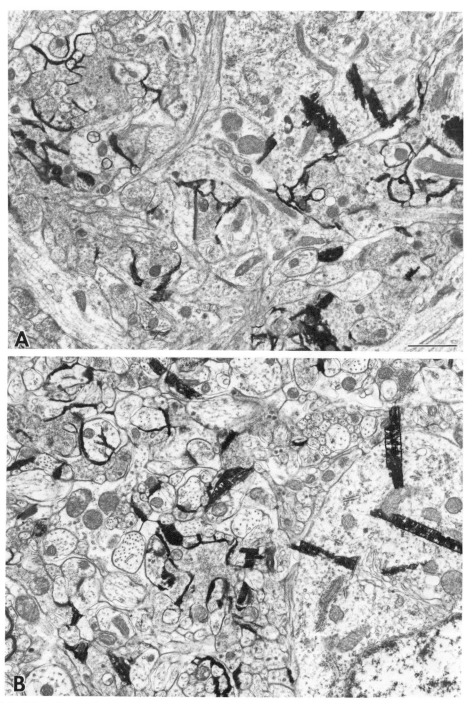

FIG. 23.8. A and **B:** Low-power electron microscopic fields illustrate the extracellular and transneuronal labeling present in lamina II after injection of WGA-HRP in the sciatic nerve followed by transection of the nerve distal to the injection. In both A and B reaction product is often sparse in terminals but outlines them. Reaction product is also present in dendrites and cell bodies. Calibration: 1 μm. (Courtesy of Dr. J. Valtschanoff.)

are likely to have developmental significance (16); their role in the adult nervous system remains uncertain.

Although WGA-HRP reaction product was in many cases confined within the terminal, it could also be seen to occupy the extracellular space (Fig. 23.6) resulting in a partial or almost complete outlining of the labeled terminal. Labeling of dendrites, neuronal somata, and glial cells was also very common (see also ref. 45). As a rule, when present around a synaptic ending it did not extend into the synaptic cleft (Fig. 23.6C and D). We are now investigating whether extracellular labeling may be correlated with injury: WGA-HRP in DMSO was injected bilaterally into the sciatic nerve of anesthetized rats. Immediately following the injection, the sciatic nerve of one side was crushed or cut proximal to the injection. Perfusion and histology were as described above. At the light microscope, labeling in all cases was largely limited to lamina II, regardless of the presence of a peripheral injury. However, labeling was denser on the side of the injury (Fig. 23.7). At the electron microscope extracellular labeling dominated the field on the injured side, while unequivocally labeled terminals were relatively sparse, most terminals of primary afferent origin containing only traces of reaction product (Fig. 23.8). Profuse transneuronal labeling could also be observed.

The present observation of extracellular labeling after WGA-HRP injection suggests that a normal physiological process may release endogenous peptides and/or glycoproteins from nerve terminals away from the active zone, diffusing for some distance before binding to their receptors (12,23). These substances may be excluded from the synapse itself. That extracellular labeling may be enhanced after sciatic nerve lesion raises the possibility that high levels of some endogenous agent released from terminals into the extracellular space may act as a central signal of peripheral injury and may be involved in various postlesion phenomena, including plasticity and hyperalgesia.

REFERENCES

1. Aanonsen, L. M., Lei, S., and Wilcox, G. L. (1990): Excitatory amino acid receptors and nociceptive neurotransmission in rat spinal cord. *Pain,* 41:309–321.
2. Andres, K. H. (1961): Untersuchungen über den Feinbau von Spinalganglien. *Z. Zellforsch.,* 55:1–48.
3. Battaglia, G., and Rustioni, A. (1988): Co-existence of glutamate and substance P in dorsal root ganglion neurons of the rat and monkey. *J. Comp. Neurol.,* 277:302–312.
4. Brushart, T. M., and Mesulam, M. M. (1980): Transganglionic demonstration of central sensory projections from skin and muscle with HRP-lectin conjugates. *Neurosci. Lett.,* 17:1–6.
5. Cangro, C. B., Sweetnam, P. M., Wrathall, J. R., Haser, W. B., Curthoys, N. P., and Neale, J. H. (1985): Localization of elevated glutaminase immunoreactivity in small DRG neurons. *Brain Res.,* 336:158–161.
6. Conti, F., De Biasi, S., Fabri, M., Abdullah, L., Manzoni, T., and Petrusz, P. Substance P-containing pyramidal neurons in the cat somatic sensory cortex *(submitted).*
7. Curras, M. C., and Dingledine, R. J. (1990): The selectivity of amino acid neurotransmitters acting at NMDA and AMPA receptors expressed in Xenopus oocytes. *Soc. Neurosci. Abstr.,* 16:619.
8. Davies, S. N., and Lodge, D. (1987): Evidence for involvement of N-methylaspartate receptors in "wind-up" of class 2 neurones in the dorsal horn of the rat. *Brain Res.,* 424:402–406.
9. De Biasi, S., and Rustioni, A. (1988): Glutamate and substance P coexist in primary afferent terminals in the superficial laminae of spinal cord. *Proc. Natl. Acad. Sci. USA,* 85:7820–7824.
10. De Biasi, S., and Rustioni, A. (1990): Ultrastructural immunocytochemical localization of excitatory amino acids in the somatosensory system. *J. Histochem. Cytochem.,* 38:1745–1754.
11. Duggan, A. W., and Johnston, G. A. R. (1970): Glutamate and related amino acids in cat spinal roots, dorsal root ganglia and peripheral nerves. *J. Neurochem.,* 17:1205–1208.
12. Fuxe, K., and Agnati, L. F. (1991): Two principal modes of electrochemical communication in the brain: volume versus wiring transmission. In: *Volume transmission in the brain,* edited by K. Fuxe and L. F. Agnati, pp. 1–9. Raven Press, New York.

13. Giuffrida, R., Rustioni, A. (1989): Dorsal root ganglion neurons projecting to the dorsal column nuclei of rats. *Soc. Neurosci. Abstr.*, 15:441.
14. Hepler, J. R., Toomim, C. S., McCarthy, K. D., et al. (1988): Characterization of antisera to glutamate and aspartate. *J. Histochem. Cytochem.*, 36:13–22.
15. Jahr, C. E., and Jessel, T. M. (1985): Synaptic transmission between dorsal root ganglion and dorsal horn neurons in culture: antagonism of monosynaptic excitatory postsynaptic potentials and glutamate excitation by kyurenate. *J. Neurosci.*, 4:2281–2289.
16. Jessel, T. M., Hynes, M. A., and Dodd, J. (1990): Carbohydrates and carbohydrate-binding proteins in the nervous system. *Annu. Rev. Neurosci.*, 13:227–255.
17. Jessel, T. M., Yoshioka, K., and Jahr, C. E. (1986): Amino acid receptor-mediated transmission at primary afferent synapses in rat spinal cord. *J. Exp. Biol.*, 124:239–258.
18. Johnson, J. L., and Aprison, M. H. (1970): The distribution of glutamic acid, a transmitter candidate, and other amino acids in the dorsal sensory neuron of the cat. *Brain Res.*, 24:285–292.
19. Kawagoe, R., Onodera, K., and Takeuchi, A. (1986): The release of endogenous glutamate from the newborn rat spinal cord induced by dorsal root stimulation and substance P. *Biomed. Res.*, 7:253–259.
20. Kowalski, M. M., Cassidy, M., Namboodiri, M. A. A., and Neale, J. H. (1987): Cellular organization of N-acetylaspartylglutamate in amphibian retina and spinal sensory ganglia. *Brain Res.*, 406:397–401.
21. LaMotte, C. C., Kapadia, S. E., and Kocol, C. M. (1989): Comparison of spinal and brainstem projections of rat median, ulnar, sciatic and saphenous nerves using either injections of WGA-HRP or B-HRP. *Soc. Neurosci. Abstr.*, 15:105.
22. Maslany, S., Crockett, D. P., and Egger, M. D. (1990): The projection of cutaneous primary afferents to the dorsal column nuclei and the dorsal horn in the rat: WGA-HRP vs B-HRP. *Anat. Rec.*, 226:66A.
23. Matteoli, M., Reetz, A. T., and De Camilli, P. (1990): Small synaptic vesicles and large dense-core vesicles: secretory organelles involved in two modes of neuronal signaling. In: *Volume transmission in the brain*, edited by K. Fuxe and L. F. Agnati, pp. 180–193. Raven Press, New York.
24. Maxwell, D. J., Christie, W. M., Short, A. D., Storm-Mathisen, J., and Ottersen, O. P. (1990): Central boutons of glomeruli in the spinal cord of the cat are enriched with L-glutamate-like immunoreactivity. *Neuroscience*, 36:83–104.
25. Merighi, A., Polak, J. M., and Theodosis, D. T. (1991): Ultrastructural visualization of glutamate and aspartate immunoreactivities in the rat dorsal horn, with special reference to the co-localization of glutamate, substance P and calcitonin-gene related peptide. *Neuroscience*, 40:67–80.
26. Miller, K. E., Clements, J. R., Larson, A. A., and Beitz, A. J. (1988): Organization of glutamate-like immunoreactivity in the rat superficial dorsal horn: light and electron microscopic observations. *Synapse*, 2:28–36.
27. Molander, C., and Grant, G. (1985): Cutaneous projections from the rat hindlimb foot to the substantia gelatinosa of the spinal cord studied by transganglionic transport of WGA-HRP conjugate. *J. Comp. Neurol.*, 237:476–484.
28. Ory-Lavollée, L., Blakely, R. D., and Coyle, J. T. (1987): Neurochemical and immunocytochemical studies on the distribution of N-acetyl-aspartylglutamate and N-acetyl-aspartate in rat spinal cord and some peripheral tissue. *J. Neurochem.*, 48:895–899.
29. Partneau, D. K., and Mayer, M. L. (1990): Structure-activity relationships for amino acid transmitter candidates acting at N-methyl-D-aspartate and quisqualate receptors. *J. Neurosci.*, 10:2385–2399.
30. Phend, K. D., Weinberg, R. J., and Rustioni, A. (1990): Optimizing immunogold E.M. double-labeling for amino acids. *Soc. Neurosci. Abstr.*, 16:221.
31. Plenderleith, M. B., Haller, C. J., and Snow, P. J. (1990): Peptide coexistence in axon terminals within the superficial dorsal horn of the rat spinal cord. *Synapse*, 6:344–350.
32. Potashner, S. J., and Dymczyk, L. (1986): Amino acid levels in the guinea pig spinal gray matter after axotomy of primary sensory and descending tracts. *J. Neurochem.*, 47:412–422.
33. Ribeiro-Da-Silva, A., and Coimbra, A. (1982): Two types of synaptic glomeruli and their distribution in laminae I–III of the rat spinal cord. *J. Comp. Neurol.*, 209:176–186.
34. Robertson, B., and Arvidsson, J. (1985): Transganglionic transport of wheat germ agglutinin-HRP and choleragenoid-HRP in rat trigeminal primary sensory neurons. *Brain Res.*, 348:44–51.
35. Robertson, B., and Grant, G. (1985): A comparison between wheat germ agglutinin-and choleragenoid-horseradish peroxidase as anterogradely transported markers in central branches of primary sensory neurones in the rat with some observations in the cat. *Neuroscience*, 14:895–905.
36. Rustioni, A., and Weinberg, R. J. (1989): The somatosensory system. In: *Handbook of chemical neuroanatomy, vol. 7: integrated systems of the CNS, part II*, edited by A. Björklund, T. Hökfelt, and L. W. Swanson, pp. 219–321. Elsevier, Amsterdam.
37. Schneider, S. P., and Perl, E. R. (1985): Selective excitation of neurons in the mammalian spinal dorsal horn by aspartate and glutamate in vitro: correlation with location and excitatory input. *Brain Res.*, 360:339–343.

38. Schneider, S. P., and Perl, E. R. (1988): Comparison of primary afferent and glutamate excitation of neurons in the mammalian spinal dorsal horn. *J. Neurosci.*, 8:2062–2073.
39. Skilling, S. R., Smullin, D. H., Beitz, A. J., and Larson, A. A. (1988): Extracellular amino acid concentrations in the dorsal spinal cord of freely moving rats following veratridine and nociceptive stimulation. *J. Neurochem.*, 51:127–132.
40. Storm-Mathisen, J., Leknes, A. K., Bore, A. T., et al. (1983): First visualization of glutamate and GABA in neurones by immunocytochemistry. *Nature*, 301:517–520.
41. Tracey, D. J., De Biasi, S., Phend, K., and Rustioni, A. (1991): Aspartate-like immunoreactivity in primary afferent neurons. *Neuroscience*, 40:673–686.
42. Trojanowski, J. Q. (1983): Native and derivatized lectins for in vivo studies of neuronal connectivity and neuronal cell biology. *J. Neurosci. Meth.*, 9:185–204.
43. Verhage, M., McMahon, H. T., Ghijsen, W. E. J. M., et al. (1991): Differential release of amino acids, neuropeptides, and catecholamines from isolated nerve terminals. *Neuron*, 6:517–524.
44. Weinberg, R. J., Conti, F., Van Eyck, S. L., Petrusz, P., and Rustioni, A. (1987): Glutamate immunoreactivity in superficial laminae of rat dorsal horn and spinal trigeminal nucleus. In: *Excitatory amino acid transmission*, edited by T. P. Hicks, D. Lodge, and H. McLennan, pp. 173–176. Alan R. Liss, New York.
45. Weinberg, R. J., Tracey, D. J., and Rustioni, A. (1990): Extracellular labeling of unmyelinated dorsal root terminals after WGA-HRP injections in spinal ganglia. *Brain Res.*, 523:351–355.
46. Weinberg, R. J., and Van Eyck, S. L. A tetramethylbenzidine/tungstate reaction for horseradish peroxidase histochemistry. *J. Histochem. Cytochem.*, 39:1143–1148.
47. Westlund, K. N., McNeill, D. L., and Coggeshall, R. E. (1989): Glutamate immunoreactivity in rat dorsal root axons. *Neurosci. Lett.*, 96:13–17.
48. Westlund, K. N., McNeill, D. L., Patterson, J. T., and Coggeshall, R. E. (1989): Aspartate immunoreactive axons in normal rat L4 dorsal roots. *Brain Res.*, 489:347–351.
49. Willard, A. L. (1990): Substance P mediates synaptic transmission between rat myenteric neurones in cell culture. *J. Physiol. (Lond.)*, 426:453–471.
50. Woolf, C. J., and Thompson, S. W. N. (1991): The induction and maintenance of central sensitization is dependent on N-methyl-D-aspartic acid receptor activation; implications for the treatment of post-injury pain hypersensitivity states. *Pain*, 44:293–299.
51. Yoshimura, M., and Jessel, T. (1990): Amino acid-mediated EPSPs at primary afferent synapses with substantia gelatinosa neurones in the rat spinal cord. *J. Physiol. (Lond.)*, 430:315–335.
52. Zhu, P. C., Thureson-Klein, Å., and Klein, R. L. (1986): Exocytosis from large dense cored vesicles outside the active synaptic zones of terminals within the trigeminal subnucleus caudalis: a possible mechanism for neuropeptide release. *Neuroscience*, 19:43–54.

Hyperalgesia and Allodynia,
edited by W. D. Willis, Jr.
Raven Press, Ltd., New York © 1992.

24

Involvement of Excitatory Amino Acids and Peptides in the Spinal Mechanisms Underlying Hyperalgesia

Jane E. Haley and George L. Wilcox

Department of Pharmacology, Graduate Program in Neuroscience, University of Minnesota, Minneapolis, Minnesota 55455

Hyperalgesia has been defined as a state of enhanced responsiveness to noxious stimuli. Although this can be measured quantitatively in human psychophysical studies, it can only be inferred from behavioral and electrophysiological studies in animals. This enhanced responsiveness to noxious stimuli may result from changes in either the peripheral or central nervous system. In the periphery, numerous chemical mediators forming part of a complex "inflammatory soup" (Handwerker and Reeh, Chapter 7) may act to sensitize nociceptors and/or encourage tissue inflammation. Whereas sensitization of peripheral nociceptors has been clearly demonstrated (13), there is accumulating evidence indicating that hypersensitivity events can also be rapidly elicited within the spinal cord (20,46,94,95,101). This phenomenon was first demonstrated following an acute, peripheral thermal injury; enhanced flexor reflex responses and expanded receptive fields were observed that appeared to result from central mechanisms (101). More recently, recordings of superficial projection neurons during peripheral inflammatory events have yielded similar results. Thus sensory pathways appear to be involved in this centrally mediated expansion of receptive fields (46).

Peripherally mediated hyperalgesia probably involves events originating from both neural and non-neural tissue. For instance, decreased reaction times in rodent tail flick studies can result from both sensitization of peripheral nerve endings and increases in tissue temperature resulting from increased blood flow (91). Central hyperalgesia, on the other hand, probably involves mostly neuronal events. These events can be separated into those taking place on primary afferent sensory fibers (e.g., an increase in the release of excitatory neurotransmitters) and those events occurring at the level of secondary dorsal horn neurons (e.g., an increase in a neuron's responsiveness to synaptically released neurotransmitters). Both events may be manifest as expanded receptive fields, decreased thresholds, and increased slope of stimulus–response curves. This chapter examines the kinds of stimulation that can produce hyperalgesia by a central site of action and attempts to identify the excitatory transmitters involved in such centrally mediated hyperalgesia.

PEPTIDERGIC MECHANISMS

The involvement of peptides in hyperalgesia has been hypothesized repeatedly during the past two decades following the isolation and characterization of substance P (SP). SP was the first transmitter candidate examined for possible hyperalgesic effects, and recent evidence supports the participation of neurokinins in the enhancement of neuronal responses to other modes of excitation. Early work showed that iontophoretically applied SP selectively facilitated the responses of nociceptive neurons in cat spinal dorsal horn (43); such an action *in vivo* would be expected to result in increased perception or reaction to painful stimuli. More recently, it has been observed that a single iontophoretic application of SP increases responses of nociceptive spinothalamic tract neurons *in vivo* to iontophoretic application of the selective glutamate receptor agonist N-methyl-D-aspartate (NMDA) for up to 2 hr (31). This result indicates that peptidergic transmitters may enhance responses to short-acting neurotransmitters for periods of time substantially longer than the half-life of the peptide itself. Similarly, SP *in vitro* can increase the responses of isolated dorsal horn neurons to NMDA (75). This latter observation suggests that a postsynaptic mechanism may be sufficient to account for the enhanced responsiveness observed *in vivo*.

Behavioral evidence supports the involvement of neurokinins in centrally mediated hyperalgesia. In animal behavioral studies, one is forced to infer hyperalgesia by observing decreased latencies and thresholds in response to noxious stimuli. Carrageenan, for example, after intraplantar injection in rats, induces edema and hyperalgesia to noxious thermal stimulation (41); a substantial part of this effect is probably mediated in the periphery. On the other hand, the appearance of hyperalgesia or counterirritative behavior after intrathecal injection of various excitatory compounds probably indicates that central neural events are involved (98). Intrathecally administered SP (45) and agonists selective for NK-1 or NK-2 receptor subtypes (55,68) elicit counterirritative behavior in mice. Although the nature of this behavior suggests enhanced nociceptive perception, the relevance of this behavioral syndrome to nociception has been challenged (35). Enhanced responsiveness in thermal nociceptive tests supports the putative hyperalgesic effects of SP more strongly than the counterirritative behaviors. Intrathecally administered SP (105) and related tachykinins (21) produce a short-lived decrease in the tail flick latency in rats. This enhanced responsiveness to noxious stimuli strongly supports the idea that these agents produce hyperalgesia, and the most reasonable explanation of this effect is that it takes place centrally. Cutaneously administered chemical stimuli, which may or may not elicit hyperalgesia, produce similar counterirritative behavior that can be blocked by intrathecally administered neurokinin antagonists (44,69). Thus, activation of receptors for these peptides appears to be a requirement for nociceptive responses. This evidence taken together indicates that enhanced nociceptive transmission can be induced by centrally administered SP.

Other peptides have also been proposed as mediators that enhance the responsiveness of spinal cord neurons to various stimuli. For example, calcitonin gene-related peptide (CGRP) has been localized in fine-diameter primary afferent fibers that synapse on dorsal horn projection neurons (18). Some behavioral studies suggest CGRP has hyperalgesic effects after intrathecal administration (36), and *in vitro* studies support this role (77,103). In addition, other peptides such as somatostatin (53,96) and bombesin (66) have been suggested to play a role in spinal hyperalgesic events. However, the direct participation of these peptides in hyperalgesia awaits further study (37).

EXCITATORY AMINO ACIDS

Recently, particular interest has focused on a possible neurotransmitter role for excitatory amino acids (EAAs) within the spinal cord, both in nociceptive processing and in the neuronal plasticity associated with centrally mediated hypersensitivity. Early investigations supported the idea that glutamate is a neurotransmitter involved in nociceptive transmission from primary afferent fibers to secondary neurons; iontophoretically applied glutamate increased the size of cutaneous receptive fields of spinal cord nociceptive neurons (107). Moreover, the nonselective EAA antagonist cis-PDA reduced responses to noxious mechanical stimuli, reinforcing this view (79). EAAs have been implicated in plasticity events occurring in other regions of the central nervous system such as the development of long-term potentiation (LTP) within the hippocampus. In particular, the NMDA subtype of EAA receptor appears to be pivotal in the development of the enhanced synaptic transmission observed in hippocampal LTP since it can be blocked by selective NMDA antagonists (15). In behavioral studies in mice, intrathecal administration of the nonselective excitatory amino acid antagonist D-glutamyl glycine (DGG) results in an increase in the latency to response in the tail flick test and a reduction in the response to pinch (74). Unfortunately the doses of DGG that produced antinociception also resulted in motor impairment, and this may obscure the results obtained in these behavioral studies. However, vocalization elicited by electrical stimulation of the tail is not dependent on intact motor function, and this was also reduced by DGG (74). More selective antagonists provide an opportunity to determine which receptor subtypes may be involved in nociceptive neurotransmission in the spinal cord. Behavioral studies in the rat and mouse indicate that NMDA antagonists are antinociceptive in the tail flick, hot plate, paw pressure, writhing, and formalin tests as well as reducing NMDA-induced biting and hyperalgesia (1,17,34,65,70,72,74,76,89,104). Unfortunately, the concentrations of these antagonists required to produce antinociception (0.01–1 mM) are very similar to those that induce motor paralysis (0.1–1 mM) following intrathecal administration. However, AP5 has also been shown to be antinociceptive in vocalization studies that do not rely on an intact spinal motor system (17,73,74).

Agonists for glutamate-activated cation channels, which include both the NMDA and non-NMDA subtype of EAA receptors, also produce signs of hyperalgesia when administered intrathecally. Of several agonists tested, only NMDA decreased the tail flick and hot plate latency in mice (2). This effect was short-lived, lasting less than 5 min. Like NMDA, the non-NMDA agonists quisqualate and kainate elicited caudally directed biting, licking, and scratching behavior similar to that evoked by SP. Hyperalgesia was suggested by the decreased tail flick latency, the nature of the behaviors elicited, and the occurrence of vocalization at the higher doses of NMDA and quisqualate used. Kainate differs from the other EAA agonists in two respects: first, higher doses of kainate elicited seizures rather than vocalization, suggesting that motor effects were predominant for this agonist (1); second, repeated administration of kainate produces sensitization (twofold increases in the number of behaviors elicited) in contrast to the desensitization seen with repeated administration of

SP, NMDA, and quisqualate (88). This sensitization may be an important clue to centrally mediated hyperalgesia. Recently, behavior similar to that elicited by SP and NMDA has been observed after intrathecal administration of 1s, 3R-1-aminocyclopentane-1,3-dicarboxylic acid (ACPD), an agonist selective for the G-protein-coupled metabotropic EAA receptor (52).

ELECTROPHYSIOLOGICAL STUDIES

Because electrophysiological recording of dorsal horn neuronal activity eliminates the problems associated with motor impairment in behavioral experiments, it is a useful technique for investigating the mechanisms underlying central hyperalgesia. Iontophoretic application of selective EAA agonists has been shown to activate nociceptive projection neurons in the rat (3) and primate (31), suggesting the participation of EAAs in synaptic transmission of nociceptive information. In addition to these short-duration effects, EAAs may also contribute to long-term changes in transmission. Synaptic plasticity has been observed within the spinal cord where dorsal horn neurons often respond to repetitive electrical stimulation of their receptive fields with a sequential increase in firing. This augmented response following a constant peripheral stimulation has been termed "windup" (60) and is of short duration, lasting only a few minutes. This phenomenon is dependent on the frequency of the peripheral stimulation, being observed at 0.5 Hz or greater. In addition the windup of dorsal horn neurons is probably mediated by C-fiber inputs since Aβ-fiber stimulation does not induce windup even at stimulation intensities and frequencies that elicit windup after C-fiber stimulation (29). Interestingly windup has also been observed in humans in whom repetitive constant heat (71) or electrical (49) stimulation results in increased pain ratings.

The role of EAAs in the transmission of nociception within the dorsal horn has only recently become the subject of investigation. However, both *in vitro* and *in vivo* studies now implicate these amino acids in nociceptive events. *In vitro* studies have demonstrated that superficial dorsal horn neurons, which often receive nociceptive input from C fibers, are excited by endogenous as well as exogenous EAAs (80,81). *In vivo* electrophysiological studies support the participation of endogenous EAAs in synaptic transmission between primary afferent fibers and secondary dorsal horn neurons: the nonselective NMDA and non-NMDA antagonist DGG reduced both the acute Aβ- and C-fiber-evoked activity of dorsal horn neurons resulting from stimulation of either the dorsal root or the cutaneous receptive field in the rat (30,82). This is in contrast to the actions of opioids that selectively reduce the C-fiber-evoked responses (27,87). In addition, intrathecally applied DGG has also been shown to abolish both the early and late phases of the activity of dorsal horn neurons evoked by intraplantar injections of formalin *in vivo* (40). Thus the nonselective blockade of both NMDA and non-NMDA receptors by DGG appears antinociceptive against the short duration responses elicited in dorsal horn neurons. However, the parallel reductions in Aβ-fiber responses would imply severe tactile difficulties as well.

NMDA RECEPTORS IN HYPERALGESIA

Using an *in vitro* neonatal rat spinal cord with the tail attached and measuring ventral root depolarizations, Dray and Perkins (32) demonstrated inhibition of responses to capsaicin and bradykinin administered to the tail by antagonists selective for the NMDA receptor. However, responses elicited by electrical stimulation of the tail were unaffected, and heat-evoked responses were only partially reduced. These results indicated that, although activation of NMDA receptors occurred during the neuronal response to chemical cutaneous stimulation, the responses to the electrical stimuli used in this study required some other EAA receptor subtype. However, with relatively high-frequency electrical stimulation of C fibers (enough to elicit windup), NMDA-receptor involvement is observed. The selective NMDA antagonists AP5 and ketamine clearly reduced the electrically evoked, C–fiber-mediated windup of dorsal horn neurons *in vivo* (24,29,30) and ventral horn neurons *in vitro* (90). In addition several groups have demonstrated that dorsal horn neuronal responses to noxious heat and pinch *in vivo* are reduced by AP5 and ketamine, whereas the responses to touch are unaltered (19,51,54,73). However, one *in vivo* study in rats and cats failed to show any effect of ketamine on dorsal horn neurons (42); this result may have resulted from the moderate intensities of stimulation used in this study (99), which may not have recruited the participation of NMDA receptors sufficiently. In addition to being voltage sensitive, NMDA receptors are constantly under the modulatory influence of other substances. Glycine, for example, can potentiate EAA action at a modulatory site on the NMDA receptor (48). Interestingly, an antagonist at this site, 7-chlorokynurenic acid, blocks windup (26), and glycine enhances NMDA responses of nociceptive dorsal horn neurons *in vivo* (16).

The NMDA antagonists, AP5, ketamine, and MK-801, administered either systemically or intrathecally, also markedly reduce the prolonged activity evoked in dorsal horn neurons by peripheral administration of formalin *in vivo*. The response is reduced following administration of these antagonists both prior to formalin administration and during the spontaneous activity elicited by the chemical (40). Peripheral administration of formalin elicits the generation c-Fos (a protein marker of gene activation) within neurons in the spinal cord. Interestingly, this expression of c-Fos following intraplantar injection of formalin can be inhibited by the intrathecal administration of MK-801 (50), confirming the involvement of NMDA receptors in the spinal events evoked by noxious chemical stimuli. In addition, other neuromediators may also be involved in the activation of dorsal horn neurons to prolonged noxious stimuli; for example, blockade of nitric oxide synthesis by nitro-L-arginine methyl ester (L-NAME) decreases behavioral (63) and neuronal (39) responses to noxious chemical stimuli.

The induction and maintenance of the central component of the enhanced flexion reflex response, originally observed by Woolf (101), are also likely to involve NMDA receptors. Systemic administration of NMDA antagonists can block this enhanced response when given both prior to and following the induction of the hypersensitivity state (102). Whereas this hypersensitivity lasts several hours, a hyperalgesic state lasting several days has recently been described in rats following unilateral sciatic nerve ligation (11). Prophylactic treatment with MK-801 prevents the development of this hyperalgesic state (22) and *post hoc* treatment with MK-801 partially reverses it (Yaksh et al., Chapter 20), indicating this phenomenon may also have an NMDA component, possibly involving an excitotoxic injury to inhibitory interneurons (85; Bennett and Laird, Chapter 26).

In this laboratory, we have observed enhanced responses of dorsal horn projection neurons to peripheral stimuli when subthreshold currents of EAA agonists are iontophoresed near the neuron. An important observation in these studies indicates a contrast between the non-NMDA receptor agonist alpha-amino-3-hydroxy-5-methyl-4-isoxazole-propionic acid (AMPA) and NMDA (54). Although AMPA increased responses to all intensities of stimulation (non-noxious and noxious), NMDA, on the other hand, enhanced responses to noxious stimuli more than it enhanced responses to non-noxious stimuli. This distinction was evident for both mechanical and thermal stimuli. Apparently, NMDA enhanced the gain of the responding neuron (i.e., increased the slope of the stimulus–response curve), whereas AMPA lowered its threshold. An action such as this would be expected to be important in the intensity of perceived pain and is consistent with the participation of NMDA receptors in hyperalgesia (99).

NMDA antagonists appear to have antinociceptive actions at the level of the spinal cord since intrathecal administration *in vivo* is effective, as is systemic administration in spinalized animals (1,29,40,54,102). A recent study by Skilling and colleagues (84) supports the hypothesis that EAAs are involved in nociceptive responses at the spinal level. Using *in vivo* microdialysis techniques in conscious rats, they have demonstrated release of both glutamate and aspartate within the lumbar dorsal horn following formalin administration into the paw. Release occurred during the second peak of the response and was associated with periods of intense biting and licking of the injected paw by the animal. Thus the profile of release of these amino acids within the spinal cord following formalin administration correlates with both the nociceptive behavior of the animals and the responses of dorsal horn neurons. Whether the EAAs are released from primary afferent fibers or secondary neurons could not be determined from this study; however, localization of glutamate-like immunoreactivity in primary afferent fibers (9) suggests that at least part of this released glutamate and aspartate originated from primary afferent fibers.

The location of NMDA receptors within the spinal cord has been examined using anatomical techniques (4,38), and electrophysiological experiments have corroborated these findings. The NMDA receptor antagonist AP5 is unable to alter the afferent fiber compound action potential (73), indicating that it is probably exerting its effects after the arrival of peripheral inputs. In recordings of dorsal horn neurons, motoneurons, and ventral root depolarizations both *in vitro* and *in vivo*, NMDA receptor antagonists reduce the polysynaptic component of the responses whereas the nonselective antagonist DGG reduced the monosynaptic component (8,23,56,57,83,90). Thus, non-NMDA receptors may be located on postsynaptic sites that do not differentiate between A- and C-fiber inputs, perhaps on the cell bodies of the spinothalamic tract neurons themselves. However, NMDA receptors are also likely to be present on interneurons forming part of the pathway for the transmission of C-fiber inputs. Indeed, binding studies have shown NMDA receptors localized within the interneuron-rich substantia gelatinosa region (4,10,38,47,62,92).

The dissociative anesthetic ketamine has been studied as an analgesic for many years but has only recently been identified as an NMDA receptor channel blocker (7). Consequently, the analgesic properties of this NMDA antagonist (which occur at lower doses than its anesthetic effects) have been assessed in humans since ketamine was already clinically in use as an anesthetic. Ketamine has been administered intramuscularly, intravenously, and subcutaneously and is an effective analgesic in experimental and postoperative pain (59,78). Although the duration of action of ketamine is short, ranging between 10 and 100 min depending on the route of administration, both intravenous and subcutaneous infusion appear effective against cancer pain (61,67). The effectiveness of intrathecally administered ketamine (14) implies that a site of action for its nociceptive effects lies within the spinal cord. Thus the involvement of EAAs in nociception appears to extend from rodents to humans. The utility of ketamine in postoperative pain suggests that early application after traumatic injury may be an appropriate therapy to minimize development of long-duration pain.

PRIMING NMDA RECEPTORS VIA NON-NMDA RECEPTORS

The NMDA receptor is unique in that it is both ligand and voltage gated; these characteristics result from a resting block of the ion channel by magnesium (58). Thus depolarization of the neuron is required in order for the magnesium ions to leave the channel and allow receptor-activated ion flux to occur. These voltage- and ligand-gated properties of NMDA receptors have led to their implication in a variety of excitability changes in central nervous system function including epilepsy (33) and LTP in the hippocampus (15).

In the spinal cord, there are at least two means by which NMDA receptors might be "primed" by depolarization. First, rapid depolarization mediated by non-NMDA receptors could precede successful activation of NMDA receptors by several milliseconds. Neurons possessing non-NMDA as well as NMDA receptors could be depolarized initially via the non-NMDA receptors, briefly and unconditionally, following glutamate release. It is therefore likely that these neurons would be depolarized synaptically by most glutamatergic inputs. Studies in this laboratory have found that approximately half of the projection neurons in rat spinal cord are in fact activated by both NMDA and AMPA (54). Thus, one would expect that most projection neurons in the rat could be activated by sufficiently intense synaptic input from glutamatergic terminals to result in NMDA receptor activation. Neurons lacking non-NMDA receptors may require additional depolarization by other substances before NMDA receptors can be fully activated by EAAs. Indeed, about 40% of projection neurons in the rat are activated by iontophoretically applied NMDA but not AMPA, implying that short-term exposure to glutamate alone may be insufficient to allow substantial NMDA receptor activation to occur (54).

PRIMING NMDA EVENTS WITH PEPTIDERGIC EVENTS

Second, slower depolarizing influences preceding glutamate release by seconds or minutes could assist in the activation of neurons lacking non-NMDA receptors. These influences include glutamate acting at metabotropic receptors activated by quisqualate and ACPD, and SP acting at NK-1 receptors. Both of these metabotropic receptors share the same intracellular signaling pathway. Activation of these receptors is thought to activate phospholipase C (PLC), producing inositol triphosphate (IP_3) and diacyl glycerol (DAG) (86,106). IP_3 in turn is thought to act at receptors on intracellular calcium stores, releasing calcium into the cytoplasm (12); this intracellular calcium may promote depolarizing inward calcium currents observed in spinal cord slices (64). DAG is thought to activate protein kinase C (12), which may phosphorylate ion channels, including perhaps potassium channels. Potassium channel phosphorylation (5) and dephosphorylation (6) have been inferred to decrease and increase, respectively, potassium conductance in central nervous system neurons. Therefore, phosophorylation of potassium channels by protein kinase C would be expected to contribute to the slow SP-induced depolarization observed in spinal cord neurons (64). We have recently shown that ACPD, injected intrathecally in mice, elicits behavior similar to that elicited by SP and similar in its susceptibility to analgesic substances (52). Similarly, agonists at 5-HT$_2$ receptors, which similarly couple to PLC, also elicit counterirritative behaviors after intrathecal injection (100). Thus, there is evidence that receptors, coupling through IP$_3$ and DAG, may promote slow excitatory events contributing to spinal cord neuronal and behavioral excitation.

Glutamate and SP have been shown to coexist in small dorsal root ganglia (25), and double labeling has indicated that fine primary afferent terminals in the dorsal horn contain glutamate and SP in separate synaptic vesicles (Rustioni and Weinberg, Chapter 23). Activation of these fine afferent fibers by nociceptive stimuli would promote the simultaneous release of glutamate and/or aspartate (97) together with SP or other peptides. Any of these substances may produce depolarization via the non-NMDA and/or metabotropic receptors (93), perhaps removing the magnesium block of the NMDA-receptor complex. This could allow NMDA receptors to be activated by prolonged afferent barrages of action potentials such as those evoked by subcutaneous injection of formalin (40) or after traumatic injury to peripheral nerve (Bennett and Laird, Chapter 26).

CONCLUSIONS

The involvement of spinal NMDA receptors in the amplification of dorsal horn neuron responses to peripheral inputs, as observed in windup and the formalin response, makes this receptor a very attractive candidate for other hypersensitivity states resulting from peripheral disease or injury. Other pharmacological manipulations may recruit NMDA-mediated hyperalgesic events. For example, allodynia following intrathecal injections of strychnine is blocked by MK-801, but not by most opioid or adrenergic analgesic agents (104). Similarly, opioids are less effective at inhibiting both the windup of neurons and their responses to formalin once the response has begun (27,28). Thus, mechanisms such as these, many involving EAA receptors, may be associated with the problems encountered in the treatment of some chronic pain states. That the NMDA receptor antagonists appear effective at reducing windup and established strychnine allodynia, formalin hyperalgesia, and enhanced flexion reflex responses indicates that they may provide a new approach to developing effective analgesics.

The neurotransmission of nociceptive inputs across synapses in the spinal cord dorsal horn appears to involve a temporal cascade of events that collaborate to produce many of the facets of excitation, temporal summation, recruitment, and sensitization that characterize the phenomenon of pain (99). Short-term events possibly mediated by EAAs may contribute to rapid transmission of information to secondary neurons in the spinal cord. Other EAA receptors may mediate short-term temporal summation under conditions of rapid repeated stimulation or abnormal prolonged discharges from sites of injury. Peptidergic transmitters, possibly released differentially under different afferent activation conditions, may contribute to this temporal cascade by increasing the effect of EAAs. These events, lasting seconds to minutes, may lay the groundwork for long-term changes that permanently alter spinal cord connectivity in such a way as to encourage subsequent excitatory transmission.

Such long-term retention of excitability may participate in the long-lived hyperalgesic states observed in the clinic. Thus, interruption of the early events accompanying prolonged intense excitation may prove to be useful clinical strategies to prevent the development of chronic pain states close to the precipitating event.

REFERENCES

1. Aanonsen, L. M., and Wilcox, G. L. (1986): Phencyclidine selectively blocks a spinal action of N-methyl-D-aspartate in mice. *Neurosci. Lett.*, 67:191–197.
2. Aanonsen, L. M., and Wilcox, G. L. (1987): Nociceptive action of excitatory amino acids in the mouse: effects of spinally administered opioids, phencyclidine and sigma agonists. *J. Pharmacol. Exp. Ther.*, 243:9–19.
3. Aanonsen, L. M., Lei, S., and Wilcox, G. L. (1990): Excitatory amino acid receptors and nociceptive neurotransmission in rat spinal cord. *Pain*, 41:309–321.
4. Aanonsen, L. M., and Seybold, V. S. (1989): Phencyclidine and sigma receptors in rat spinal cord: binding characterization and quantitative autoradiography. *Synapse*, 4:1–10.
5. Aghajanan, G. K. (1985): Modulation of a transient outward current in serotonergic neurones by alpha 1-adrenoceptors. *Nature*, 315:501–503.
6. Andrade, R., and Aghajanian, G. K. (1985): Opiate- and alpha 2-adrenoceptor-induced hyperpolarizations of locus ceruleus neurons in brain slices: reversal by cyclic adenosine 3':5'-monophosphate analogues. *J. Neurosci.*, 5:2359–2364.
7. Anis, A., Berry, S. C., Burton, N. R., and Lodge, D. (1983): The dissociative anaesthetics, ketamine and phencyclidine, selectively reduce excitation of central mammalian neurons by N-methyl-aspartate. *Br. J. Pharmacol.*, 79:565–575.
8. Bagust, J., Kerkut, G. A., and Rakkah, N. I. A. (1989): Differential sensitivity of dorsal and ventral root activity to magnesium and 2-amino-5-phosphonovalerate (APV) in an isolated mammalian spinal cord preparation. *Brain Res.*, 479:138–144.
9. Battaglia, G., and Rustioni, A. (1988): Coexistence of glutamate and substance P in dorsal root ganglion neurons of the rat and monkey. *J. Comp. Neurol.*, 277:302–312.
10. Beal, J. A. (1983): Identification of presumptive long axon neurons in the substantia gelatinosa of the rat lumbosacral spinal cord: a Golgi study. *Neurosci. Lett.*, 41:9–14.
11. Bennett, G. J., and Xie, Y.-K. (1988): A peripheral neuropathy in rat that produces disorders of pain sensation like those seen in man. *Pain*, 33:87–107.
12. Berridge, M. J. (1987): Inositol trisphosphate and diacylglycerol: two interacting second messengers. *Annu. Rev. Biochem.*, 56:159–193.
13. Besson, J. M., and Chaouch, A. (1987): Peripheral and spinal mechanisms of nociception. *Physiol. Rev.*, 67:167–186.
14. Bion, J. F. (1984): Intrathecal ketamine for war surgery. A preliminary study under field conditions. *Anaesthesia*, 39:1023–1028.
15. Bliss, T. V. P., and Lynch, M. A. (1988): Long-term potentiation of synaptic transmission in the hippocampus: properties and mechanisms. In: *Long term potentiation: from biophysics to behaviour*, pp. 3–72. Alan R. Liss, New York.
16. Budai, D., Wilcox, G. L., and Larson, A. (1992): Enhancement of NMDA-evoked neuronal activity by glycine in vivo. *Neurosci. Lett. (in press)*.
17. Cahusac, P. M. B., Evans, R. H., Hill, R. G., Rodriquez, R. E., and Smith, D. A. S. (1984): The behavioral effects of an *N*-methylaspartate receptor antagonist following application to the lumbar spinal cord of conscious rats. *Neuropharmacology*, 23:719–724.
18. Carlton, S. M., Westlund, K. N., Zhang, D. X., Sorkin, L. S., and Willis, W. D. (1990): Calcitonin gene-related peptide containing primary afferent fibers synapse on primate spinothalamic tract cells. *Neurosci. Lett.*, 109:76–81.
19. Conseiller, C., Benoist, J. M., Hamann, K.-F., Maillard, M. C., and Besson, J. M. (1972): Effects of ketamine (CI 581) on cell responses to cutaneous stimulations in laminae IV and V in the cat's dorsal horn. *Eur. J. Pharmacol.*, 18:346–352.
20. Cook, A. J., Woolf, C. J., and Wall, P. D. (1986): Prolonged C-fibre mediated facilitation of the flexion reflex in the rat is not due to changes in afferent terminal or motoneuron excitability. *Neurosci. Lett.*, 70:91–96.
21. Cridland, R. A., and Henry, J. L. (1986): Comparison of the effects of substance P, neurokinin A, physaelamin and eledoisin in facilitating a nociceptive reflex in the rat. *Brain Res.*, 381:93–99.
22. Davar, D., and Maciewitz, R. (1989): MK-801 blocks thermal hyperalgesia in a rat model of neuropathic pain. *Neurosci. Soc. Abstr.*, 15:472.

23. Davies, J., and Watkins, J. C. (1983): Role of amino acid receptors in mono- and polysynaptic excitation in the cat spinal cord. *Exp. Brain Res.*, 49:280–290.
24. Davies, S. N., and Lodge, D. (1987): Evidence for involvement of N-methylaspartate receptors in 'wind up' of class 2 neurons in the dorsal horn of the rat. *Brain Res.*, 424:402–406.
25. De Biasi, S., and Rustioni, A. (1988): Glutamate and substance P coexist in primary afferent terminals in the superficial laminae of spinal cord. *Proc. Natl. Acad. Sci. USA*, 85:7820–7824.
26. Dickenson, A. H., and Aydar, E. (1991): Antagonism at the glycine site on the NMDA receptor reduces spinal nociception in the rat. *Neurosci. Lett.*, 121:263–266.
27. Dickenson, A. H., and Sullivan, A. F. (1986): Electrophysiological studies on the effects of intrathecal morphine on nociceptive neurons in the rat dorsal horn. *Pain*, 24:211–222.
28. Dickenson, A. H., and Sullivan, A. F. (1987): Subcutaneous formalin-induced activity of dorsal horn neurons in the rat: differential response to an intrathecal opiate administered pre or post formalin. *Pain*, 30:349–360.
29. Dickenson, A. H., and Sullivan, A. F. (1987): Evidence for a role of the NMDA receptor in the frequency dependent potentiation of deep rat dorsal horn nociceptive neurons following C-fibre stimulation. *Neuropharmacology*, 26:1235–1238.
30. Dickenson, A. H., and Sullivan, A. F. (1990): Differential effects of excitatory amino acid antagonists on dorsal horn nociceptive neurons in the rat. *Brain Res.*, 506:31–39.
31. Dougherty, P., and Willis, W. D. Enhancement of spinothalamic neuron responses to chemical and mechanical stimuli following combined microiontophoretic application of NMDA and substance P. *Pain*, 47:85–93.
32. Dray, A., and Perkins, M. N. (1987): Blockade of nociceptive responses in neonatal rat spinal cord *in vitro* by excitatory amino acid antagonists. *J. Physiol. (Lond.)*, 382:177P.
33. Fagg, G. E., Foster, A. C., and Ganong, A. H. (1986): Excitatory amino acid synaptic mechanisms and neurological function. *Trends Pharmacol. Sci.*, 7:357–363.
34. Fratta, W., Casu, M., Balestrieri, A., Loviselli, A., Biggio, G., and Gessa, G. L. (1980): Failure of ketamine to interact with opiate receptors. *Eur. J. Pharmacol.*, 61:389–391.
35. Frenk, H., Bossut, D., Urca, G., and Mayer, D. J. (1988): Is substance P a primary afferent neurotransmitter for nociceptive input? I. Analysis of pain-related behaviors resulting from intrathecal administration of substance P and six excitatory compounds. *Brain Res.*, 455:223–231.
36. Gamse, R., and Saria, A. (1986): Nociceptive behavior after intrathecal injections of substance P, neurokinin A and calcitonin gene-related peptide in mice. *Neurosci. Lett.*, 70:143–147.
37. Gaumann, D. M., Yaksh, T. L., Post, C., Wilcox, G. L., and Rodriguez, M. (1989): Intrathecal somatostatin in cat and mouse: studies on pain, motor behavior and histopathology. *Anesth. Analg.*, 68:623–632.
38. Greenamyre, J. T., Olson, J. M., Penney, Jr., J. B., and Young, A. B. (1985): Autoradiographic characterization of N-methyl-D-aspartate-, quisqualate- and kainate-sensitive glutamate binding sites. *J. Pharmacol. Exp. Ther.*, 233:254–263.
39. Haley, J. E., Dickenson, A. H., and Schachter, M. (1992): Electrophysiological evidence for a role of nitric oxide in prolonged chemical nociception in the rat. *Neuropharmacology (in press)*.
40. Haley, J. E., Sullivan, A. F., and Dickenson, A. H. (1990): Evidence for spinal N-methyl-D-aspartate receptor involvement in prolonged chemical nociception in the rat. *Brain Res.*, 518:218–226.
41. Hargreaves, K., Dubner, R., Brown, F., Flores, C., and Joris, J. (1988): A new and sensitive method for measuring thermal nociception in cutaneous hyperalgesia. *Pain*, 32:77–88.
42. Headley, P. M., Parsons, C. G., and West, D. C. (1987): The role of N-methylaspartate receptors in mediating responses of rat and cat spinal neurons to defined sensory stimuli. *J. Physiol. (Lond.)*, 385:169–188.
43. Henry, J. L. (1976): Effects of substance P on functionally identified units in cat spinal cord. *Brain Res.*, 114:439–451.
44. Hwang, A. S., and Wilcox, G. L. (1986): Intradermal hypertonic saline-induced behavior as a nociceptive test in mice. *Life Sci.*, 38:2389–2396.
45. Hylden, J. L. K., and Wilcox, G. L. (1981): Intrathecal substance P elicits a caudally-directed biting and scratching behavior in mice. *Brain Res.*, 217:212–215.
46. Hylden, J. L. K., Nahin, R. L., Traub, R. J., and Dubner, R. (1989): Expansion of receptive fields of spinal lamina I projection neurons in rats with unilateral adjuvant-induced inflammation: the contribution of dorsal horn mechanisms. *Pain*, 37:229–243.
47. Jansen, K. L. R., Faull, R. L. M., Dragunow, M., and Waldvogel, H. (1990): Autoradiographic localisation of NMDA, quisqualate and kainic acid receptors in human spinal cord. *Neurosci. Lett.*, 108:53–57.
48. Johnson, J. W., and Ascher, P. (1987): Glycine potentiates the NMDA response in cultured mouse neurons. *Nature*, 325:529–531.
49. Jorum, E., Holm, E., Lundberg, L., and Torebjörk, H. E. (1990): Temporal summation in nociceptive systems. *Pain*, Suppl. 5:S314.

50. Kehl, L. J., Lichtblau, L., Gogas, K. R., Pollock, C. H., Mayes, M., Basbaum, A. I., and Wilcox, G. L. (1990): The NMDA antagonist MK801 reduces noxious stimulus-evoked Fos expression in the spinal cord dorsal horn. In: *Pain research and clinical management: proceedings of the sixth world congress on pain,* edited by M. Bond, C. J. Woolf, and J. E. Charlton, pp. 307–311. Elsevier, Amsterdam.

51. Kitahata, L. M., Taub, A., and Kosaka, Y. (1973): Lamina-specific suppression of dorsal-horn unit activity by ketamine hydrochloride. *Anesthesiology,* 38:4–11.

52. Kitto, K., and Wilcox, G. L. (1991): Behavioral effects of intrathecally administered ACPD and AP4, agonists for novel EAA receptors. *Soc. Neurosci. Abstr.,* 17:71.

53. Kuraishi, Y., Hirota, N., Sato, Y., Hino, Y., Satoh, M., and Takagi, H. (1985): Evidence that substance P and somatostatin transmit separate information related to pain in the spinal dorsal horn. *Brain Res.,* 325:294–298.

54. Lei, S., and Wilcox, G. L. (1990): Excitatory amino acid receptor regulation of spinal nociceptive neurotransmission. *Eur. J. Pharmacol.,* 183:1438.

55. Lei, S., and Wilcox, G. L. (1991): Opioid and neurokinin activities of substance P fragments and their analogs. *Eur. J. Pharmacol.,* 193:209–215.

56. Lodge, D., and Anis, N. A. (1984): Effects of ketamine and three other anaesthetics on spinal reflexes and inhibitions in the cat. *Br. J. Anaesth.,* 56:1143–1151.

57. Long, S. K., Evans, R. H., Cull, L., Krijzer, F., and Bevan, P. (1988): An *in vitro* mature spinal cord preparation from the rat. *Neuropharmacology,* 27:541–546.

58. MacDermott, A. B., and Dale, N. (1987): Receptors, ion channels and synaptic potentials underlying the integrative actions of excitatory amino acids. *Trends Neurosci.,* 10:280–284.

59. Maurset, A., Skoglund, L. A., Hustveit, O., and Øye, I. (1989): Comparison of ketamine and pethidine in experimental and postoperative pain. *Pain,* 36:37–41.

60. Mendell, L. M. (1966): Physiological properties of unmyelinated fiber projection to the spinal cord. *Exp. Neurol.,* 16:316–332.

61. Mizuno, K., Kanamaru, T., Ogawa, S., and Suzuki, H. (1990): Ketamine infusions for treatment of pain in patients with advanced cancer. *Pain, Suppl.* 5:S375.

62. Monaghan, D. T., and Cotman, C. W. (1985): Distribution of *N*-methyl-D-aspartate-sensitive L-[³H]glutamate-binding sites in rat brain. *J. Neurosci.,* 5:2909–2919.

63. Moore, P. K., Oluyomu, A. O., Babbedge, R. C., Wallace, P., and Hart, S. L. (1991): L-N^G-Nitro arginine methyl ester exhibits antinociceptive activity in the mouse. *Br. J. Pharmacol.,* 102:198–202.

64. Murase, K., Ryu, P. D., and Randic, M. (1989): Tachykinins modulate multiple ionic conductances in voltage-clamped rat spinal dorsal horn neurons. *J. Neurophysiol.,* 61:854–865.

65. Murray, C. W., Cowen, A., Larson, A. A. (1991): Neurokinin and NMDA antagonists (but not a kainic acid antagonist) are antinociceptive in the mouse formalin model. *Pain,* 44:179–185.

66. O'Donohue, T. L., Massari, Y. J., Pazoles, C.-J., et al. (1984): A role for bombesin in sensory processing in the spinal cord. *J. Neurosci.,* 4:2956–2962.

67. Oshima, E., Tei, K., Kayazawa, H., and Urabe, N. (1990): Continuous subcutaneous injection of ketamine for cancer pain. *Can. J. Anaesth.,* 37:385–386.

68. Papir-Kricheli, D., Frey, J., Laufer, R., et al. (1987): Behavioral effects of receptor-specific substance P agonists. *Pain,* 31:263–276.

69. Piercey, M. F., Schroeder, L. A., Folkers, K., Xu, J.-C., and Horig, J. (1981): Sensory and motor functions of spinal cord substance P. *Science,* 215:1361–1363.

70. Post, C., and Arweström, E. (1986): Antinociception and motor blocking effects of a glutamate antagonist. *Soc. Neurosci. Abstr.,* 12:622.

71. Price, D. D., Hu, J. W., Dubner, R., and Gracely, R. H. (1977): Peripheral suppression of first pain and central summation of second pain evoked by noxious heat pulses. *Pain,* 3:57–68.

72. Raigorodsky, G., and Urca, G. (1987): Intrathecal *N*-methyl-D-aspartate (NMDA) activates both nociceptive and antinociceptive systems. *Brain Res.,* 422:158–162.

73. Raigorodsky, G., and Urca, G. (1990): Involvement of *N*-methyl-D-aspartate receptors in nociception and motor control in the spinal cord of the mouse: behavioral, pharmacological and electrophysiological evidence. *Neuroscience,* 36:601–610.

74. Raigorodsky, G., and Urca, G. (1990): Spinal antinociceptive effects of excitatory amino acid antagonists: quisqualate modulates the action of N-methyl-D-aspartate. *Eur. J. Pharmacol.,* 182:37–47.

75. Randic, M., Hecimovic, H., and Ryu, P. D. (1990): Substance P modulates glutamate-induced currents in acutely isolated rat spinal dorsal horn neurons. *Neurosci. Lett.,* 117:74–80.

76. Ryder, S., Way, W. L., and Trevor, A. J. (1978): Comparative pharmacology of the optical isomers of ketamine in mice. *Eur. J. Pharmacol.,* 49:15–23.

77. Ryu, P. D., Gerber, G., Murase, K., and Randic, M. (1988): Calcitonin gene-related peptide enhances calcium current of rat dorsal root ganglion neurons and spinal excitatory synaptic transmission. *Neurosci. Lett.,* 89:305–312.

78. Sadove, M. S., Shulman, M., Hatano, S., and Fevold, N. (1971): Analgesic effects of ketamine administered in subdissociative doses. *Anesth. Analg.*, 50:452–457.
79. Salt, T. E., and Hill, R. G. (1983): Pharmacological differentiation between responses of rat medullary dorsal horn neurons to noxious mechanical and noxious thermal cutaneous stimuli. *Brain Res.*, 263:167–171.
80. Schneider, S. P., and Perl, E. R. (1985): Selective excitation of neurons in the mammalian spinal dorsal horn by aspartate and glutamate in vitro: correlation with localization and excitatory input. *Brain Res.*, 360:339–343.
81. Schneider, S. P., and Perl, E. R. (1988): Comparison of primary afferent and glutamate excitation of neurons in the mammalian spinal dorsal horn. *J. Neurosci.*, 8:2062–2073.
82. Schouenborg, J., and Sjölund, B. H. (1986): First order nociceptive synapses in rat dorsal horn are blocked by an amino acid antagonist. *Brain Res.*, 379:394–398.
83. Sjölund, B. H., Hao. J.-X., and Larsson, J. (1990): Low dose ketamine inhibits spinal nociceptive reflex—mediated via glutamate receptors? *Pain*, Suppl. 5:S226.
84. Skilling, S. R., Smullin, D. H., Beitz, A. J., and Larson, A. A. (1988): Extracellular amino acid concentrations in the dorsal spinal cord of freely moving rats following veratridine and nociceptive stimulation. *J. Neurochem.*, 51:127–132.
85. Sugimoto, T., Bennett, G. J., and Kajander, K. C. (1989): Strychnine-enhanced transsynaptic degeneration of dorsal horn neurons in rats with an experimental painful peripheral neuropathy. *Neurosci. Lett.*, 98:139–143.
86. Sugiyama, H., Ito, I., and Hirono, C. (1987): A new type of glutamate receptor linked to inositol phospholipid metabolism. *Nature*, 325:531–533.
87. Sullivan, A. F., Dickenson, A. H., and Roques, B. P. (1989): δ-Opioid mediated inhibitions of acute and prolonged noxious-evoked responses in rat dorsal horn neurons. *Br. J. Pharmacol.*, 98:1039–1049.
88. Sun, X., and Larson, A. A. (1991): Behavioral sensitization to kainic acid and quisqualic acid in mice: comparison to NMDA and substance P responses. *J. Neurosci.*, 11:3111–3123.
89. Takahashi, R. N., Morato, G. S., and Rae, G. A. (1987): Effects of ketamine on nociception and gastrointestinal motility in mice are unaffected by naloxone. *Gen. Pharmacol.*, 18:201–203.
90. Thompson, S. W. N., King, A. E., and Woolf, C. J. (1990): Activity-dependent changes in rat ventral horn neurons in vitro; summation of prolonged afferent evoked postsynaptic depolarizations produce a D-2-amino-5-phosphonovaleric acid sensitive windup. *Eur. J. Neurosci.*, 2: 638–649.
91. Tjolsen, A., Lund, A., Eide, P. K., Berge, O. G., and Hole, K. (1989): The apparent hyperalgesic effect of a serotonin antagonist in the tail flick test is mainly due to increased tail skin temperature. *Pharmacol. Biochem. Behav.*, 32:601–605.
92. Todd, A. J., and Lewis, S. G. (1986): The morphology of Golgi-stained neurons in Lamina II of the rat spinal cord. *J. Anat.*, 149:113–119.
93. Urbán, L., and Randic, M. (1984): Slow excitatory transmission in rat dorsal horn: possible mediation by peptides. *Brain Res.*, 290:336–341.
94. Wall, P. D. (1984): Mechanisms of acute and chronic pain. In: *Advances in pain research and therapy, vol. 6,* edited by L. Kruger and J. C. Liebeskind, pp. 95–104. Raven Press, New York.
95. Wall, P. D., Coderre, T. J., Stern, Y., and Wiesenfeld-Hallin, Z. (1988): Slow changes in the flexion reflex of the rat following arthritis or tenotomy. *Brain Res.*, 447:215–222.
96. Weisenfeld-Hallin, Z. (1985): Intrathecal somatostatin modulates spinal sensory and reflex mechanisms: behavioral and electrophysiological studies in the rat. *Neurosci. Lett.*, 62:69–74.
97. Westlund, K. N., McNeill, D. L., Patterson, J. T., and Coggeshall, R. E. (1989): Aspartate immunoreactive axons in normal rat L_4 dorsal roots. *Brain Res.*, 489:347–351.
98. Wilcox, G. L. (1988): Pharmacological studies of grooming and scratching behavior elicited by spinal substance P and excitatory amino acids. *Ann. NY Acad. Sci.*, 525:228–236.
99. Wilcox, G. L. (1991): Excitatory neurotransmitters and pain. In: *Pain research and clinical management: proceedings of the sixth world congress on pain,* edited by M. Bond, C. J. Woolf, and J. E. Charlton, pp. 97–117. Elsevier, Amsterdam.
100. Wilcox, G. L., and Alhaider, A. A. (1990): Nociceptive and antinociceptive action of serotonin agonists administered intrathecally. In: *Serotonin and pain* edited by J.-M. Besson, pp. 205–219. *(Excerpta Medica International Congress Series* no. 879).
101. Woolf, C. J. (1983): Evidence for a central component of post-injury pain hypersensitivity. *Nature* 306:686–688.
102. Woolf, C. J., and Thompson, S. W. N. (1991): The induction and maintenance of central sensitization is dependent on *N*-methyl-D-aspartic acid receptor activation; implications for the treatment of post-injury pain hypersensitivity states. *Pain*, 44:293–299.
103. Woolf, C. J., and Wiesenfeld-Hallin, Z. (1986): Substance P and calcitonin gene-related peptide synergistically modulate the gain of the nociceptive flexor withdrawal reflex in the rat. *Neurosci. Lett.*, 66:226–230.

104. Yaksh, T. L. (1989): Behavioral and autonomic correlates of the tactile evoked allodynia produced by spinal glycine inhibition: effects of modulatory receptor systems and excitatory amino acid antagonists. *Pain*, 37:111–123.
105. Yashpal, K., Wright, D. M., and Henry, J. L. (1982): Substance P reduces tail flick latency: implication for chronic pain syndromes. *Pain*, 15:155–167.
106. Yokota, Y., Sasai, Y., Tanaka, K., et al. (1989): Molecular characterization of a functional cDNA for rat substance P receptor. *J. Biol. Chem.*, 264:17649–17652.
107. Zieglgänsberger, W., and Herz, A. (1971): Changes of cutaneous receptive fields of spinocervical tract neurones and other dorsal horn neurons by microelectrophoretically administered amino acids. *Exp. Brain Res.*, 13:111–126.

Hyperalgesia and Allodynia,
edited by W. D. Willis, Jr.
Raven Press, Ltd., New York © 1992.

25

Peripheral and Central Contribution to the Persistent Expression of the C-fos Proto-oncogene in Spinal Cord After Peripheral Nerve Injury

*†Allan I. Basbaum, *Shu-Ing Chi, and *‡§Jon D. Levine

*Departments of *Anatomy, †Physiology, ‡Medicine, and §Oral and Maxillofacial Surgery and Keck Center for Integrative Neurosciences, University of California, San Francisco, California 94143*

Nerve injury in humans can precipitate a variety of chronic pain syndromes, many of which are associated with a hyperalgesic state. The mechanism underlying the generation of these pains is, however, poorly understood, which in part explains why many of these pain syndromes are very difficult to treat. Our studies of the factors that contribute to altered pain sensation are directed at the changes in the spinal cord that occur after peripheral nerve injury. As described below, we use the sciatic nerve neuroma model. Since any pain arising from complete nerve section is, of course, spontaneous or can only be evoked by peripheral stimulation of innervated tissue bordering the area of denervation, it may not be appropriate to refer to nerve–injury-induced hyperalgesia. In spite of this limitation, our results provide new information as to the nature of the long-term activity changes in the spinal cord that occur after peripheral nerve injury. It is likely that comparable anatomical and physiological spinal cord changes arise after *partial* nerve injury and that these changes contribute to the hyperalgesia that is often associated with partial nerve injury, as for example, in causalgic states.

The approach that we are taking involves the use of immunocytochemistry to evaluate the molecular changes that occur in neurons that have been activated by peripheral stimuli (14,19,23,30). We follow these changes in order to monitor the activity of a large population of spinal cord neurons. The particular molecular marker that we localize is the protein product of the c-fos proto-oncogene. C-fos is the cellular homologue of a retroviral transforming factor that induces osteosarcoma in mice. When the viral gene was cloned, it was determined that normal tissue, including neurons, contains what is presumed to be the original or "proto" gene, hence, the term "proto-oncogene." The c-fos gene is activated under a variety of conditions that are known to increase neural activity. The c-fos message appears within 10 min of stimulation and the Fos protein within another 10 to 20 min. The protein is rapidly translocated to the nucleus of neurons where it can be marked immunocytochemically with an antibody directed against this protein (21).

Although there are numerous *in vitro* studies that have demonstrated that the c-fos gene is induced just prior to cellular differentiation and growth, its function in neurons (which are postmitotic) is unclear. It has been suggested that the c-fos gene acts as a "third messenger," through which peripheral inputs, via a complicated cascade, regulate numerous additional genes. Based on *in vitro* studies, it has been demonstrated that the Fos protein is a transacting factor that regulates the transcription of a host of other genes. Which genes are regulated by the c-fos protein in adult neurons has not been established. A temporal relationship between increased Fos expression and increased dynorphin in response to peripheral tissue injury has been demonstrated and regulation of dynorphin expression via interaction of the Fos protein with a noncanonical transcriptional regulatory element has been reported (10,22).

Regardless of the specific molecular function of the c-fos gene in the mammalian neuron, it is clear that by monitoring the level of expression of the Fos protein, either by *in situ* hybridization methods to localize the Fos message or immunocytochemistry to monitor the Fos protein, it is possible to evaluate patterns of activity in large populations of neurons in the CNS. This approach has proven especially useful for studies in the spinal cord, where, in contrast with many brain areas (20), the basal levels of Fos expression are very low. Thus, it is easy to detect increases in activity of the gene, from which increases in neural activity can be deduced.

Initially we studied the changes in Fos expression that were evoked by various noxious somatic, articular, and visceral stimuli (12,19,23). Maximal numbers of Fos-like immunoreactive neurons were recorded when rats were killed 2 to 4 hr after the noxious stimulus was administered. Within 24 hr the number of labeled cells returned to prestimulation levels. Consistent with the electrophysiological studies that have identified the location of nociresponsive neurons, we found that noxious stimulation of tissue in the rat evokes Fos-like immunoreactivity in neurons of the superficial dorsal horn, laminae I and II, in the region of lamina V, around the central canal, lamina X, and in ventral horn laminae VII and VIII. Differences between the pattern of staining after somatic and visceral stimulation, including a more restricted labeling of cells in the marginal zone after the latter stimulus, were also consistent with electrophysiological studies and provided further data in support of the use of Fos immunocytochemistry to monitor the activity of large populations of neurons. Finally, in double-label studies we demonstrated that a considerable number of the Fos-positive neurons are at the origin of major ascending pathways, including the spinoreticular and spinothalamic tracts (19).

These studies provided valuable information about the topological distribution of neurons that are activated by tissue injury. There is of course considerable evidence that spinal cord neurons are also profoundly activated by injury to peripheral nerve (8,28). These studies are particularly important because they provide insights into the changes in the nervous system that may contribute to the neuropathic pains associated with injury to the nervous system. To date, most studies have been directed at one of two models, the neuroma model produced by section and ligation of the sciatic nerve (29) or the multiple-ligature model, produced by placing several ligatures around the sciatic nerve (4).

The neuroma model has received considerable attention in physiological, pharmacological, and behavioral studies. Of particular interest is the evidence that axonal sprouts within the neuroma become hyperactive, mechanically sensitive, and responsive to alpha-adrenergic agonists (29). Thus, within days of nerve section and ligation, it has been demonstrated that spontaneous activity increases in the injured nerve. In general the first fibers to become active are myelinated; unmyelinated axons develop abnormal spontaneous activity somewhat later (13). These persistent changes in the peripheral nerve are associated with persistent changes in the spinal cord (8,28). Thus, spinal neurons connected to a neuroma have abnormal spontaneous activity (29), and the dorsal root potential (a reflection of activity in second-order neurons in the spinal dorsal horn) is abnormal, or in some animals absent, within days of nerve section (28,34).

Since it is not possible to evoke sensations by somatic stimulation of the denervated area of the limb, it is difficult to determine whether the changes in the neuroma contribute to a true hyperalgesic state. On the other hand, it has been demonstrated that autotomy is present after peripheral nerve section, and, based on a variety of studies, it has been argued that autotomy is indicative of a central pain state, somewhat analogous to the neuropathic pains that are observed in humans after peripheral nerve injury. Regardless of the relationship of autotomy to neuropathic pain, it is clear that there are profound changes produced in the CNS after peripheral nerve injury, and thus the neuroma model provides a useful way to produce and to assess central changes.

In our studies we evaluated the changes in Fos expression that occur at different times after a sciatic nerve neuroma is produced (5). We hypothesized that if there is chronic pain associated with this model, then it should be possible to demonstrate a persistent increase in Fos expression in the spinal cord. In our studies, the sciatic nerve of adult male rats was sectioned and ligated. At different times after the lesion, the rats were perfused with aldehydes and the spinal cord tissue processed for c-fos immunocytochemistry. We used an antibody directed against an *in vitro* translated Fos gene. Although there are many Fos-related antigens (which have amino acid sequences often recognized by antisera raised against the Fos protein), the antibody that we have used only recognizes the Fos protein. This proved to be of particular value in our studies because in response to noxious stimuli the fos-related antigens are typically expressed later in time than the Fos protein (30).

To quantify the expression of Fos in neurons of different laminae of the spinal cord, we first counted the number of labeled cells through the lumbar enlargement using a camera lucida attachment to the light microscope. The gray matter was divided into three different regions: the superficial dorsal horn (laminae I and II), the nucleus proprius (laminae III and IV), the remaining gray matter (laminae V, VI, and VII). As expected, the highest number of Fos-immunoreactive cells was found within hours of the nerve section. The largest number of labeled cells was found in the superficial laminae, as we observed after tissue injury. Considerable numbers of cells, however, were also found in regions of the cord associated with processing of non-nociceptive and nociceptive information. This was expected from the fact that nerve section cuts *all* classes of afferent fiber.

As described above, within 24 hr of tissue stimulation, almost no cells are found in the dorsal horn. It was thus of great interest that in contrast to the short-lived expression of Fos observed after tissue injury, we found a persistent, albeit varying expression of Fos after peripheral nerve injury. Note that the half-life of the Fos protein is very limited, from 2 to 4 hr. Since it is hypothesized that Fos expression is a reflection of neuronal activity, this persistent expression of the gene was suggestive of persistent activity. The most constant level of Fos expression after nerve injury occurred in laminae V to VII. The increase in Fos expression was highly significant when compared to the level of expression in sham-operated rats, which underwent the same surgical procedure to expose the sciatic nerve but did not have the nerve sectioned. Sham-operated rats had approximately five cells per 50-μm section in laminae V to VII. Sciatic nerve-lesioned rats had approximately 35 cells per 50-μm section in these laminae. This level was maintained up to 1 month after the surgery.

The relatively stable level of Fos expression in the deeper laminae of the dorsal horn differed from that observed in the superficial laminae (I and II). In these latter regions we found an oscillatory pattern of labeling. After the initial peak of expression recorded 2 hr after the surgery, there was a progressive decrease in the number of labeled neurons. By 24 hr, the number of cells in the superficial laminae approached that seen in the sham controls. Another 24 hr later, however, i.e., 48 hr after sciatic nerve section, there was a striking reappearance of the Fos expression in the superficial laminae. Over the next week, there was again a decline in the numbers of labeled cells; however, another peak of labeling was observed 2 weeks after nerve section. Compared to sham-operated rats, the increase persisted up to 1 month after surgery. In contrast to the maintained, albeit oscillatory increase in Fos expression in the superficial laminae and the deeper laminae, the staining in cells of the nucleus proprius of rats with sciatic nerve lesions was more variable. There was some delayed increase in staining in the experimental animals; however, the variability of staining in the sham-operated controls was also high and thus no statistically significant difference was detected.

Having shown that nerve injury is indeed associated with increased and persistent staining of Fos-labeled neurons in the dorsal horn in a pattern consistent with there being a tonic nociceptive input, we next addressed the factors that contribute to the altered pattern of staining. As described above, it has been shown that soon after the neuroma develops, there is an increased activity of the injured afferent fibers. It was thus of interest to evaluate whether local anesthetic blockade of the neuroma at different times after surgery would affect the pattern of staining observed. To this end we examined the pattern of Fos-immunoreactive neurons 2 days and 2 weeks after nerve section, at which times there were increased Fos expression in laminae V to VII and peaks of increased staining in the superficial dorsal horn. The experimental protocol involved percutaneous injection of bupivacaine in the region of the injured nerve; this approach avoided direct contact with the nerve. Although this local anesthetic has a very prolonged action in humans (>10 hr), we found that bupivacaine only blocked conduction in the injured nerve for a period of approximately 90 min. To block Fos expression beyond the half-life of the Fos, the anesthetic was administered three to four times, at 60- to 90-min intervals. To control for systemic absorption following direct application of the local anesthetic to the nerve, another group of animals received the same dose and volume of anesthetic subcutaneously at the back of the neck.

Consistent with the hypothesis that activity within the neuroma contributes to the increased expression of Fos in the dorsal horn, we found that local anesthetic blockade of the nerve significantly reduced the number of labeled cells in laminae V to VII. In contrast, the control injection had no effect on the expression of Fos in these regions. Based on these results, we conclude that activity within laminae V to VII at 2 days after nerve injury is largely generated by activity arising within the neuroma itself. In contrast, we found significantly reduced labeling of Fos-immunoreactive neurons in the superficial dorsal horn both after direct nerve injection of the anesthetic and after injection at the back of the neck. Since a systemic action of the local anesthetic was effective, we cannot conclude that the increased dorsal horn expression of Fos was exclusively due to increased activity in the injured afferents. It is possible that the anesthetic acted centrally, at the level of the spinal cord. Alternatively, if the injured, sprouting peripheral nerve small-diameter afferents (which probably provide most of the input that activates neurons in the superficial dorsal horn) became sensitized to the action of the local anesthetic, there might still be a predominant peripheral site of action of the blocking agent. Importantly, at 2 days after surgery, we found no effect of the local anesthetic on the Fos expression in the nucleus proprius.

The effect of local anesthetic on the pattern of Fos expression at 2 weeks was very different. We found similar results with direct nerve injection and subcutaneous injection at the back of the neck, for all regions examined. In other words, the increased expression in the superficial laminae, the nucleus proprius, and the deeper laminae (V–VII) was significantly reduced, regardless of the route of administration of the local anesthetic. This indicates that between 2 days and 2 weeks, additional changes occur in the neuroma and/or spinal cord. It is conceivable that the peripheral sprouts have become particularly sensitive to local anesthetic such that they respond to even low systemic doses of the drug. Alternatively, or possibly in addition, central neurons throughout the dorsal horn may become susceptible to local anesthetic administration. In fact, there is evidence that dorsal horn neurons that were activated by intense noxious stimuli have a persistent spontaneous activity that is unusually sensitive to low doses of local anesthetic administered systemically (32,35).

As described above, since the axons in the neuroma are disconnected from the periphery, it is difficult to correlate the changes in Fos expression with readily identified pain behaviors or with hyperalgesic/neuropathic pain conditions. (We did not follow animals that displayed autotomy.) Our results, however, are consistent with previous studies that have reported increased activity of injured primary afferents and profound changes in the firing of spinal cord neurons.

In addition to the contribution of increased activity in the injured nerve, the massive barrage generated by the nerve section itself may also contribute to the persistent expression of Fos in the spinal cord. There is, in fact, considerable evidence that intense noxious stimulation provokes long-term changes in spinal neurons, changes that probably contribute to prolonged hyperalgesic states. For example, Woolf (31) demonstrated that heat injury of the skin can sensitize the flexor reflex responses in the ipsilateral limb. It is proposed that the nerve injury sets up barrages of impulses that result in sustained sensitization of central circuits, such that the flexor reflex can subsequently be evoked by stimuli that are typically below threshold for the reflex. That, of course, could have resulted from a peripheral sensitization, i.e., a lowering of the threshold of the C-fiber afferents, through injury-evoked production of hyperalgesic prostaglandins. Although that almost certainly occurs, it was further demonstrated that the reflex could not only be activated by low-threshold stimuli ipsilaterally, but that stimulation of the *contralateral* limb also became effective. Most interestingly, local anesthetic blockade of the original, i.e., ipsilateral, injury site, did not prevent the lowered threshold for activation of the reflex from the contralateral limb. It was concluded that the unilateral peripheral nerve injury evoked prolonged changes in the spinal cord, which contributed to the hyperalgesic responses that could be elicited from both sides of the body.

These injury inputs (including the barrage associated with nerve section) may have important clinical consequences. Thus, for example, it was demonstrated that the incidence of postoperative pain can be reduced if surgical procedures are performed under combined general and local anesthesia (18). The latter was intended to prevent the spinal cord from "experiencing" the insult of the surgical procedure. In another study it was reported that if the spinal cord was "shut down," with repeated spinal epidural injections of morphine several days prior to limb amputation, the incidence of postamputation phantom limb pain was significantly reduced in the year following surgery (2). Taken together with the present results, it appears that the massive barrage associated with nerve section contributes to long-term changes in the spinal cord neurons and that these changes contribute to the persistent reorganization of the cord that follows the injury. Presumably, the changes provoked by the massive barrage interact with the increased spontaneous activity that arises from within the neuroma. Interfering with the massive barrage, by preblock with local anesthetic, or with the hyperactivity of the injured afferents, by postblock of the neuroma, can prevent the persistent activity that is presumed to contribute to the prolongation of postoperative pain and possibly to the neuropathic pains that are often associated with nerve injury.

It was of interest, however, that preblock anesthetic in our model only reduced the expression of Fos in the superficial dorsal horn. The activity in the more ventral regions, which could be readily reduced by postblock local anesthetic administration was unaffected. This result indicates that one can dissociate some of the factors that contribute to the long-term expression of Fos in the different regions of the spinal cord. Activity located in the superficial dorsal horn apparently results not only from the increased spontaneous activity of the neuroma, but also from the massive barrage that occurs with nerve injury. By contrast, the activity of the more ventral regions of the spinal cord appears to be independent of the initial injury discharge.

Several factors might contribute to the differential sensitivity of the superficial dorsal horn neurons to the massive barrage. The most likely factor is the particular afferent that terminates in the superficial dorsal horn. Although nociresponsive neurons in the superficial dorsal horn, laminae V, and the ventral horn are activated by unmyelinated afferents, it is likely that only the superficial neurons receive a significant monosynaptic input (27). These small-diameter afferents are relatively unique in their transmitter phenotype. They contain a variety of neuropeptides, including substance P and calcitonin gene-related peptide, either of which may provoke long-term changes in second-order neurons. Perhaps more important is that these same afferents also contain the excitatory amino acid neurotransmitter glutamate (7). Through an N-methyl-D-aspartate- (NMDA) mediated receptor, it is likely that glutamate release from the unmyelinated afferents during the massive barrage provokes a type of long-term potentiation in neurons of the superficial laminae (33). In fact, there is evidence that the phenomenon of windup, which results from strong and repeated activation of fine afferent fibers, can be blocked by NMDA antagonists (9). It will obviously be of interest to evaluate the effect of NMDA antagonists on the long-term expression of Fos in the nerve injury model.

That these antagonists may indeed have effects on Fos expression is indicated from our studies of the effects of the noncompetitive NMDA antagonist MK801 on the induction of Fos in the spinal dorsal horn by formalin injection into the hindpaw (15). We found that intrathecal injection of MK801, at doses that did not block the behavioral response to formalin injection, significantly reduced, by about 35%, the number of Fos-immunoreactive neurons in laminae I and II, without affecting Fos expression in more ventral laminae. This result indicates that C-fiber stimulation activates Fos expression in the superficial laminae, in part through an NMDA–receptor-mediated primary afferent volley. It is likely, therefore, that the effect of local anesthetic preblock on the long-term changes in Fos expression of the superficial dorsal horn reflect a predominant blockade of the small-diameter, peptide/amino acid-containing primary afferents that terminate directly on neurons of laminae I and II. Interestingly, the incidence of nerve–lesion-evoked autotomy can also be attenuated by pretreatment with MK801 (25).

Another interesting possibility relates to the excitotoxicity that can be produced by sudden and massive release of glutamate from primary afferent fibers. Thus, for example, Sugimoto and colleagues (26) reported that after section of the trigeminal nerve, cell death occurs in the superficial laminae of the trigeminal nucleus caudalis, predominantly in small neurons of the substantia gelatinosa. Conceivably, the massive discharge provoked by sciatic nerve section produces comparable injury and/or death of small cells of the same region of the spinal dorsal horn. Although this has not been reported after sciatic nerve section, it has been seen in the ligature model described by Bennett and Xie (4). If some or all of the neurons are inhibitory interneurons of the substantia gelatinosa, this could result in a disinhibition of other cells within the superficial dorsal horn. This, of course, might be manifested by a persistent Fos expression. Indeed the transient reduction in Fos expression in the superficial dorsal horn at 24 hr after nerve injury might be the "calm before the storm." Loss of inhibitory control during that period might precede the reappearance of Fos expression at the 2-day time point. The fact that Fos expression in the deeper laminae of the cord is not affected by blockade of the injury discharge and the fact that there is little evidence for excitotoxicity after peripheral nerve injury in these regions are consistent with our conclusion that the persistent Fos expression in the deeper laminae is related more to the hyperactivity of the axons in the neuroma.

Having established several factors that contribute to the persistence of Fos expression in the spinal cord after development of a sciatic nerve neuroma, we next asked whether it is possible to pharmacologically regulate nerve–injury-provoked increases in the expression of Fos. In other studies, we had established that tissue–injury-evoked increases in Fos expression in the spinal cord can be dose dependently blocked by either morphine (23) or by the gamma-aminobutyric–acid-B (GABA-B) agonist baclofen (6). Since neuropathic pains are generally less responsive to narcotics than are nociceptive pains (1,3), it was of particular interest to evaluate whether the effects of these different drugs on nerve–injury-evoked Fos expression were comparable to their effects on tissue–injury-evoked Fos expression. To this end we examined the effect of these drugs, at doses that not only produced an analgesic response in the formalin test but that also blocked Fos expression by at least 50%.

In these studies we chose to evaluate the effects of drugs on Fos expression 2 weeks after nerve injury. This time was chosen because it was the point at which we found evidence for both central and peripheral contributions to the persistent Fos expression. We reasoned that the likelihood of finding a suppressive effect of the putative analgesic would be greatest at this time point. Somewhat surprisingly, therefore, we found that 5.0 mg/kg morphine, administered intraperitoneally, was absolutely without effect on the numbers of Fos-immunoreactive neurons in each of the regions of the spinal cord examined. In contrast, baclofen produced a profound reduction in the number of labeled neurons, in all regions of the spinal cord, the superficial dorsal horn, the nucleus proprius, and the more ventral laminae (V, VI, and VII).

The failure of morphine to modify nerve–injury-evoked Fos expression was surprising. Although there is evidence of a loss of opioid binding sites on the presynaptic terminals of primary afferent fibers that have been sectioned distally (11), there should be considerable targets postsynaptically. Thus, approximately 30% to 50% of the opioid binding persists after dorsal rhizotomy, and opiates can block the glutamate-evoked excitation of dorsal horn neurons (36), indicating a postsynaptic action. The presence of enkephalin-immunoreactive synapses presynaptic to spinothalamic projection neurons also argues for a considerable postsynaptic action of opioids (24). Indeed, although there is evidence for a reduction of the inhibitory effect of opioids on the spontaneous activity of deafferented dorsal horn neurons (17), the effect is not completely eliminated in the deafferented rat. On the other hand, the failure of morphine to inhibit Fos expression is remarkably consistent with the clinical observation that opiates are often ineffective in the treatment of neuropathic pains (1,3). It is likely that the mechanisms through which spinal neurons become refractory to the effects of opiates under conditions of peripheral nerve injury contribute to the clinical observations.

It was, however, of great interest that the GABA-B ligand baclofen exerted a profound inhibitory effect on nerve–injury-evoked Fos expression in all regions of the spinal cord gray matter. One important difference between opioids and GABA reflects the diameter of the primary afferents that are subject to presynaptic inhibition. Thus, opioids probably exert a relatively selective inhibitory regulation of small-diameter afferents. By contrast, GABAergic presynaptic inhibition is exerted on both large- and small-diameter afferents. Since the peripheral nerve injury results in hyperactivity of all categories of afferent fibers, it is likely that the central effects of injury reflect activity in a broad class of afferent. The reduction of Fos expression by baclofen may be due to this broad action. Importantly, there is no evidence that GABAergic binding sites are affected by peripheral nerve injury (16); thus both pre- and postsynaptic mechanisms continue to operate in the normal and nerve-injury animals.

Given the powerful effect of baclofen on Fos expression in both the formalin, i.e., tissue injury model, and in the nerve injury model, it is surprising that baclofen is not that effective in clinical pain conditions (with the exception of trigeminal neuralgia). One possibility is that the dose of baclofen necessary to block pain (including neuropathic pains) is such that the effects of the drug on motoneurons (i.e., inhibition with subsequent paralysis) cannot be avoided. Our results, however, indicate that the development of GABAergic compounds that act more selectively on dorsal horn neurons may be useful in the clinical treatment of some pain states, including those that arise from peripheral nerve injury.

In summary, we have shown that by monitoring the activity of large populations of spinal cord neurons by their expression of the Fos protein it is possible to characterize important features of the changes that occur after peripheral nerve injury. Our results indicate that activity in the injured afferent fibers is an important contributor to the persistence of activity in the spinal cord. There is also evidence, however, for central changes that affect the activity of spinal cord neurons, independent of the activity that arises in the periphery. We also provide evidence that the injury discharge that arises when a peripheral nerve is cut evokes long-lasting changes in the properties of spinal neurons, especially those in the superficial laminae of the cord. Interfering with the development of those changes may have significant consequences for pain that arises after injury. These changes almost certainly contribute to the hyperalgesic phenomena that are precipitated by nerve injury in animals and humans. Finally, we demonstrated that although both morphine and baclofen profoundly inhibit the expression of Fos in spinal neurons when the peripheral stimulus is to tissue, only baclofen was effective when the Fos induction was provoked by injury to nerve. These results provide an important laboratory correlate of the differential effectiveness of opiates and baclofen for the treatment of neuropathic pain in patients. It is hoped that understanding the mechanisms that contribute to the differential effectiveness of these different analgesics will provide useful information toward the development of new approaches to treating hyperalgesic conditions that appear in the presence of injury to the nervous system.

ACKNOWLEDGMENT

This work was supported by USPHS grants NS14627, NS21647, and DE/NIDA 08973.

REFERENCES

1. Arner, S., and Meyerson, B. A. (1988): Lack of analgesic effect of opioids on neuropathic and idiopathic pain. *Pain,* 33:11–23.
2. Bach, S., Noreng, M. F., and Tjéllden, N. U. (1988): Phantom limb pain in amputees during the first 12 months following limb amputation, after preoperative lumbar epidural blockade. *Pain,* 33:297–301.
3. Basbaum, A. I., and Besson, J. M. (1991): *Towards a new pharmacotherapy of pain.* Wiley and Sons, London.
4. Bennett, G. J., and Xie, Y.-K. (1988): A peripheral mononeuropathy in rat that produces disorders of pain sensation like those seen in man. *Pain,* 33:87–107.
5. Chi, S.-I., Levine, J. D., and Basbaum, A. I. (1989): Time course of peripheral neuroma-induced expression of Fos protein immunoreactivity in spinal cord of rats and effects of local anesthetics. *Neurosci. Abstr.,* 15:155.
6. Chi, S.-I., Levine, J. D., and Basbaum, A. I. (1990): Effects of baclofen and morphine on the persistent expression of c-fos in rat spinal cord following peripheral nerve injury. *Neurosci. Abstr.,* 16:566.
7. DeBiasi, S., and Rustioni, A. (1988): Glutamate and substance P coexist in primary afferent terminals in the superficial laminae of spinal cord. *Proc. Natl. Acad. Sci. USA,* 85:7820–7824.
8. Devor, M., and Rappaport, Z. H. (1990): Pain and the pathophysiology of damaged nerve. In: *Pain syndromes in neurology,* edited by H. L. Fields, pp. 47–84. Butterworths, London.
9. Dickenson, A. H. (1990): A cure for wind up: NMDA receptor antagonists as potential analgesics. *Trends Pharmacol Sci.,* 11:307–309.
10. Draisci, G., and Iadarola, M. J. (1989): Temporal analysis of increase in c-fos, preprodynorphin and preproenkephalin mRNA's in rat spinal cord. *Mol. Brain Res.,* 6:31–37.
11. Fields, H. L., Emson, P. C., Leigh, B. K., Gilbert, R. F. T., and Iverson, L. L. (1980): Multiple opiate receptor sites on primary afferent fibres. *Nature,* 284:351–353.
12. Gogas, K. R., Presley, R. W., Levine, J. D., and Basbaum, A. I. (1991): The antinociceptive action of supraspinal opioids results from an increase in descending inhibitory control: correlation of nociceptive behavior and c-fos expression. *Neuroscience,* 42:617–628.
13. Gorvin-Lippmann, R., and Devor, M. (1978): Ongoing activity in severed nerves: source and variation with time. *Brain Res.,* 159:406–410.
14. Hunt, S. P., Pini, A., and Evan, G. (1987): Induction of c-fos-like protein in spinal cord neurons following sensory stimulation. *Nature,* 328:632–634.
15. Kehl, L. J., Basbaum, A. I., Pollock, C. H., Mayes, M., and Wilcox, G. L. (1990): The NMDA receptor antagonist MK801 reduces noxious stimulus-evoked Fos expression in the mammalian spinal dorsal horn. *Pain,* suppl. 5:S165.
16. Jessell, T., Tsunoo, A., Kanazawa, I., and Otsuka, M. (1979): Substance P: depletion in the dorsal horn of rat spinal cord after section of the peripheral processes of primary sensory neurons. *Brain Res.* 168:247–259.
17. Lombard, M.-C., and Besson, J.-M. (1989): Electrophysiological evidence for a tonic activity of the spinal cord intrinsic opioid systems in a chronic pain model. *Brain Res.,* 477:48–56.

18. McQuay, H. J., Carroll, D., and Moore, R. A. (1988): Postoperative orthopaedic pain—the effect of opiate premedication and local anaesthetic blocks. *Pain,* 33:291–295.

19. Menétrey, D., Gannon, A., Levine, J. D., and Basbaum, A. I. (1989): Expression of c-fos protein in interneurons and projection neurons of the rat spinal cord in response to noxious somatic, articular and visceral stimulation. *J. Comp. Neurol.,* 258:177–195.

20. Morgan, J., Cohen, D., Hempstead, J., and Curran, T. (1987): Mapping patterns of c-fos expression in the central nervous system after seizure. *Science,* 237:192–197.

21. Morgan, J. I., and Curran, T. (1989): Stimulus-transcription coupling in neurons: role of cellular immediate-early genes. *Trends Neurosci.,* 12:459–462.

22. Naranjo, J. R., Mellström, B., Achaval, M., and Sassone-Corsi, P. (1991): Molecular pathways of pain: Fos/Jun-mediated activation of a noncanonical AP-1 site in the prodynorphin gene. *Neuron,* 6:607–617.

23. Presley, R. W., Menétrey, D., Levine, J. D., and Basbaum, A. I. (1990): Systemic morphine suppresses noxious stimulation-evoked Fos protein-like immunoreactivity in the rat spinal cord. *J. Neurosci.,* 10:323–335.

24. Ruda, M. A., Coffield, J., and Dubner, R. (1984): Demonstration of postsynaptic opioid modulation of thalamic projection neurons by the combined techniques of retrograde horseradish peroxidase and enkephalin immunocytochemistry. *J. Neurosci.,* 4:2117–2132.

25. Seltzer, Z., Cohn, S., Ginzburg, R., and Beilin, B. Z. (1991): Modulation of neuropathic pain behavior in rats by spinal disinhibition and NMDA receptor blockade of injury discharge. *Pain,* 45:69–76.

26. Sugimoto, T., Takemura, M., Sakai, A., and Ishimaru, M. (1987): Rapid transneuronal destruction following peripheral nerve transection in the medullary dorsal horn is enhanced by strychnine, picrotoxin and bicuculline. *Pain,* 30:385–393.

27. Sugiura, Y., Lee, C. L., and Perl, E. R. (1986): Central projections of identified, unmyelinated (C) afferent fibers innervating mammalian skin. *Science,* 234:358–361.

28. Wall, P. D., and Devor, M. (1981): The effect of peripheral nerve injury on dorsal root potentials and on transmission of afferent signals into the spinal cord. *Brain Res.,* 209:95–111.

29. Wall, P. D., and Gutnick, M. (1974): Properties of afferent nerve impulses originating from a neuroma. *Nature,* 248:740–743.

30. Williams, S., Evan, G. I., and Hunt, S. P. (1990): Changing patterns of c-fos induction in spinal neurons following thermal cutaneous stimulation in the rat. *Neuroscience,* 36:73–81.

31. Woolf, C. J. (1983): Evidence for a central component of post-injury pain hypersensitivity. *Nature,* 306:686–688.

32. Woolf, C. J., and McMahon, S. B. (1985): Injury-induced plasticity of the flexor reflex in chronic decerebrate rats. *Neuroscience,* 16:395–404.

33. Woolf, C. J., and Thompson, S. W. N. (1991): The induction and maintenance of central sensitization is dependent on N-methyl-D-aspartic receptor activation; implications for the treatment of post-injury pain hypersensitivity states. *Pain,* 44:293–300.

34. Woolf, C. J., and Wall, P. D. (1982): Chronic peripheral nerve section diminishes the primary afferent A-fibre mediated inhibition of rat dorsal horn neurones. *Brain Res.,* 242:77–85.

35. Woolf, C. J., and Wiesenfeld-Hallin, Z. (1985): The systemic administration of local anaesthetics produces a selective depression of C-afferent fibre evoked activity in the spinal cord. *Pain,* 23:361–374.

36. Zieglgansberger, W., and Bayeri, H. (1976): The mechanism of inhibition of neuronal activity by opiates in the spinal cord of the cat. *Brain Res.,* 115:111–125.

Hyperalgesia and Allodynia,
edited by W. D. Willis, Jr.
Published by Raven Press, Ltd.,
New York, 1992.

26

Central Changes Contributing to Neuropathic Hyperalgesia

Gary J. Bennett and Jennifer M. A. Laird

Neurobiology and Anesthesiology Branch, National Institute of Dental Research,
National Institutes of Health, Bethesda, Maryland 20892

It is well-known that changes in the sensitivity of primary afferent neurons inner-vating injured tissue contribute to the perceptual state that we call hyperalgesia. During the past few years a great deal of experimental data have been provided showing that the injury-evoked activation of primary afferent nociceptors also gives rise to changes in the responsiveness of pain-processing neurons in the spinal cord dorsal horn. It is now clear that both of these phenomena, primary afferent sensiti-zation and central hyperexcitability, contribute to the state of hyperalgesia. These phenomena are the body's normal response to tissue damage: they are initiated by the injury and disappear as the damage heals; in fact, it is reasonable to presume that hyperalgesia is part of the healing process itself.

In rare instances, tissue injury, especially if it includes injury to a peripheral nerve, produces a hyperalgesic state that is considered to be abnormal. This neuropathic hyperalgesia is abnormal because its severity is disproportionately great and it does not disappear as the injury heals. It has been hypothesized (2,5) that neuropathic hyperalgesia represents a pathological expression of the same mechanisms that un-derlie the normal hyperalgesic state.

Both the initiation and the maintenance of the hyperalgesia that normally follows injury have been shown to depend, at least in part, on neurotransmission at synapses with N-methyl-D-aspartate (NMDA) receptors (for review, see ref. 14). It is known that high levels of NMDA-receptor activation can damage the postsynaptic neuron (9). We review here recent work with an experimental painful peripheral neuropathy that suggests that excitotoxicity contributes to neuropathic hyperalgesia by damag-ing inhibitory interneurons in the spinal cord dorsal horn. The resulting disinhibition would be expected to contribute to a state of central hyperexcitability.

DAMAGE TO SPINAL CORD INTERNEURONS

Sugimoto and colleagues (12) have shown that transection of the rat's inferior al-veolar nerve produces transsynaptic degeneration in neurons in the superficial lam-inae of the medullary dorsal horn (trigeminal nucleus caudalis). However, this effect appeared only if the proximal stump was returned to the nerve's bony canal and the animal was given small doses of a convulsant drug like strychnine. It was hypothesized that within the confines of the canal, pulsations from the nerve's companion artery would constantly activate the axonal sprouts within the stump (unlike normal axons, sprouts are known to be mechanosensitive); the effect of the strychnine was presumed to exacerbate the injurious effects of this primary afferent input by blocking afferent-evoked inhibitory effects. In turn, this hypothesis suggested that a high level of primary–afferent-evoked postsynaptic excitation was required for the production of transsynaptic degeneration. This idea was supported by the demonstration of transsynaptic degeneration following a rapid series of nerve–transection-evoked injury discharges in animals pretreated with a subconvulsive dose of strychnine (13).

Using an experimental painful peripheral neuropathy that is created by damage to the rat's sciatic nerve (3), Kajander and colleagues (6,7) demonstrated that many of the primary afferent neurons in the damaged nerve were discharging spontaneously at high rates (20–40 Hz) as early as 24 hr after the nerve injury. At 1 to 3 days postinjury, a period that brackets the onset of behavioral signs of hyperalgesia in this model, spontaneous discharge was found in approximately one-third of the primary afferents with Aβ axons and one-fifth of those with Aδ axons, but not in any significant percentage of the primary afferent C fibers. However, Xie and Xiao (15) subsequently showed that C fibers contribute to the primary afferent barrage at 7 to 40 days postinjury. In view of these observations, we hypothesized that animals with the experimental neuropathy would exhibit transsynaptic degeneration in the spinal dorsal horn of the lumbar segments innervated by the damaged sciatic nerve.

The experiments summarized in Fig. 26.1 show that at 8 days postinjury the ex-

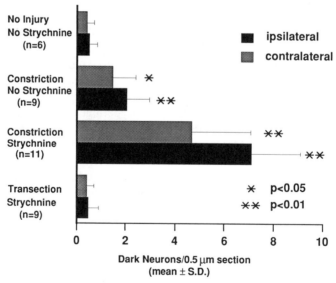

FIG. 26.1. The effects of the chronic constriction injury, strychnine (subconvulsive dose, 1 mg/kg, i.p.; daily for 7 days), and complete sciatic transection on the average incidence of degenerating/atrophic neurons ("dark neurons") in the ipsilateral and contralateral dorsal horn of segment L4 at 8 days postinjury. *, **, significantly different from control (no injury, no strychnine); also significantly different in a within-subject comparison to the incidence of dark neurons in the dorsal horn of C6. (Data from ref. 11.)

perimental neuropathy created by constricting the sciatic nerve does produce trans-synaptic degeneration (10,11). In thin (0.5 μm) sections of plastic-embedded tissue stained with toluidine blue, the cytoplasm of normal neurons stains lightly and the nucleoplasm stains even more lightly. Normal neurons also have nuclear and cellular outlines that are smooth, i.e., they appear to be turgid. In contrast, in the nerve-injured animals many neurons show a greatly increased affinity for the stain in both the cytoplasm and nucleoplasm (hence the label "dark neurons"). Moreover, their nuclear and cellular margins are wrinkled, indicating that they have shriveled. In rats without nerve injury (Fig. 26.1, top row), the incidence of dark neurons is less than one per section (it is not clear why the incidence is not zero; it may be a fixation artefact or an indication of normal cell loss due to aging). Rats with the neuropathy (Fig. 26.1, second row) have a fourfold higher incidence of dark neurons on the side of the nerve injury and, surprisingly, a threefold increase on the opposite side; the increase on the ipsilateral side was significantly greater. The appearance of dark neurons on the contralateral side may be related to a recently described contralateral sensory abnormality seen in some animals with this injury (1). Combining the con-striction injury with strychnine administration (Fig. 26.1, third row) causes a further increase in the incidence of transsynaptic degeneration (14-fold ipsilaterally and 11-fold contralaterally, a statistically significant difference). It is apparent that trans-synaptic degeneration does not follow every nerve injury; as shown in Fig. 26.1 (fourth row), a complete transection of the sciatic nerve did not produce dark neu-rons, even when the animals were administered strychnine.

The dark neurons found in these experiments were mostly small- or medium-sized neurons in laminae I to III and confined to the sciatic nerve's territory (on both sides). It is thus very likely that many of these cells were inhibitory interneurons that were innervated by primary afferents in the damaged nerve. The increase caused by strychnine (which had no effect on its own) could be reasonably ascribed to an increase in primary afferent-evoked postsynaptic depolarization due to block-ade of afferent-evoked inhibition. It is difficult to gauge the severity of functional impairment associated with the anatomical changes seen in dark neurons. We do not know whether these cells die, remain in an atrophic state, or eventually recover. Nevertheless, it is reasonable to hypothesize that the alteration in appearance is associated with at least some degree of dysfunction. If this is true, then one might be able to detect abnormalities in the inhibitory systems that are mediated by the damaged interneurons. Such an abnormality should be significantly greater ipsilat-eral to the nerve injury.

ABNORMAL PRESYNAPTIC INHIBITION

A primary afferent volley in the spinal dorsal horn leads to both excitatory and inhibitory effects in pain-processing circuitry. The magnitude of the pain signal sent to the brain is a function of the interaction between this afferent-evoked excitation and inhibition. There are two general classes of spinal inhibitory mechanisms: pre- and postsynaptic inhibition; both are mediated by primary afferent synapses on in-terneurons. Synapses issued by the inhibitory interneurons that mediate postsyn-aptic inhibition are found on the neurons that transmit information to the brain (and also on other cells). These synapses generate hyperpolarizing potentials, i.e., the classical inhibitory postsynaptic potentials (IPSPs). The second inhibitory mechanism, presynaptic inhibition, also involves primary–afferent-evoked activation of inhibitory interneurons, but the inhibition is produced by a different mechanism. Presynaptic inhibition is a result of primary afferent depolarization (PAD), which operates as follows.

When a nerve impulse reaches one of its axon's terminals, the terminal is depolarized; this leads to the release of neurotransmitter and, in turn, to activation of the postsynaptic neuron. The amount of neurotransmitter released, and hence the magnitude of activation in the postsynaptic neuron, is a function of the magnitude of the depolarization of the terminal that is evoked by the arriving impulse, with greater release following greater depolarization. In the spinal cord dorsal horn, the terminals of primary afferent axons not only form synapses on other neurons, they also receive synapses (so-called presynaptic synapses) on themselves from inhibitory interneurons (it is probable that the latter are distinct from the inhibitory interneurons that mediate postsynaptic inhibition). Activity at the synapse that is on the terminal causes depolarization. If an impulse from the terminal's own axon arrives while the terminal is already depolarized, the magnitude of the depolarization caused by the arriving impulse will be reduced, and hence the amount of neurotransmitter released will be reduced, as will the postsynaptic effect evoked subsequent to that impulse.

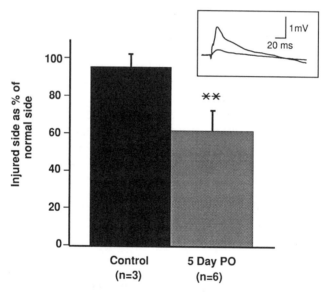

FIG. 26.2. Maximum dorsal root potentials (DRPs) recorded from control rats (unoperated) and rats with unilateral painful neuropathy at 5 days postoperatively (5 Day PO) in response to a maximal ipsilateral A-fiber volley. For the control animals, the maximum DRP magnitude from the left side is expressed as a percentage of that from the right side; the deviation from 100% represents the normal side-to-side variability. For the nerve-injured rats (5 Day PO), the maximum DRP on the injured side is significantly smaller ($p<0.01$). The DRPs were recorded from the L4 dorsal root, which was sectioned distally (i.e., passive DRP). The input volley was recorded from the distal portion of the severed L4 root and initiated by bipolar stimulating electrodes on the sciatic nerve, about 1 cm proximal to the constriction injury in the nerve-injured case and at a comparable location in the control case. Inset: DRPs evoked by maximal ipsilateral A-fiber volleys (upper trace: normal side; lower trace: nerve-injured side) from a rat at 5 days postinjury. (Data from ref. 8.)

Thus, PAD results in presynaptic inhibition, a process that constantly modulates the activity evoked in the spinal cord by primary afferent input. A reduction in presynaptic inhibition will lead to greater than normal primary–afferent-evoked postsynaptic depolarization, in other words, central hyperexcitability due to disinhibition. Synchronous PAD in large numbers of primary afferents can be recorded as a passive wave of depolarization that spreads from the primary afferent terminals, up the intraspinal portion of their axons, and out into the portion of the axons in the dorsal root (the dorsal root potential, DRP).

As shown in Figs. 26.2 and 26.3, presynaptic inhibition, as inferred from the magnitude of the DRP, is significantly reduced in rats with the experimental painful neuropathy as early as 5 days after the injury (8). This reduction is demonstrated in two ways. First, as shown in Fig. 26.2, when one side of the rat is compared to its other side, the largest DRP that can be evoked by a maximal, ipsilateral A-fiber input volley is smaller on the side of the neuropathy (and this is true whether the DRP magnitude is quantified as peak amplitude or area under the curve). Second, as shown in Fig. 26.3, a similar side-to-side comparison using ipsilateral A-fiber volleys of graded intensity shows that the DRP on the neuropathy side is always smaller for any given input volley. The DRP abnormality indicates that there is a deficit of presynaptic inhibition ipsilateral to the neuropathy. This finding is consistent with the hypothesis that at least some dark neurons are inhibitory interneurons whose functional impairment results in a reduction in the inhibitory processes that normally regulate the spinal cord's pain-processing circuitry.

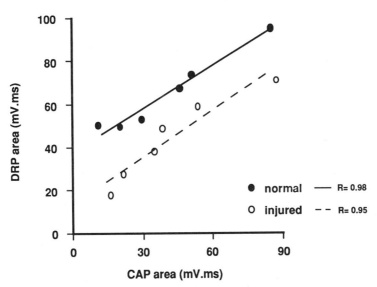

FIG. 26.3. The effects of ipsilateral A-fiber input volleys of increasing intensity (ranging from about 25% to 100% of the maximum) on the magnitude of the dorsal root potential (DRP) recorded on the same side. Normal side (sham-operated control) and the injured side (chronic constriction injury) in a rat at 5 days postinjury. The magnitudes of the input volley (CAP, compound action potential) and DRP are expressed in arbitrary units (millivolt × milliseconds, mV.ms) denoting the areas under the respective curves. The regression coefficients (R) show that the data from both sides are described satisfactorily by linear functions. (Data from ref. 8.)

CONCLUSIONS

If our hypothesis is correct, then we see that spontaneous discharge in damaged (and, perhaps, sensitized) primary afferents is doubly deleterious: it gives rise to painful and/or dysesthetic sensations and contributes to a transsynaptic, excitotoxic injury process in the spinal cord dorsal horn that leads to central hyperexcitability. If this is true, then blockade of the NMDA receptor ought to reduce or eliminate neuropathic hyperalgesia and prevent the appearance of dark neurons. The second half of this prediction has not been tested yet, but it has been shown that MK-801, an NMDA-receptor blocker, prevents neuropathic hyperalgesia in the chronic constriction model when it is given for the first few days postinjury (4). NMDA-receptor antagonists are being developed by several pharmaceutical companies, and one can hope that these drugs will be useful, therapeutically and prophylactically, for those suffering from neuropathic pain; animal data already indicate that such drugs will be useful for the control of the hyperalgesia that ordinarily follows trauma and surgery.

REFERENCES

1. Attal, N., Jazat, F., Kayser, V., and Guilbaud, G. (1990): Further evidence for "pain-related" behaviors in a model of unilateral peripheral mononeuropathy. *Pain,* 41:235–251.
2. Bennett, G. J. (1991): Evidence from animal models on the pathogenesis of painful peripheral neuropathy: relevance for pharmacotherapy. In: *Towards a new pharmacotherapy of pain,* edited by A. I. Basbaum and J.-M. Besson, pp. 365–379. John Wiley and Sons, Chichester.
3. Bennett, G. J., and Xie, Y.-K. (1988): A peripheral mononeuropathy in rat that produces disorders of pain sensation like those seen in man. *Pain,* 33:87–107.
4. Davar, G., and Maciewicz, R. (1988): MK-801 blocks thermal hyperalgesia in a rat model of neuropathic pain. *Soc. Neurosci. Abstr.,* 15:472.
5. Dubner, R. (1991): Neuronal plasticity and pain following peripheral tissue inflammation or nerve injury. In: *Proceedings of the VIth World Congress on Pain,* edited by M. R. Bond, J. E. Charlton, and C. J. Woolf, pp. 263–276. Elsevier, Amsterdam.
6. Kajander, K. C., and Bennett, G. J. (1988): Analysis of the activity of primary afferent neurons in a model of neuropathic pain in the rat. *Soc. Neurosci. Abstr.,* 14:912.
7. Kajander, K. C., Wakisaka, S., and Bennett, G. J. (1989): Early ectopic discharges are generated at the dorsal root ganglion in rats with a painful peripheral neuropathy. *Soc. Neurosci. Abstr.,* 15:816.
8. Laird, J. M. A., and Bennett, G. J. Dorsal root potentials and afferent input to the spinal cord in a rat model of experimental peripheral neuropathy (*submitted*).
9. Rotham, S. M., and Olney, J. W. (1987): Excitotoxicity and the NMDA receptor. *Trends Neurosci.,* 10:299–302.
10. Sugimoto, T., Bennett, G. J., and Kajander, K. C. (1989): Strychnine-enhanced transsynaptic degeneration of dorsal horn neurons in rats with an experimental painful peripheral neuropathy. *Neurosci. Lett.,* 98:139–143.
11. Sugimoto, T., Bennett, G. J., and Kajander, K. C. (1990): Transsynaptic degeneration in the superficial dorsal horn after sciatic nerve injury: effects of a chronic constriction injury, transection, and strychnine. *Pain,* 42:205–213.
12. Sugimoto, T., Takemura, M., Sakai, A., and Ishimaru, M. (1987): Strychnine-enhanced transsynaptic destruction of medullary dorsal horn neurons following transection of the trigeminal nerve in adult rats including evidence of involvement of the bony environment of transection neuroma in the peripheral mechanism. *Arch. Oral Biol.,* 32:623–629.
13. Sugimoto, T., Takemura, M., Sakai, A., and Ishimaru, M. (1987): Rapid transneuronal destruction following peripheral nerve transection in the medullary dorsal horn is enhanced by strychnine, picrotoxin and bicuculline. *Pain,* 30:385–393.
14. Woolf, C. J., and Thompson, S. W. N. (1991): The induction and maintenance of central sensitization is dependent on N-methyl-D-aspartic acid receptor activation: implications for the treatment of post-injury pain hypersensitivity states. *Pain,* 44:293–300.
15. Xie, Y.-K., and Xiao, W.-H. (1990): Electrophysiological evidence for hyperalgesia in the peripheral neuropathy. *Sci. China [B],* 33:663–672.

Hyperalgesia and Allodynia,
edited by W. D. Willis, Jr.
Published by Raven Press, Ltd.,
New York, 1992.

27

Molecular and Biochemical Events Mediate Neuronal Plasticity Following Inflammation and Hyperalgesia

Mary Ann Ruda and Ronald Dubner

*Neurobiology and Anesthesiology Branch, National Institute of Dental Research,
National Institutes of Health, Bethesda, Maryland 20892*

The increase in responsiveness to stimulation at sites of peripheral tissue damage produced by traumatic injury, infection, or surgery is commonly referred to as hyperalgesia and is characterized by an increase in sensitivity to suprathreshold noxious stimuli and a lowered threshold to pain. The pain can persist for long periods of time and may outlast the duration of the acute inflammatory process. The pathophysiological mechanisms underlying inflammation and hyperalgesia are not completely understood. Peripheral mechanisms such as sensitization of nociceptors appear to play a role, but recent evidence indicates that altered central nervous system processing or neuronal plasticity in the spinal dorsal horn and elsewhere contributes to the pathophysiology. This central hyperexcitability appears to involve the three major classes of chemical mediators participating in nociceptive processing: neuropeptides including the opioid peptides dynorphin and enkephalin, excitatory amino acids, and monoamines. This chapter presents evidence on the role of some of these chemical mediators in spinal dorsal horn hyperexcitability produced by inflammation. We can view the whole process as a model of activity-dependent plasticity in which alterations in gene expression and neural function are evoked by afferent input relevant to the survival of the organism. The findings have more general implications, since it is likely that similar mechanisms of neuronal plasticity occur in development and learning (21).

CORRELATION OF BEHAVIORAL HYPERALGESIA AND SPINAL DORSAL HORN HYPEREXCITABILITY

The injection of complete Freund's adjuvant (CFA), carrageenan, or other irritative chemicals into the rat's hindpaw can produce an intense inflammation characterized by erythema, edema, and hyperalgesia limited to the injected paw (25,34). We assess the hyperalgesia by exposing the rat's hindpaw to a radiant heat stimulus and measure the paw withdrawal latency. The reduction in paw withdrawal latency as compared to the control hindpaw is used as a measure of hyperalgesia. Other measures of integrative behavior involving supraspinal processing, such as duration of paw withdrawal and paw licking behavior, are highly correlated with the paw withdrawal latency. Using this model, we find that the hyperalgesia peaks within 2 to 6 hr and can persist for 5 to 10 days. There is no change in the paw withdrawal latency of the contralateral foot as compared to control animals, indicating that the noninjected paw can be used as a control.

The response properties of projection neurons in lamina I of the superficial dorsal horn of the anesthetized rat have been studied during these same time periods following the administration of CFA (30). Most of the neurons in dorsal horn lamina I of the rat respond exclusively to noxious stimulation. The projection neurons in lamina I travel via the dorsolateral funiculus to the midbrain or thalamus, or both (29,68). Five days after the administration of CFA, many of these neurons exhibit an enlargement of their receptive fields and may have discontinuous fields in response to noxious stimulation. Some of the receptive fields included the entire surface of the foot. The receptive fields from the inflamed paws were on the average 2.4 times larger than the receptive fields of control animals. There also was a significant increase in the number of cells exhibiting spontaneous activity as compared to control animals (87% to 24%). Other studies, in addition, have reported decreased thresholds of dorsal horn neurons to mechanical stimulation following inflammation and injury (6,46,74).

When the response properties of these neurons are studied between 4 and 8.5 hr after CFA administration, changes in receptive field size parallel the time course of development of the hyperalgesia (30). Neurons studied early in this time period (less than 6 hr) have receptive fields that resemble those in control animals. In the 6- to 8.5-hr period, the receptive fields are enlarged and resemble lamina I neurons in the 5-day CFA-injected animals. A few neurons were observed for 2 hr beginning approximately 5 hr after CFA injection (Fig. 27.1). The receptive fields first included a few of the digits as in control animals, but with time, the fields enlarged and included almost the entire surface of the foot.

The finding that inflammatory agents or repeated tissue injury leads to expansion of receptive fields of spinal dorsal horn neurons has also been reported by others (26,44–46,74). How does the expansion of the receptive fields of nociceptive neurons lead to hyperalgesia? One hypothesis (18) is that expanded receptive fields will result in greater overlap of receptive fields and, therefore, will lead to a greater number of neurons activated by a stimulus applied to a hyperalgesic zone than the same stimulus applied to a normal zone. The increase in neuronal activity may ultimately be perceived as more intense pain.

These receptive field changes could represent altered processing in the peripheral or central nervous system, or both. Hylden et al. (30) tested whether the observed increase in receptive field size could be explained by sensitization of peripheral nociceptors or by physical changes in the edematous paw. The possible effects of physical changes leading to mechanical deformation of tissue at a distance from the site of stimulation were ruled out by showing that the enlarged fields were sensitive to electrical and noxious heat stimuli. Electrical stimulation proximal to the receptor region ruled out a role for sensitized nociceptors. In addition, peripheral nociceptors did not show expanded receptive fields. The effects of central summation of activity from spontaneously active, sensitized nociceptors, possibly leading to threshold input at previously ineffective synapses, were tested by locally anesthetizing most of the receptive fields. There was no change in the response to electrical, mechanical, or thermal stimuli following local anesthesia. Thus, the expansion of the receptive fields of dorsal horn lamina I neurons following inflammation likely involves altered

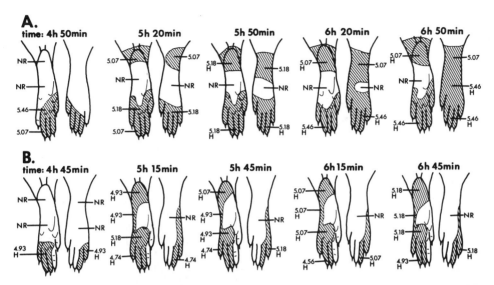

FIG. 27.1. The receptive field properties of two lamina I neurons (**A** and **B**) were observed for over 2 hr (from approximately 5–7 hr after CFA). Each pair of sketches of the hindpaw represents a dorsal (right) and ventral (left) view of the injected hindpaw. The apparent receptive field to mechanical and thermal stimuli at each time point is shaded. Mechanical thresholds were determined with von Frey filaments and are indicated by the numbers near the shaded regions [values expressed as $\log_{10}(10 \times$ force in mg)]. H, response to radiant heat; NR, no response. (From ref. 30.)

processing in the dorsal horn itself and may provide a mechanism for the behavioral hyperalgesia observed in the animals.

CORRELATION OF OPIOID PEPTIDE SYNTHESIS AND GENE EXPRESSION WITH BEHAVIORAL HYPERALGESIA

Unilateral peripheral inflammation results in an increase in the spinal dorsal horn levels of mRNA coding for dynorphin peptide precursor proteins. RNA blot analysis using a cDNA probe reveals an inflammation-induced increase in preprodynorphin mRNA as early as 4 hr (Fig. 27.2), with the peak, eightfold increase occurring between 2 and 5 days and returning to control levels by 10 to 14 days (16,34,35). The changes in dynorphin gene expression parallel the changes in behavioral hyperalgesia induced by CFA and other inflammatory agents (16,34). An increase in dynorphin peptide [dynorphin A(1–8)] content occurs later; it is apparent by 2 days and a threefold increase can be found by 4 days after the induction of inflammation (34,48). An increase in preproenkephalin mRNA is also induced by inflammation, but the elevation is only about 50% above control levels (35). The changes in preprodynorphin and preproenkephalin mRNA levels and dynorphin peptide levels are segmentally specific and only occur in that part of the spinal cord dorsal horn receiving input from the inflamed hindpaw. The contralateral, noninjected side is the same as control animals and serves as an appropriate control.

Using *in situ* hybridization histochemistry, the neurons showing increases in preprodynorphin mRNA can be localized autoradiographically with a synthetic oligo-

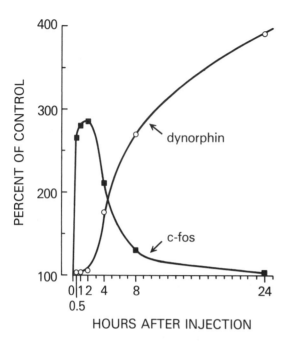

FIG. 27.2. Quantification of increases in rat c-*fos* mRNA and preprodynorphin mRNA. The curves are the average of two separate RNA blots performed after the administration of carrageenan. The blots were reprobed with beta-actin, which codes for a structural protein that does not change with inflammation and is used to standardize the amount of RNA applied to each lane of the blot. The ordinate, therefore, is the ratio of c-*fos* or preprodynorphin mRNA levels to that of beta-actin using densitometric analyses. (From ref. 16.)

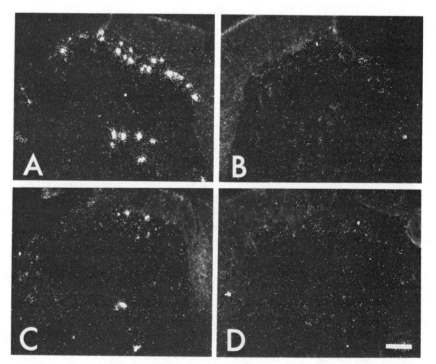

FIG. 27.3. Dark-field photomicrographs of the rat lumbar dorsal horn in control (**A** and **B**) and capsaicin-treated (**C** and **D**) animals at 4 days after CFA-induced inflammation. A and C indicate the inflamed sides and B and D the control sides. Tissue is labeled by *in situ* hybridization histochemistry using an ^{35}S-labeled preprodynorphin oligonucleotide probe. Scale bar = 100 μm. (From ref. 33.)

nucleotide probe to a partial sequence of the preprodynorphin gene (58). Figure 27.3 shows the high density of silver grains overlying neurons in the dorsal horn on the experimental side (Fig. 27.3A) as compared to the uninjected side (Fig. 27.3B), 4 days after a CFA injection into the hindpaw. There is an increase in the number of cells (approximately a threefold increase) with a higher intensity of labeling on the experimental as compared to the control side. The increase in labeling is concentrated in the medial part of the superficial laminae of the dorsal horn, the area that receives innervation from the inflamed hindpaw. Neurons in the neck of the dorsal horn (laminae V and VI) also exhibited increases in preprodynorphin mRNA (compare Fig. 27.3A and B). An increase in neuronal labeling for immunoreactive dynorphin peptide was observed ipsilateral to the inflammation in the same regions of the superficial layers and neck of the dorsal horn (58). Therefore, the neurons that undergo an increase in preprodynorphin mRNA and dynorphin peptide levels are located in the two regions of the dorsal horn that contain projection neurons as well as local circuit neurons and convey nociceptive information. The dynorphin neurons in the superficial dorsal horn are both local circuit neurons and projection neurons (50). Recent studies have shown that dynorphin immunoreactivity is released into the superficial dorsal horn following high-frequency activation of unmyelinated primary afferent fibers (28). Dynorphin immunoreactive neurons receive direct monosynaptic input from unmyelinated afferents (69). It should be noted that the increased expression and release of dynorphin peptide occur in the same superficial zone where neurons with expanded receptive fields were induced by CFA injection.

MOLECULAR MECHANISMS THAT REGULATE DYNORPHIN GENE TRANSCRIPTION FOLLOWING INFLAMMATION

Cellular immediate-early genes code for protein products that act as transcription factors. They bind to DNA or to DNA binding proteins in the promotor region of target genes and are thought to regulate initial genetic events leading to prolonged functional changes in the nervous system (10,49,60). C-*fos* codes for one such nuclear phosphoprotein and is the cellular homolog of the viral oncogene, v-*fos,* the transforming gene of mouse osteogenic sarcoma viruses (11). RNA blot analysis using a c-*fos* cDNA probe shows that the content of c-*fos* mRNA increases within 30 min after injection of an inflammatory agent into the rat hindpaw (16) (Fig. 27.2). There was a peak elevation at 2 hr, a decrease to one-half maximal levels by 4 hr, and nearly complete recovery to control levels by 8 hr after injection. Several studies have described the activation of the proto-oncogene c-*fos* in the spinal cord by examining tissue sections for the distribution of Fos protein-like and Fos-related protein-like immunoreactivity (Fos-IR) (4,5,27,47,53–56,70,72,73). There is a rapid and robust elevation in the number of neurons that express Fos-IR in their nuclei in the dorsal horn following activation of nociceptive primary afferents with electrical or chemical stimulation or following inflammation. Figure 27.4 shows the laminar distribution of Fos-IR in nuclei in spinal neurons 3 days after CFA-induced inflammation. The most numerous Fos-IR nuclei were found in the superficial laminae (I and II) and in the neck of the dorsal horn (V–VI) ipsilateral to the affected limb (54). Thus, neurons exhibiting Fos-IR had a distribution similar to the neurons exhibiting preprodynorphin mRNA increased labeling on the side receiving input from the inflamed hindpaw.

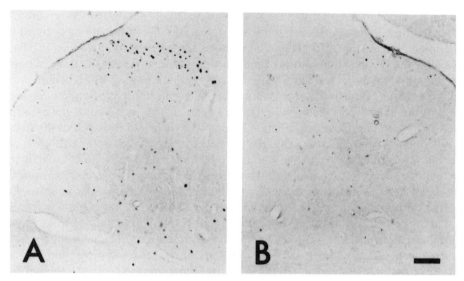

FIG. 27.4. Fos-IR neurons in the lumbar spinal cord ipsilateral (**A**) and contralateral (**B**) to carrageenan-induced inflammation at day 3. The immunocytochemical reaction product, which indicates the presence of Fos protein, is limited to the nucleus of the cells. The most densely labeled cells are concentrated in the superficial laminae and the neck of the dorsal horn. Note the few nuclei labeled on the contralateral side. Scale bar = 100 μm. (From ref. 54.)

The colocalization of Fos-IR and preprodynorphin mRNA in dorsal horn neurons has been demonstrated by double-labeling neurons with anti-Fos antibody and a dynorphin synthetic oligonucleotide probe (51,54). Double-labeled neurons exhibited an aggregation of silver grains overlying the cell body, indicating the presence of preprodynorphin mRNA, and a brown chromagen in the nucleus, indicating Fos-IR (Fig. 27.5). Double-labeling was found in both the superficial laminae and in the neck of the dorsal horn on the side receiving input from the inflamed hindpaw (54). Very few double-labeled neurons were found on the side contralateral to the inflamed hindpaw. Over 80% of the neurons in the superficial laminae and neck of the dorsal horn expressing preprodynorphin mRNA colocalized Fos-IR, although the number of neurons expressing Fos-IR was substantially greater than the subpopulation of double-labeled neurons. Unilateral inflammation also resulted in increased levels of preproenkephalin mRNA colocalized with Fos-IR. Over 80% of neurons in the superficial laminae and the neck of the dorsal horn exhibiting preproenkephalin mRNA labeling also colocalized Fos-IR (53). However, the two opioid genes appear to be differentially regulated following noxious stimulation since increases in preproenkephalin mRNA transcripts were slight in comparison to the dramatic increase in preprodynorphin transcripts. The high percentage of dynorphin and enkephalin gene expression colocalized with Fos and Fos-related proteins suggests that Fos-phosphoprotein signaling may be coupled to dynorphin and enkephalin gene transcription. Fos protein is thought to bind cooperatively with Jun protein at an AP-1 DNA recognition site in the promotor region of target genes and subsequently to affect transcriptional control (10,49,60). Recently, an AP–1-like binding site in the promotor region of the rat preprodynorphin gene has been shown to bind Fos and Jun protein and to induce dynorphin gene transcription (51). However, several immedi-

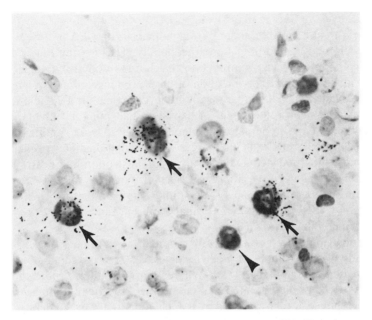

FIG. 27.5. Neurons in the superficial dorsal horn that colocalize Fos-IR and preprodynorphin mRNA. *Arrows* indicate the double-labeled neurons that show reaction product for Fos-IR in the cell nucleus and silver grains from the *in situ* hybridization autoradiography reaction over-lying the cytoplasm of the cells. Arrowhead indicates a neuron single-labeled for Fos-IR. The cells have been lightly counterstained with cresyl violet. (From ref. 54.)

ate-early genes have now been identified, and there appears to be a convergence of signal transduction pathways in the nucleus of neurons leading to the regulation of target genes (10,49,60,73). The interaction of different transcription factors and DNA recognition elements in the promotor region indicates that one or more factors may be rate limiting in the regulation of genes whose protein products are associated with neuronal plasticity in response to peripheral tissue injury.

SYNAPTIC PROCESSES THAT INITIATE INCREASES IN DYNORPHIN PEPTIDE BIOSYNTHESIS

The role of different classes of nociceptive afferents in the events leading to Fos protein and dynorphin peptide expression following inflammation can be examined by destroying subpopulations of primary afferent fibers. Capsaicin is a neurotoxin that, when administered neonatally to rats, destroys almost all the unmyelinated primary afferent fibers, most of which are nociceptive afferents. In addition, the content of several neuropeptides, including substance P (SP) and calcitonin gene-related peptide (CGRP) in the dorsal root ganglia and spinal dorsal horn are reduced (23,24,62). Within 1 hr after administration, capsaicin produces an increase in the expression of mRNA coding for SP and CGRP in the dorsal root ganglia. However, 2 weeks after capsaicin administration, there are few SP-containing neurons and a reduced number of CGRP neurons remaining in the dorsal root ganglion. Six to eight weeks after capsaicin, there is still no detectable recovery of SP or CGRP.

Based on the above finding that SP and CGRP have not recovered by 6 to 8 weeks after capsaicin treatment, inflammation was induced with CFA in 8-week-old rats in which capsaicin had been administered neonatally. The distribution of Fos-IR and preprodynorphin mRNA was compared to that found in control animals with CFA-induced inflammation (33). The injection of CFA produced edema and decreases in paw withdrawal latencies of similar magnitude in capsaicin- and vehicle-treated rats, indicating that the neurotoxic effect of capsaicin had minimal effects on CFA-induced inflammation and hyperalgesia. In contrast, there were significant decreases in immunoreactive SP terminals in all areas where small-diameter primary afferents terminate, suggesting that neonatal capsaicin administration had destroyed most of the small-diameter nociceptive afferents. Further evidence that SP-containing primary afferent fibers are lost comes from studies showing that those afferents colocalizing SP and CGRP (found only in primary afferent fibers) are destroyed by neonatal capsaicin administration (63).

When the distribution of Fos-IR was examined in capsaicin-treated rats with an inflamed hindpaw, the number of labeled nuclei was greatly reduced in comparison to vehicle-treated animals (Fig. 27.6). Whereas inflammation produced a rapid increase in Fos-IR in vehicle-treated animals in the superficial laminae within 2 hr, with a peak response at 6 hr followed by a delayed increase in the deeper laminae at 24 hr, no such pattern emerged in the capsaicin-treated animals. Only transient and

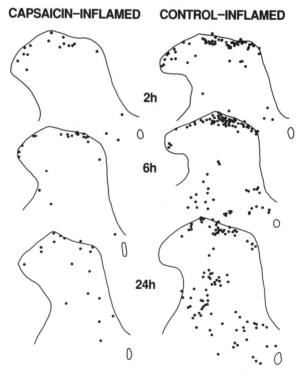

CAPSAICIN–INFLAMED   CONTROL–INFLAMED

2h

6h

24h

FIG. 27.6. Camera lucida drawings of tissue sections from the lumbar spinal cord of capsaicin- and vehicle-treated rats showing the distribution of Fos-IR nuclei on the CFA-injected side at 2, 6, and 24 hr. Each drawing shows the nuclei labeled in one 24-μm section. (From ref. 33.)

slight increases were observed. Similarly, *in situ* hybridization histochemistry revealed that the number of neurons exhibiting preprodynorphin mRNA expression was reduced by over 80% in the superficial laminae and by 50% in the neck of the dorsal horn, in capsaicin-treated as compared to vehicle-treated rats (Fig. 27.3C and D). It appears that Fos protein and dynorphin gene expression are both dependent on input from capsaicin-sensitive primary afferents. The concomitant loss of SP- and CGRP-containing primary afferents in these animals suggests that these neuropeptides participate in the initiation of synaptic events that lead to Fos protein and dynorphin gene expression. The direct input of CGRP terminals onto dynorphin-containing neurons has already been demonstrated (69). We conclude that the increased activity of unmyelinated primary nociceptive afferents induced by inflammation is primarily, but not exclusively, responsible for activation of the cellular immediate-early gene c-*fos* and the ultimate regulation of its protein product on target gene transcription.

EFFECT OF DYNORPHIN OR KAPPA-OPIOID RECEPTOR AGONISTS ON THE RECEPTIVE FIELD SIZE OF SUPERFICIAL DORSAL HORN NEURONS

Evidence has been presented above that both the observed changes in receptive field size of superficial dorsal horn neurons and the alterations in dynorphin gene expression were closely correlated with the development of behavioral hyperalgesia. These findings led us to test whether the receptive field size changes and the increase in dynorphin peptide levels were related. The effects of spinally administered dynorphin, or a nonpeptidergic kappa-opioid agonist (U-50,488H), on the receptive fields and other response properties of superficial dorsal horn neurons in rats without inflammation were examined (31).

Neuronal activity was recorded from 15 superficial dorsal horn neurons before and after the application of dynorphin to the surface of the spinal cord (50 nmol dose). In five of these cells there was an expansion of the receptive field using mechanical stimulation onto an adjacent toe or the footpad at 5 min after dynorphin treatment (Fig. 27.7A). The average increase in receptive field size was about 50%. A separate group of 23 cells was examined after administration of the active isomer of the kappa-opioid receptor agonist U-50,488H. Eight of these cells exhibited an average expansion of their receptive fields of about 30%, 5 to 10 min after spinal administration (0.19 to 1.9 μmol) (Fig. 27.7B). One cell showed a decrease in receptive field size. After the administration of U50,488H, there also were changes in the responsiveness of cells to mechanical and thermal stimuli. Eight cells exhibited enhanced responses to mechanical stimuli (five of them also had expanded receptive fields), whereas four exhibited a suppression of activity. Nine cells demonstrated a facilitation of their heat-evoked response, but five of them exhibited suppression of activity at higher doses. Seven other cells only exhibited suppression of the thermal response.

These results suggest that dynorphin and kappa-opioid agonists have dual effects in the spinal dorsal horn. They result in expanded receptive fields of some neurons accompanied often by increased sensitivity to mechanical and thermal stimuli; in other neurons there is a suppression of responsiveness to mechanical and thermal stimuli that often occurs at higher doses. Other studies have also reported facilitation or inhibition of dorsal horn neuronal activity after the administration of kappa-opioid

A DYNORPHIN

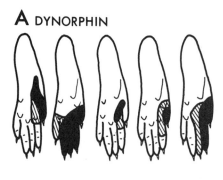

B U-50,488H

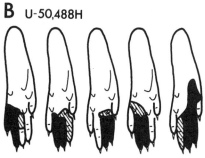

FIG. 27.7. Receptive fields of superficial dorsal horn neurons before and after the spinal administration of dynorphin (**A**) or U-50,488H (**B**). *Filled areas* represent apparent receptive fields prior to drug injection and *shaded areas* indicate the maximum extent of the expanded portion of the receptive field after drug injection. (From ref. 31.)

agonists (7,43). The two types of responses may represent activation of two functionally different populations of neurons, or, alternatively, the two responses may reflect interaction of the agonists at more than one receptor type. The observed effects of U-50,488H were not reversed by naloxone, suggesting that the effects may have not been mediated by classical opioid receptors or that the large doses used could not be sufficiently displaced by postadministration of the antagonist. Alternatively, Caudle and Isaac (7) suggest that dynorphin-induced potentiation and the subsequent loss of C-fiber reflexes involve excitotoxicity mediated at *N*-methyl-D-aspartate (NMDA) receptor sites and ultimately leads to cell dysfunction (see below). Administration of opioid antagonists after the initiation of such a mechanism would have little or no effect.

SELECTIVE OPIOID RECEPTOR AGONISTS EXHIBIT ENHANCED ANALGESIC EFFECTS FOLLOWING INFLAMMATION AND HYPERALGESIA THAT MAY BE DEPENDENT ON SPINAL ADRENERGIC MECHANISMS

Unilateral inflammation and polyarthritis in rats result in enhanced analgesic effects to systemically administered opioid agonists (36,40,41,52,64–66). These effects in animal models of peripheral inflammation have been attributed to a pharmacological action at receptor sites within inflamed tissue (37,64). However, using the carrageenan model of inflammation and thermal hyperalgesia, it recently has been shown that an increase in sensitivity to opioid agonists and alpha-2 adrenergic agonists takes place at the spinal level (32). Such enhanced sensitivity suggests that spinal cord neuronal plasticity following inflammation may involve biochemical alterations at the receptor level with possible changes in receptor affinity or in receptor upregulation.

The mu-selective opioid agonist DAMGO and the delta-selective opioid agonist DPDPE were administered intrathecally to rats at the peak of their response to carrageenan-induced inflammation and hyperalgesia (32). DAMGO had little effect on the paw withdrawal latency of noninflamed paws at doses less than 1 μg. However, the inflamed paws of these same rats exhibited a dose-dependent increase in paw withdrawal latency at doses as low as 33 ng. Subcutaneous injections of DAMGO in this dose range did not attenuate the hyperalgesia of the inflamed paws. Thus, the attenuation of hyperalgesia produced by DAMGO was due to a local action at the level of the spinal cord and could not be attributed to a systemic or peripheral effect. The intrathecal administration of DPDPE also revealed a dose-dependent increase in paw withdrawal latency of inflamed paws at low doses (5–50 μg) but did not have any effect on noninflamed paws. Intrathecally administered clonidine (1–10 μg) also produced dose-related attenuation of the hyperalgesia of inflamed paws but was ineffective in this dose range on noninflamed paws.

The opioid antagonist naloxone and the alpha-2 adrenergic antagonist idazoxan were tested for their ability to reverse agonist-induced attenuation of hyperalgesia. Intrathecally administered naloxone and idazoxan blocked the effect of intrathecal morphine (5 μg) on both inflamed and noninflamed paws. The effects of clonidine in attenuating the hyperalgesia of inflamed paws were blocked by idazoxan but not by naloxone.

These experiments indicate that both mu- and delta-opioid agonists and alpha-2 adrenergic agonists exhibit supersensitivity following inflammation. The ability of an alpha-2 adrenergic antagonist to block opioid attenuation of hyperalgesia suggests that the enhanced opioid effect may be dependent on spinal adrenergic mechanisms.

NMDA RECEPTOR ACTIVATION AND NEURONAL PLASTICITY IN THE SPINAL DORSAL HORN

Excitatory amino acids such as glutamate and aspartate act at NMDA receptor sites and participate in the activation of dorsal horn nociceptive neurons (1,14, 15,42,59,61,71). The phenomenon of "windup" (increased responsiveness of dorsal horn nociceptive neurons with frequency-dependent stimulation) is prevented by the administration of NMDA antagonists (12,13). The hyperexcitability of dorsal horn nociceptive neurons produced by formalin is also blocked by NMDA antagonists (22). In addition, the hypersensitivity of the rat flexion reflex following electrical stimulation or chemical stimulation with mustard oil is also blocked or eliminated by the administration of either competitive or noncompetitive NMDA antagonists (75). The hypersensitivity of the flexion reflex likely is a measure of dorsal horn hyperexcitability since the effects parallel changes produced in dorsal horn neurons by electrical stimulation or by mustard oil (9,74). Finally, the expanded receptive fields of neurons in the superficial laminae or the neck of the dorsal horn following inflammation and hyperalgesia also can be reduced by the administration of an NMDA antagonist (57). It appears, then, that dorsal horn neuronal plasticity and hyperexcitability following tissue injury involve the release of excitatory amino acids and their effects at NMDA receptor sites. The findings suggest that NMDA antagonists may have potential utility as analgesics (19,75).

The release of excitatory amino acids in the spinal dorsal horn is enhanced by neuropeptides such as SP and CGRP. Glutamate and SP coexist in some primary afferent terminals in the superficial dorsal horn (2). SP and CGRP also potentiate the dorsal root stimulation-evoked release of glutamate and aspartate from spinal cord *in vitro* preparations (39). The corelease of excitatory amino acids and neuropeptides potentiates the depolarization of dorsal horn neurons. SP has been found to enhance the responses of spinothalamic tract neurons in the monkey to NMDA, and these responses are blocked by an NMDA antagonist (15). These effects may be important in the strengthening of synaptic connections in the spinal cord and likely participate in the long-lasting hyperexcitability found following inflammation and hyperalgesia.

A PROPOSED MODEL OF DORSAL HORN MECHANISMS OF HYPEREXCITABILITY THAT LEADS TO BEHAVIORAL HYPERALGESIA

We have shown that there is a large increase in dynorphin gene expression and dynorphin peptide levels in the spinal cord associated with peripheral inflammation and hyperalgesia. Other studies have shown increases in dynorphin expression following partial nerve damage (17,38), total peripheral nerve transection (8), or spinal cord injury (20). It has been postulated (18,31) that dynorphin levels are related to enhanced excitability and development of expanded receptive fields following various types of injury that affect spinal cord neuronal input. A model has been proposed in which increased nociceptive activity in the periphery (tissue damage or nerve injury) leads to excessive depolarization via excitation at NMDA receptor sites (18). Dynorphin and other neuropeptides such as SP and CGRP enhance this excitability via their facilitation of NMDA receptor agonist activity. The excessive depolarization promotes excitotoxicity and neuronal dysfunction, possibly leading to cell death (7). The model proposes that neurons most sensitive to this neurotoxicity are small local circuit neurons that likely are inhibitory. Recently, it has been found that small neurons in the superficial dorsal horn exhibit morphological changes following partial nerve injury (67). Abnormal function of such neurons could lead to a loss of inhibitory mechanisms in the spinal dorsal horn. This hypothesized sequence of events would have important consequences. The increased depolarization and loss of inhibitory mechanisms would contribute to the expansion of receptive fields and neuronal hyperexcitability, ultimately leading to behavioral hyperalgesia.

The findings presented above are also important because they suggest that pain is not a passive symptom but an aggressive one that produces central nervous system changes that underlie the pathophysiology leading to persistent pain. Such pain leads to changes in behavior, often with resulting depression and maladaptive personal relationships. John Bonica (3) was prophetic when he referred to chronic pain as a "malefic force" than can ruin a person's life. We now have strong evidence of the effect of excessive nociceptive input in the central nervous system and the need to eliminate or reduce such input as soon as possible.

REFERENCES

1. Aanonsen, L. M., Lei, S., and Wilcox, G. L. (1990): Excitatory amino acid receptors and nociceptive neurotransmission in rat spinal cord. *Pain*, 41:309–321.

2. Battaglia, G., and Rustioni, A. (1988): Co-existence of glutamate and substance P in dorsal root ganglion neurons of the rat and monkey. *J. Comp. Neurol.*, 277:302–312.
3. Bonica, J. J. (1990): Definitions and taxonomy of pain. *The management of pain*, 2nd ed., pp. 18–27. Lea and Febiger, Philadelphia.
4. Bullitt, E. (1989): Induction of c-*fos* protein within the lumbar spinal cord and thalamus of the rat following peripheral stimulation. *Brain Res.*, 493:391–397.
5. Bullitt, E. (1990): Expression of c-*fos*-like protein as a marker for neuronal activity following noxious stimulation in the rat. *J. Comp. Neurol.*, 296:517–530.
6. Calvino, B., Villanueva, L., and LeBars, D. (1987): Dorsal horn (convergent) neurons in the intact anaesthetized arthritic rat. I. Segmental excitatory influences. *Pain*, 28:81–98.
7. Caudle, R. M., and Isaac, L. (1988): Influence of dynorphin(1–13) on spinal reflexes in the rat. *J. Pharmacol. Exp. Ther.*, 246:508–513.
8. Cho, H. J., and Basbaum, A. I. (1988): Increased staining of immunoreactive dynorphin cell bodies in the deafferented spinal cord of the rat. *Neurosci. Lett.*, 84:125–130.
9. Cook, A. J., Woolf, C. J., Wall, P. D., and McMahon, S. B. (1987): Dynamic receptive field plasticity in rat spinal cord dorsal horn following C-primary afferent input. *Nature*, 325:151–153.
10. Curran, T., and Morgan, J. I. (1987): Memories of *fos*. *Bioessays*, 7:255–258.
11. Curran, T., and Teich, N. M. (1982): Candidate product of the FBJ murine osteosarcoma virus oncogene: characterization of a 55,000-dalton phosphoprotein. *J. Virol.*, 42:114–122.
12. Davies, S. N., and Lodge, D. (1987): Evidence for involvement of N-methylaspartate receptors in 'wind-up' of class 2 neurons in the dorsal horn of the rat. *Brain Res.*, 424:402–406.
13. Dickenson, A. H., and Sullivan, A. F. (1987): Evidence for a role of the NMDA receptor in the frequency dependent potentiation of deep dorsal horn neurons following C-fibre stimulation. *Neuropharmacology*, 26:1235–1238.
14. Dickenson, A. H., and Sullivan, A. F. (1990): Differential effects of excitatory amino-acid antagonists on dorsal horn nociceptive neurones in the rat. *Brain Res.*, 506:31–39.
15. Dougherty, P. M., and Willis, W. D. (1991): Enhancement of spinothalamic neuron responses to chemical and mechanical stimuli following combined microiontophoretic application of N-methyl-D-aspartic acid and substance P. *Pain*, 47:85–93.
16. Draisci, G., and Iadarola, M. J. (1989): Temporal analysis of increases in c-fos, preprodynorphin and preproenkephalin in mRNAs in rat spinal cord. *Mol. Brain Res.*, 6:31–37.
17. Draisci, G., Kajander, K. C., Dubner, R., Bennett, G. J., and Iadarola, M. J. (1991): Up-regulation of opioid gene expression in spinal cord evoked by experimental nerve injuries and inflammation. *Brain Res.*, 560:186–192.
18. Dubner, R. (1991): Neuronal plasticity and pain following peripheral tissue inflammation or nerve injury. In: *Proceedings of the VIth World Congress on Pain*, edited by M. R. Bond, J. E. Charlton, and C. J. Woolf, pp. 263–276. Elsevier, Amsterdam.
19. Dubner, R. (1991): Pain and hyperalgesia following tissue injury: new mechanisms and new treatments. *Pain*, 44:213–214.
20. Faden, A. I., Molineaux, C. J., Rosenberger, J. G., Jacobs, T. P., and Cox, B. M. (1985): Endogenous opioid immunoreactivity in rat spinal cord following traumatic injury. *Ann. Neurol.*, 17:386–390.
21. Goelet, P., Castellucci, V. F., Schacher, S., and Kandel, E. R. (1986): The long and short of long-term memory—a molecular framework. *Nature*, 322:419–422.
22. Haley, J. E., Sullivan, A. F., and Dickenson, A. H. (1990): Evidence for spinal N-methyl-D-aspartate receptor involvement in prolonged chemical nociception in the rat. *Brain Res.*, 518:218–226.
23. Hammond, D. L., and Ruda, M. A. (1989): Developmental alterations in thermal nociceptive threshold and the distribution of immunoreactive calcitonin gene-related peptide and substance P after neonatal administration of capsaicin in the rat. *Neurosci. Lett.*, 97:57–62.
24. Hammond, D. L., and Ruda, M. A. (1991): Developmental alterations in the distribution of immunoreactive calcitonin gene-related peptide, substance P and fluoride-resistant acid phosphatase in the spinal cord of the rat after neonatal administration of capsaicin: relationship to nociceptive threshold. *J. Comp. Neurol.*, 312:436–450.
25. Hargreaves, K., Dubner, R., Brown, F., Flores, C., and Joris, J. (1988): A new and sensitive method for measuring thermal nociception in cutaneous hyperalgesia. *Pain*, 32:77–88.
26. Hu, J. W., Sessle, B. J., Raboisson, P., Dallel, R., and Woda, A. (1992): Stimulation of craniofacial muscle afferents induces prolonged facilitatory effects in trigeminal nociceptive brainstem neurones. *Pain*, 48:53–60.
27. Hunt, S. P., Pini, A., and Evan, G. (1987): Induction of c-*fos*-like protein in spinal cord neurons following sensory stimulation. *Nature*, 328:632–634.
28. Hutchinson, W. D., Morton, C. R., and Terenius, L. (1990): Dynorphin A: in vivo release in the spinal cord of the cat. *Brain Res.*, 532:299–306.
29. Hylden, J. L. K., Anton, F., and Nahin, R. L. (1989): Spinal lamina I projection neurons in the rat: collateral innervation of parabrachial area and thalamus. *Neuroscience*, 28:27–37.

30. Hylden, J. L. K., Nahin, R. L., Traub, R. J., and Dubner, R. (1989): Expansion of receptive fields of spinal lamina I projection neurons in the rats with unilateral adjuvant-induced inflammation: the contribution of dorsal horn mechanisms. *Pain,* 37:229–243.

31. Hylden, J. L. K., Nahin, R. L., Traub, R. J., and Dubner, R. (1991): Effects of spinal kappa-opioid receptor agonists on the responsiveness of nociceptive superficial dorsal horn neurons. *Pain,* 44:187–193.

32. Hylden, J. L. K., Thomas, D. A., Iadarola, M. J., Nahin, R. L., and Dubner, R. (1991): Spinal opioid analgesia effects are enhanced in a model of unilateral inflammation/hyperalgesia: possible involvement of noradrenergic mechanisms. *Eur. J. Pharmacol.,* 194:135–143.

33. Hylden, J. L. K., Noguchi, K., and Ruda, M. A. Neonatal capsaicin treatment attenuates spinal *Fos* activation and dynorphin gene expression following peripheral tissue inflammation and hyperalgesia. *J. Neurosci. (in press).*

34. Iadarola, M. J., Brady, L. S., Draisci, G., and Dubner, R. (1988): Enhancement of dynorphin gene expression in spinal cord following experimental inflammation: stimulus specificity, behavioral parameters and opioid receptor binding. *Pain,* 35:313–326.

35. Iadarola, M. J., Douglass, J., Civelli, O., and Naranjo, J. R. (1988): Differential activation of spinal cord dynorphin and enkephalin neurons during hyperalgesia: evidence using cDNA hybridization. *Brain Res.,* 455:205–212.

36. Joris, J., Costello, A., Dubner, R., and Hargreaves, K. M. (1990): Opiates suppress carrageenan-induced edema and hyperthermia at doses that inhibit hyperalgesia. *Pain,* 43:95–103.

37. Joris, J.L., Dubner, R., and Hargreaves, K. M. (1987): Opioid analgesia at peripheral sites: a target for opioids released during stress and inflammation? *Anesth. Analg.,* 66:1277.

38. Kajander, K. C., Sahara, Y., Iadarola, M. J., and Bennett, G. J. (1990): Dynorphin increases in the dorsal spinal cord in rats with a painful peripheral neuropathy. *Peptides,* 11:719–728.

39. Kangrga, I., and Randic, M. (1990): Tachykinins and calcitonin gene-related peptide enhance release of endogenous glutamate and aspartate from the rat spinal cord dorsal horn slice. *J. Neurosci.,* 10:2026–2038.

40. Kayser, V., and Guilbaud, G. (1983): The analgesic effects of morphine, but not those of the enkephalinase inhibitor thiorphan, are enhanced in arthritic rats. *Brain Res.,* 267:131–138.

41. Kayser, V., Neil, A., and Guilbaud, G. (1986): Repeated low doses of morphine induce a rapid tolerance in arthritic rats but a potentiation of opiate analgesia in normal animals. *Brain Res.,* 383:392–396.

42. King, A. E., Thompson, S. W. N., Urban, L., and Woolf, C. J. (1988): An intracellular analysis of amino acid induced excitations of deep dorsal horn neurones in the rat spinal cord slice. *Neurosci. Lett.,* 89:286–292.

43. Knox, R. J., and Dickenson, A. H. (1987): Effects of selective and non-selective kappa-opioid receptor agonists on cutaneous C–fiber-evoked responses of rat dorsal horn neurones. *Brain Res.,* 415:21–29.

44. Laird, J. M. A., and Cervero, F. (1989): A comparative study of the changes in receptive-field properties of multireceptive and nocireceptive rat dorsal horn neurons following noxious mechanical stimulation. *J. Neurophysiol.,* 62:854–863.

45. McMahon, S. B., and Wall, P. D. (1984): Receptive fields of rat lamina I projection cells move to incorporate a nearby region of injury. *Pain,* 19:235–247.

46. Menétrey, D., and Besson, J.-M. (1982): Electrophysiological characteristics of dorsal horn cells in rats with cutaneous inflammation resulting from chronic arthritis. *Pain,* 13:343–364.

47. Menétrey, D., Gannon, A., Levine, J. D., and Basbaum, A. I. (1989): Expression of c-*fos* protein in interneurons and projection neurons of the rat spinal cord in response to noxious somatic, articular, and visceral stimulation. *J. Comp. Neurol.,* 285:177–195.

48. Millan, M. J., Czonkowski, A., Morris, B., et al. (1987): Inflammation of the hind limb as a model of unilateral, localized pain: influence on multiple opioid systems in the spinal cord of the rat. *Pain,* 35:299–312.

49. Morgan, J. I., and Curran, T. (1989): Stimulus-transcription coupling in neurons: role of cellular immediate-early genes. *Trends Neurosci.,* 12:459–462.

50. Nahin, R. L., Hylden, J. L. K., Iadarola, M. J., and Dubner, R. (1989): Peripheral inflammation is associated with increased dynorphin immunoreactivity in both projection and local circuit neurons in the superficial dorsal horn of the rat lumbar spinal cord. *Neurosci. Lett.,* 96:247–252.

51. Naranjo, J. R., Mellström, B., Achaval, M., and Sassone-Corsi, P. (1991): Molecular pathways of pain: fos/jun-mediated activation of a noncanonical AP-1 site in the prodynorphin gene. *Neuron,* 6:607–617.

52. Neil, A., Kayser, V., Gacel, G., Besson, J.-M., and Guilbaud, G. (1986): Opioid receptor types antinociceptive activity in chronic inflammation: both κ- and μ-opiate agonistic effects are enhanced in arthritic rats. *Eur. J. Pharmacol.,* 130:203–208.

53. Noguchi, K., Dubner, R., and Ruda, M. A. (1992): Preproenkephalin mRNA in spinal dorsal horn neurons is induced by peripheral inflammation and is colocalized with fos and fos-related proteins. *Neuroscience,* 46:561–570.

54. Noguchi, K., Kowalski, K., Traub, R., Solodkin, A., Iadarola, M. J., and Ruda, M. A. (1991): Colocalization of dynorphin and fos proteins in spinal cord neurons following inflammation induced hyperalgesia. *Mol. Brain Res.*, 10:227–233.
55. Noguchi, K., Morita, Y., Kiyama, H., Sato, M., Ono, K., and Tohyama, M. (1989): Preproenkephalin gene expression in the rat spinal cord after noxious stimuli. *Mol. Brain Res.*, 5:227–234.
56. Presley, R. W., Menétrey, D., Levine, J. D., and Basbaum, A. I. (1990): Systematic morphine suppresses noxious stimulus-evoked fos protein-like immunoreactivity in the rat spinal cord. *J. Neurosci.*, 10:323–335.
57. Ren, K., Hylden, J. L. K., Williams, G. M., Ruda, M. A., and Dubner, R. (1991): Effects of MK-801 on behavioral hyperalgesia and dorsal horn neuronal activity in rats with adjuvant-induced inflammation. *Soc. Neurosci. Abstr.*, 17:1208.
58. Ruda, M. A., Iadarola, M. J., Cohen, L. V., and Young, W. S. III. (1988): In situ hybridization histochemistry and immunocytochemistry reveal an increase in spinal dynorphin biosynthesis in a rat model peripheral inflammation and hyperalgesia. *Proc. Natl. Acad. Sci. USA*, 85:622–626.
59. Schneider, S. P., and Perl, E. R. (1985): Selective excitation of neurons in the mammalian spinal dorsal horn by aspartate and glutamate in vitro: correlation with location and excitatory input. *Brain Res.*, 630:339–343.
60. Sheng, M., and Greenberg, M. E. (1990): The regulation and function of c-*fos* and other immediate early genes in the nervous system. *Neuron*, 4:477–485.
61. Sher, G. D., and Mitchell, D. (1990): Intrathecal N-methyl-D-aspartate induces hyperexcitability in rat dorsal horn convergent neurones. *Neurosci. Lett.*, 119:199–202.
62. Skofitsch, G., and Jacobowitz, D. M. (1985): Quantitative distribution of calcitonin gene-related peptide in the rat central nervous system. *Peptides*, 6:1069–1073.
63. Solodkin, A., and Ruda, M. A. (1988): Effects of capsaicin on spinal cord axons that colocalize substance P and calcitonin gene-related peptide. *Soc. Neurosci. Abstr.*, 14:694.
64. Stein, C., Millan, M. J., Shippenberg, T. S., and Herz, A. (1988): Peripheral effect of fentanyl upon nociception in inflamed tissue of the rat. *Neurosci. Lett.*, 84:225–228.
65. Stein, C., Millan, M. J., Shippenberg, T. S., Peter, K., and Herz, A. (1989): Peripheral opioid receptors mediating antinociception in inflammation. Evidence for involvement of mu, delta and kappa receptors. *J. Pharmacol. Exp. Ther.*, 248:1269–1275.
66. Stein, C., Millan, M. J., Yassouridis, A., and Herz, A. (1988): Antinociceptive effects of μ- and κ-agonists in inflammation are enhanced by a peripheral opioid receptor-specific mechanism. *Eur. J. Pharmacol.*, 155:255–264.
67. Sugimoto, T., Bennett, G. J., and Kajander, K. C. (1990): Transsynaptic degeneration in the superficial dorsal horn after sciatic nerve injury: effects of a chronic constriction injury, transection, and strychnine. *Pain*, 42:205–213.
68. Swett, J. E., McMahon, S. B., and Wall, P. D. (1985): Long ascending projections to the midbrain from cells of lamina I and nucleus of the dorsolateral funiculus of the rat spinal cord. *J. Comp. Neurol.*, 238:401–416.
69. Takahashi, O., Traub, R. J., and Ruda, M. A. (1988): Demonstration of calcitonin gene-related peptide immunoreactive axons, contacting dynorphin A(1–8) immunoreactive spinal neurons in a rat model of peripheral inflammation and hyperalgesia. *Brain Res.*, 475:168–172.
70. Tolle, T. R., Castro-Lopes, J. M., Coimbra, A., and Zieglgänsberger, W. (1990): Opiates modify induction of c-*fos* proto-oncogene in the spinal cord of the rat following noxious stimulation. *Neurosci. Lett.*, 111:46–51.
71. Willcockson, W. S., Chung, J. M., Hori, Y., Lee, K. H., and Willis, W. D. (1984): Effects of iontophoretically released amino acids and amines on primate spinothalamic tract cells. *J. Neurosci.*, 4:732–740.
72. Williams, S., Evan, G. I., and Hunt, S. P. (1990): Changing patterns of c-*fos* induction in spinal neurons following thermal cutaneous stimulation in the rat. *Neuroscience*, 36:73–81.
73. Wisden, W., Errington, M. L., Williams, S., et al. (1990): Differential expression of immediate early genes in the hippocampus and spinal cord. *Neuron*, 4:603–614.
74. Woolf, C. J., and King, A. E. (1990): Dynamic alterations in the cutaneous mechanoreceptive fields of dorsal horn neurons in the rat spinal cord. *J. Neurosci.*, 10:2717–2726.
75. Woolf, C. J., and Thompson, S. W. N. (1991): The induction and maintenance of central sensitization is dependent on N-methyl-D-aspartic acid receptor activation; implications for the treatment of post-injury pain hypersensitivity states. *Pain*, 44:293–299.

Hyperalgesia and Allodynia,
edited by W. D. Willis, Jr.
Raven Press, Ltd., New York © 1992.

28

Mechanisms of Central Changes Produced by Peripheral Damage

Discussion

G. F. Gebhart, Moderator

Dr. Wilcox: First of all, I'd like to correct an error that I made. Dougherty and Willis have had success similar to our own with AP-7, I was told, and they just had a methodical problem with CNQX, so that's a correction.

Dr. Coggeshall: I'd like to ask a question to quite a few people, including Drs. Bennett, Ruda, and Basbaum. When you count things in the nervous system, what are you counting? All of you use the term and this is extremely common in nervous system work. As a matter of fact, I counted up the number of people that count things and it's over 10,000, and they make statements like 20% more cells or 15% less synapses. The point is that the things you're counting are not cells or synapses, they are cell profiles. The profile numbers are a function of cell number, cell size, cell orientation, cell arrangement, but there is no known relation by which you can predict cell numbers from profile numbers, which is what you're counting. I'm going to claim, or at least I'm suggesting mildly, that the serial unfolding techniques and the various correction factors that have been devised to do this don't work; you get errors of 50% to 100%. If you say cell numbers, you're not right. The dissector techniques are now becoming available so you can get unbiased counts. For example, in Dr. Bennett's model, it's clear to me that you have some size differences in your cells. That is to say, your cells that you think are damaged look different in size to me. So the numbers of profiles on the two sides may very well not reflect the number of cells. In order to get this very important work right, you need to do this work in an unbiased way. It's no more difficult than just counting the profiles, but you've got to get it so that it's unbiased so you can make these conclusions. Now, I understand that all these papers are accepted in the literature and in grants and that's going to last, I would say, for 2 or 3 more years, until they'll be all turned down. Most of the conclusions are probably correct, but when you're dealing with differences like 20% and 30%, there's a very good possibility that they're not correct, if you're talking about cells; they are correct for cell profiles. So I guess it's just a caution. You need to be careful about this because from your data as stated, you cannot draw your conclusions.

Dr. Basbaum: I don't disagree with you, with one caveat. In our case we're counting nuclei.

Dr. Coggeshall: It doesn't matter. Nuclei, cells, whatever, you're counting profiles, and there's no simple relation between profile number and nuclear number, or profile number and synapse number, or profile number and cell number. You've got to do tops, get the numerical densities, multiply by the volume of the system, in order to get unbiased counts. You can't use these serial unfolding techniques, the model-based systems that people are using.

Dr. Gebhart: Any other comments?

Dr. Ochoa: I was relieved to hear that the definition, the official definition, of hyperalgesia was being abused this afternoon, because I think that definition in reality is not very helpful.

We heard the use of the term hyperalgesia to define an abnormal reduction of threshold to pain, and that, by the book, is allodynia, not hyperalgesia. Again, I'm relieved to hear that because in the clinic that definition is artificial. One practically does not see allodynia without hyperalgesia. One sees hyperalgesia without allodynia, but the opposite one doesn't. I think the definition of what used to be a very useful term, hyperalgesia, reduced threshold to pain and increased response to suprathreshold pain, was excellent. Now we have one that is confusing us, and it came out of the blue. It fell down on us, a nonpeer-reviewed definition, and I think it's confusing us. I was really happy to hear that hyperalgesia was being used to define reduced thresholds to pain this afternoon.

Dr. Bullitt: I've got a question for you, Dr. Basbaum, although maybe some of the others of you interested in c-fos may have comments as well. Basically, I am uncomfortable at the moment that c-fos expression is going to be a useful marker for chronic pain, and there are a number of reasons for that. One of them is that in a number of different systems, ranging from tissue culture to looking at seizures, the gene expression follows a definite time course. Prolonged stimulation of a cell results in rapid induction of the gene, but even with continued stimulation, the gene turns off. In both tissue culture and in the seizure model, it's also been shown that if you then withdraw the stimulus from the cell for about a 4-hr period and then reapply it, the cell resets and you can once again induce c-fos. So, if you're using a chronic pain model and are looking at an animal weeks or days from the time of your stimulus that presumably is producing chronic pain, you are not, I believe, going to be able to see c-fos expression in those neurons that have been firing during most of that time period. What you may be able to identify are cells that sometimes fire and then rest for a bit and then fire again. That activity may be related to your animal's activity, if it has a neuroma and bumps it, and some more cells may fire. So what I expect you may see perhaps in this kind of model is a rather variable course of c-fos expression that is partially dependent on the animal's immediate past history. A second reason that I'm uncomfortable with it is, as you know, c-fos can be induced in cells, not just by neuronal depolarization, but by growth factors, and if you produce some form of neural injury, you may well alter the growth factor concentration within the spinal cord. So, to tell you the truth, I'm not sure what c-fos expression means. I wondered if you could interpret it. I'd love it if it were useful.

Dr. Basbaum: So would I.

Dr. Lebedev: Excuse me, I have rather the same question. There can be a big discrepancy with usage of single label marker as you use, c-fos, not c-mus, but c-fos. Maybe you have a different circadian rhythm of pain. Finally, the pain of neuroma in some respects is connected with a scar, and maybe you registered, indirectly, the organization of the scar.

Dr. Basbaum: Let me try to answer your question, Dr. Bullitt. I don't disagree with anything you said. I'll just point out the following. Number one, I don't know if these animals with neuroma have pain, and I stated that. Kingery has a very interesting paper in *Pain* recently with an injury model indicating that probably through peripheral sprouting through the saphenous nerve there actually is a mechanical hyperalgesia that one can detect. But number two, and I think it's very important, the c-fos expression in laminae V through VII was really continuous and comparable over the whole time period. It did not vary. I agree with you that it could be that the animal keeps bumping the neuroma and there's a mechanical sensor that's driving the neuroma every time. The fact is it's very continuous and stable in laminae V through VII. This is not the case in laminae I and II, where there were peaks and valleys and in fact at 24 hr there was very little there, and then it came back again. The other side of this is that if it is a growth–factor-induced change, it is a growth–factor-induced change that is susceptible to local anesthetic injection. That would be very provocative. I don't know how that comes about, but it does say that neural activity, assuming that the local anesthetic is affecting neural activity, is necessary under appropriate conditions, depending on what time you're looking at, for the expression of the gene.

Dr. Casey: I have two questions for Dr. Bennett. The first question is related to the last slide you showed about the differences in the dorsal root potential and the interpretation of that. Since the dorsal root potential is generated predominantly by large afferent fibers, and since your ligation has produced predominantly a large fiber neuropathy, even though there appears to be less involvement of large fibers proximal to the lesion, can you be sure that the difference in dorsal root potentials that you demonstrated is not due to a loss of large-diameter afferent fibers on the ligated side?

Dr. Bennett: It's not that they are largely unspared proximal to their injuries, but that they look absolutely indistinguishable from normal proximal to the injury. We see no change in them whatsoever, morphologically. The maximal activation of A-beta fibers may not be comparable in the two situations, as you suggest, but I call your attention to the next to the last slide. Less than maximal compound action potential inputs that were matched from one side to the other always evoked less DRP on the side of the nerve injury, and I think that parallel shift to the right is, to my mind at least, pretty conclusive evidence that it is really a change in the DRP and not a change in the signal which evokes the DRP, because when I equalize the signal, I still get the change in the DRP.

Dr. Casey: So you're looking at the compound action potential on both sides.

Dr. Bennett: Always.

Dr. Casey: The second question is about the difference in the models. Dr. Yaksh, I thought, used the same model. At least he said he used the ligation model, and he showed the duration of the hyperalgesia to be 12 days maximum, whereas you are showing it to last 3 months. Can either of you explain that really rather striking difference?

Dr. Bennett: I'm not at all sure what causes it. I suspect that it has something to do with very minor differences in the initial degree of tightness of the constriction. The syndrome is much more sensitive to that initial degree of tightness than we believed at first. If the initial tie is slightly too loose or slightly too tight, the syndrome is abbreviated and truncated. That, I suspect, is the reason.

Dr. Dubner: I have a comment and a question. The comment, I guess, is related to what Dr. Bullitt brought up and that is the role of c-fos as a marker of neuronal activity. I'd just like to say that it may be that c-fos can be used as a marker of neuronal activity, but I think the opposite is not true; that is, if you don't see c-fos that doesn't mean there isn't neuronal activity. I think that should be pointed out. I think you can clearly see that in an inflammation model. You induce inflammation and the c-fos changes, depending on which antibody you use, are over within 6 to 24 hr, yet we know that the inflammation and hyperalgesia are going on possibly for a week to 10 days. My question is for Dr. Basbaum. In the 2 weeks after nerve injury, your c-fos picture is very interesting. There's a total absence of c-fos in the sciatic nerve territory, which is the nerve that you transected; I would like you to comment on what that might mean. What type of activity is being expressed in that situation?

Dr. Basbaum: If I can correct your statement, it's not outside the sciatic distribution. It's on the lateral edge of the sciatic distribution. It clearly overlaps with the lateral edge of the sciatic distribution.

Dr. Casey: Yes, it's right at the border of the sciatic distribution.

Dr. Basbaum: That's right. I think that tells us something perhaps about what is driving it. Now the difficulty with these studies is that when you inject local anesthetic, you have to find a way to inject local anesthetic that doesn't induce c-fos by itself. That's technically difficult, but we came up with a way to do this. I don't want to go into the details now. However, it's an infiltration and perhaps some of that c-fos is, in fact, being induced by some saphenous input that may have sprouted into the sciatic territory, and that's what we're seeing at the overlap zone. The other possibility is that there's been a central sensitization. This may be a reflection of that. Unfortunately, in our hands, with the approach we use to block, we can't be certain what is actually driving it. If I had to put my money on it, it's something to do with the edge of the sciatic and saphenous distributions.

Dr. Casey: The other side of the coin is that in that model activity arising, let's say, from dorsal root ganglia, ectopic discharges or from a neuroma are presumably not producing changes in neuronal activity.

Dr. Basbaum: In the sciatic distribution, apparently not, if you believe that c-fos is a marker of activity. But, of course, the absence of c-fos doesn't mean that there's no activity.

Dr. Bullitt: I think that you may not be able to see it at all because your gene turned off 29½ days ago.

Dr. Wilcox: Dr. Dubner, I think a more important thing about c-fos is not whether it indicates neuronal activity, but the fact that it's a nuclear protein. I think it represents the future, knowing cells that are changing, or doing something in their nucleus. What it means now we don't know, but what's going to happen later? That could be important.

Dr. Woolf: A question for Dr. Ruda about your use of the neonatal capsaicin model. Maybe I'm putting words into your mouth that are not correct, but you've done that to remove C fibers and therefore to test whether C fibers are involved in various forms of behavior, in this case the response to inflammation. But the nervous system, when interfered with in this neonatal period, does not remain passive, and the vacated synaptic sites produced by the death of these C fibers result in the growth of A fibers into that area. Dr. Fitzgerald and I have recently shown that hair follicle afferents grow into lamina II. Whether they actually make functional synaptic contacts, I don't know, but certainly the spinal cord of an animal treated with neonatal capsaicin is quite different from that of the normal, intact animal, so I just think one has to appreciate that one's intervention has changed the system one's looking at.

Dr. Ruda: I agree with you completely, because the other half of that study that Dr. Hammond and I did that I didn't present today was concerned with the sprouting and reappearance of CGRP primary afferents after 8 weeks. That's why we did this study prior to the reappearance of the primary afferents. Things could have been going on that we're not aware of, but it's very important to keep in mind exactly what kind of changes we may be instituting. This is reflected in my comment about how much was still the same in terms of the constitutive expression, because other studies that we have going on in the laboratory right now tend to suggest that constitutive expression of some other genes has been altered in these neonatal capsaicin-treated animals. So, it's important. Thank you.

Dr. Besson: I have two questions. The first one is for Dr. Basbaum. You saw no effect of morphine on your experimental model after a peripheral lesion, but as you know you have still about 25% to 30% of opiate receptors postsynaptically. The question is, did you try to increase your dose of morphine?

Dr. Basbaum: No, your point's well taken. We did not go above 5 mg/kg because this was a dose that was very effective in a tissue injury model, and, to be honest, we were very surprised by the result. It was a knee-jerk experiment. We actually thought we'd get an effect, and I'm surprised we didn't get any. I don't know why; maybe 10 or 20 mg/kg would shut it off—it's indeed possible. Maybe something with greater efficacy like sufentanyl might be more effective, which would be interesting. Getting back to what Dr. Dubner said, perhaps one of the reasons why it's less sensitive is that a lot of these cells are being driven by larger fibers later on and that any presynaptic regulation is still baclofen susceptible, but it's not morphine susceptible. I don't know what is happening to the postsynaptic receptor under these conditions. I don't understand why a patient with neuropathic pain can't have their pain blocked by pouring opiates on the spinal cord, and I know Dr. Foley is going to tell me that it depends on how much. But the fact is that if you say you can shut off the cell with opiates at the level of the cord through a postsynaptic mechanism and if you extrapolate that to the human, you should shut off the cord. The fact is it doesn't work.

Dr. Besson: Thank you. Dr. Wilcox, I have a question related to NMDA receptors. We've heard a lot about NMDA and it's already published by various authors that very low doses of ketamine, 2 mg/kg i.v., suppress the windup phenomenon. Relatively low doses of MK801 suppress c-fos–labeling-induced formalin. Do you think that 2 mg/kg of ketamine in the rat induces an analgesic effect, because to prepare for surgery in the rat you need at least 100 mg/kg of ketamine.

Dr. Wilcox: A rhetorical question, if I've ever heard one. Right. Ketamine is not analgesic, correct? The story is that there is more than one channel coming in there. You have an AMPA channel and you have the substance P channel. You can turn off the NMDA channel to a sufficient degree to measure it, but that doesn't make the pain go away.

Dr. Gebhart: Dr. Basbaum, to follow up on what Dr. Besson asked, did you try a preemptive treatment with morphine? That is, treat the animal with morphine before the nerve was cut?

Dr. Basbaum: No.

Dr. Basbaum: Dr. Rustioni, the latter part of your talk obviously was extremely provocative. You were very circumspect in that one might have said why not just use the antibody to see if you're getting staining. You have done triple labeling in cases where you've injected WGA-HRP and therefore injured the nerve and seen extracellular labeling. Under those circumstances, did you ever see a significant level of extracellular peptide?

Dr. Rustioni: Yes, it's a question that we want to answer, of course. It's not easy to retain the peptides that are eventually released in the extracellular space. We are planning to start to work on exactly that question, but I think we'll have to revise our fixative and technical protocol to be able to retain whatever endogenous peptides or other macromolecules that may be released in the extracellular space. With WGA-HRP, the lectin has combining sites with the membrane so we have an easier time in retaining it. I think we have to work around problems with protocols in order to demonstrate directly that the endogenous material is released. So the fact that we didn't see it may be partly the fact that we didn't think about looking for it when we originally did the work, and we might have missed it, but I don't think it would be possible with the protocol that we are using now.

Hyperalgesia and Allodynia,
edited by W. D. Willis, Jr.
Raven Press, Ltd., New York © 1992.

29

Therapy and Future Directions

Overview

Kathleen M. Foley

*Department of Neurology, Memorial Sloan-Kettering Cancer Center,
New York, New York 10021*

This section on therapy and future directions points up the glaring dearth of sophisticated neurophysiologic and neuroradiologic correlates to the clinically observed signs of hyperalgesia and allodynia. Of particular interest, the chapters of Hansson and Lindblom and of Boivie propose a refinement of the definition of these two clinical phenomena, which have been formally defined by the Taxonomy Committee of the International Association for the Study of Pain. Hyperalgesia has been defined as an increased response to a stimulus that is normally painful, whereas allodynia describes pain due to a stimulus that does not normally provoke pain. Hansson and Lindblom, focusing on the pathophysiologic mechanisms that underlie these phenomena, propose that hyperalgesia results from altered amplification of the nociceptive message. Using quantitative testing combined with psychophysical pain measurements in patients with peripheral and central nervous system lesions, they demonstrate the variable response that can occur in such patients. Based on these studies, they argue for a definition of hyperalgesia that encompasses both the concept of a lower pain threshold due to sensitized nociceptors or an increased rate of growth of pain intensity with graded stimulation. Such a definition requires further validation with clinical neurophysiologic studies, but their attempts to elaborate on the underlying mechanisms of these clinical phenomena are a critical starting point in characterizing these sensory signs more rigorously.

The qualitative and quantitative sensory studies of Boivie in patients with central pain provide further support for redefinition. Boivie emphasizes the common feature of abnormal temperature and pain sensation in such patients. Using sensory evoked potentials and quantitative sensory testing, he has confirmed the presence of abnormal conduction in the spinothalamic tract and emphasized the critical role of this tract rather than the medial lemniscal pathways in generating central pain.

Bullitt's review of the current therapeutic strategies to manage patients with signs of hyperalgesia and allodynia provides an overview of a disappointing array of therapies, some of which have been partially effective in treating these painful neurologic signs and symptoms. However, the numerous therapeutic approaches described have not attempted to critically evaluate and correlate a reduction in pain with an alteration in these sensory phenomena, pointing up the need for detailed quantitative and qualitative sensory evaluation in such patients as an outcome measure concurrent with pain relief. Numerous pharmacologic approaches have been tried, and to date the best evidence supports the use of one of several tricyclic antidepressants to suppress pain with some suggestion that they may also reduce hyperalgesia in some patients.

The three clinical chapters make note of the time delay in the onset of pain for many patients following peripheral or central nervous system injury. Boivie offers an exciting concept by arguing for prophylactic therapy in patients with certain types of nerve injury who are at the greatest risk for developing central pain syndromes. Such therapy might be akin to the therapy used to prevent kindling in patients at risk to develop seizures following central nervous system injuries.

In the discussion, Chapman advocated the need for both behavioral and psychological studies to provide a systematic assessment of the common features in this population of patients following central or peripheral nervous system injury with associated hyperalgesia, allodynia, or both.

Dr. Besson's plea for the future targeted the development of animal models that can be correlated with these clinical phenomena and allow for testing of new hypotheses and for reassessment of new and old therapeutic approaches. He stressed the need for more comprehensive studies in humans using neurophysiologic, neuropharmacologic, and neuroradiographic studies such as magnetic resonance imaging and positron emission tomography to define the multiple components that underlie the pathophysiology of the hyperalgesia and allodynia.

The advances to date in our understanding of the neuroanatomy, neurophysiology, and neuropharmacology of pain have provided the impetus to focus on these very specific but common features of acute and chronic pain occurring in both the peripheral and central nervous systems. The challenge is to decipher the common mechanisms from the unique ones in order to define specific therapeutic approaches for patients with central pain and for patients with peripheral nerve pain who, at the present time, represent a largely untreated population with concomitant disability and dysfunction.

Hyperalgesia and Allodynia,
edited by W. D. Willis, Jr.
Raven Press, Ltd., New York © 1992.

30

Hyperalgesia Assessed with Quantitative Sensory Testing in Patients with Neurogenic Pain

Per Hansson and Ulf Lindblom

Department of Neurology, Karolinska Hospital, S-10401 Stockholm, Sweden

Limited attention has previously been paid to assessment of evoked pain, especially abnormal painful sensations, in patients with neurogenic pain (6,7,10,11). Analysis of evoked pain could be of relevance in understanding the pathophysiological mechanisms of neurogenic pain. It might also be used as an index of ongoing pain, if a correlation could be shown, or as a therapeutic predictor. Evoked pain has the advantage of being more objectively assessable than spontaneous pain by means of graded stimulation and psychophysical quantification. Assessment of evoked pain in patients with neurogenic pain requires, however, special methodological considerations because of associated sensibility disturbances and ongoing sensations of pain, paresthesias, and dysesthesias.

In patients with neurogenic pain one would per se expect an increased threshold for different somatosensory modalities, including pain, due to peripheral fiber loss or damage to central pathways. Despite evidence of such damage, however, the threshold for pain may be lowered, as documented by pinch algometry in the patient with an ulnar neuralgia seen in Fig. 30.1. The neuropathic basis of this finding became evident after dorsal column stimulation (DCS), which blocked the ongoing pain and changed the pain threshold to pinch, which was now increased, in conformity with neuropathic sensory loss. The low pain threshold to pinch before DCS would operationally perhaps be called hyperalgesia by some, in spite of no obvious evidence of sensitization of nociceptors. However, it was for this type of pain, evoked by mild stimuli, that the International Association for the Study of Pain (IASP) (9) launched the term allodynia. For such pain there is evidence of a central–pain-producing mechanism, disinhibition or sensory disintegration, which phenomenologically may override the neuropathic deficit resulting in decreased threshold to pinch pain. (For more detail about allodynia, see ref. 7.) In the present study we focused on sensation magnitude of graded nociceptive heat stimulation in patients with neurogenic pain.

In clinical practice we assess heat pain thresholds as well as other thermal perception thresholds with the Marstock method (4). In routine examination we use the method of limits for threshold recording, which means that we are operating with a slightly suprathreshold stimulation of heat pain due to the reaction time involved in this method. Not infrequently, and regardless of heat pain threshold level, patients

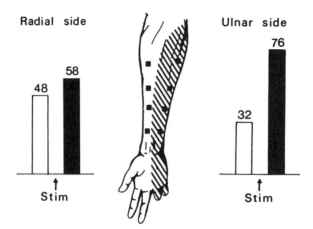

FIG. 30.1. In this patient with an ulnar neuralgia examination with pinch algometry revealed a lowered threshold to pain on the medial volar surface of the affected lower arm (right) as compared to the homologous unaffected region. Thresholds in corresponding regions of normal arm: 40–60 g/mm². After a 30-min period of dorsal column stimulation (DCS), the ongoing pain was abolished and the pain threshold to pinch was significantly increased. The pain threshold to pinch in the lateral volar part of the lower arm was unaffected by DCS.

report that the sensation magnitude of pain at threshold level is more intense in the painful area as compared to the unaffected homologous region. This empiric finding prompted further studies since the stimulus–response function of pain intensity as a function of graded nociceptive heat stimulation in patients with neurogenic pain of peripheral or central origin, to our knowledge, has not been studied in detail. Correlation of the obtained stimulus–response functions to ongoing pain, outcome of bedside sensibility testing, von Frey testing, perception levels of other thermal modalities as well as therapeutic success or failure has not yet been performed due to too small a number of patients examined so far.

METHODS

Five consecutive patients with peripheral and four with central neurogenic pain, referred to the pain unit at our department, have been included in the study. All patients completed a pain drawing at their initial visit and rated the intensity of their ongoing pain using a visual analogue scale (VAS). The VAS consisted of a 100-mm horizontal line with the words "no pain" and "worst pain ever" at the left and right extreme ends of the line, respectively. Sensory screening was then carried out with conventional bedside techniques using a camel-hair brush for touch, two metallic rollers kept at 20° and 40°C, respectively, for cold and warmth, and pinprick for mechanically evoked pain. Although not reported here, this was performed to characterize the spatial distribution and modality profile of the sensibility dysfunction in the painful area. The results of sensory screening examination must, however, be interpreted with caution since several modalities are stimulated simultaneously with these bedside techniques. For example, pins stimulate both touch and pain receptors, and warm and cold objects stimulate both mechanoreceptive and thermal receptors. Adding modality specific and graded techniques a more detailed analysis can be performed of sensory dysfunction. Methods for sensory quantification are available for touch contact, vibration, pressure, temperature, and pinprick. One method for assessment of temperature sensibility is, as previously mentioned, the Marstock method, introduced by Fruhstorfer et al. (4) in 1976. The method uses a contact thermode of Peltier elements and provides selective thermal stimulation with graded warmth and cold. The stimulating surface of the thermode could be heated or cooled depending on the direction of the current through the elements. When the direction of the current is changed by pressing a hand-held switch, operated by the patient, the temperature is reversed. The thermode included a thermocouple for instantaneous measurement of interface temperature between the thermode and the skin, connected to a pen recorder. Thresholds are in clinical routine practice determined with the method of limits, and both hypo- and hyperesthetic phenomena can be quantified as abnormal thresholds for warmth, cold, heat pain, and cold pain. A recording of thresholds for warmth, cold, cold pain, and heat pain from the anterolateral part of the thighs of a patient with paresthetic meralgia is seen in Fig. 30.2.

Using the method of limits, heat pain thresholds were first assessed with the thermode applied in the homologous unaffected skin area as a control, and then in the center of the painful region. The patient was instructed to reverse the heat stimulus by pressing the button immediately when the warm sensation became painful. Stimulus rate was 1.5°C/sec and maximum temperature was set at 55°C to avoid tissue

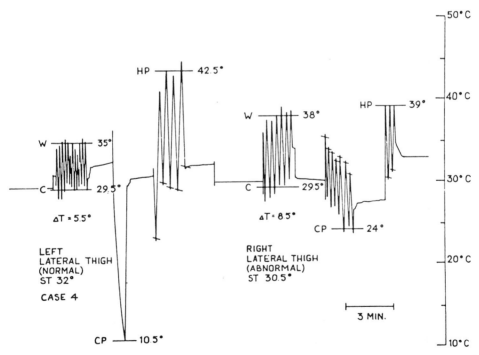

FIG. 30.2. This patient suffered from paresthetic meralgia in the right thigh. Recordings of thermal thresholds were made in the center of the painful area and in the homologous unaffected region. W, warm threshold; C, cold threshold; HP, heat pain threshold; CP, cold pain threshold. Hypoesthesia to warm stimuli was found on the affected side as well as lowered thresholds to heat pain and cold pain.

damage. Before starting, the probe and skin temperatures were adjusted to the neutral zone of absent thermal sensation. Also, the sensation of pressure from application of the thermode had adapted when recording started. The threshold was determined as the average temperature of the last two perception levels of three consecutive measurements. Thereafter, using the method of levels to avoid reaction time artefacts, the "true" heat pain threshold was titrated out by applying successive stimuli below the threshold obtained using the method of limits. Increasing suprathreshold stimuli were then applied. After each stimulus that was reported as painful, the patient rated the pain intensity on a VAS. All patients were carefully informed that they could terminate their participation in the study at any time if the given

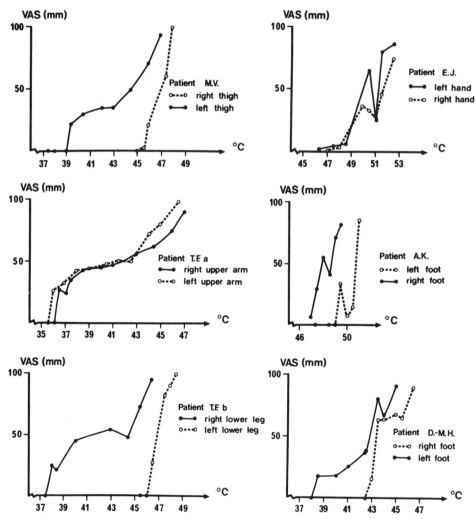

FIG. 30.3. Stimulus–response functions regarding pain intensity as a function of graded nociceptive heat stimulation for all patients referred to in the text. The *dashed curves* are obtained from the painful area in each patient, *solid curves* from control area. For patient T.F., two curves are presented (for details see text). (*Figure continues.*)

stimulus was too painful or otherwise unbearable. Stimulus intensity was increased at steps of 0.5° to 1°C until the patient terminated the experiment or when the pain intensity was rated in the right extreme end of the VAS. A minimum interstimulus interval of 3 min was allowed to avoid sensitization.

RESULTS

Patient M.V. This patient is a 41-year-old female with a brain stem infarction in the area subserved by the left posterior inferior cerebellar artery in 1989 and pain of central neurogenic type, starting within a year after the infarction, in the right arm and leg. Pain intensity at examination was rated at 35 mm using the VAS. The heat pain threshold in the painful thigh was increased, and the rate of growth of the stimulus–response function of pain intensity as a function of graded nociceptive heat stimulation was significantly increased compared to the corresponding region (Fig. 30.3).

Patient T.F. This is a 40-year-old male who had a brain stem infarction in 1988 in the area subserved by the right posterior inferior cerebellar artery. He has suffered from burning and aching pain in his left arm and leg since 1 week after the stroke. The stimulus–response function [Fig. 30.3(T.F.a)] obtained in the upper arms of this patient showed an unaltered heat pain threshold but a tendency toward a steeper slope in the upper part of the curve obtained in the painful region. At the time of examination the overall subjective intensity of ongoing pain was rated at 10 mm using the VAS. The same patient was examined in the painful leg about a week later,

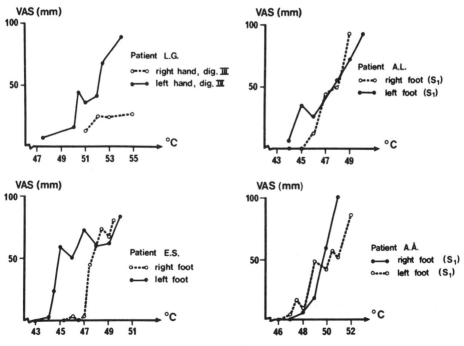

FIG. 30.3. *Continued.*

and at this visit the overall intensity of ongoing pain was rated at 40 mm using the VAS. The heat pain threshold was found to be significantly increased, and the rate of growth of the stimulus–response function was increased on the painful side [Fig. 30.3 (T.F.b)].

Patient E.J. This 71-year-old male had two subsequent infarctions in the left thalamus in 1989 and 1990. Immediately after the second stroke he complained of pain, numbness, and paresthesia in the right arm, hand, and leg. At examination the intensity of ongoing pain was rated at 10 mm on the VAS. The heat pain threshold and stimulus–response function did not differ significantly between the thenar areas in this patient (Fig. 30.3).

Patient A.K. This 45-year-old woman suffers from pain in the left lower leg and foot starting only a few weeks after surgical removal of a parasagittal meningioma. At the time of examination she rated the ongoing pain at 35 mm using the VAS. The heat pain threshold was increased, but the slope of the stimulus–response function was roughly unaltered in the painful dorsolateral part of the left foot as compared to the control region (Fig. 30.3).

Patient D.-M.H. This 50-year-old woman developed a painful neuropathic condition in the innervation territory of the right sural nerve, immediately after bilateral surgery of her Achilles tendons. VAS rating of ongoing pain intensity was 35 mm at testing. The heat pain threshold was significantly elevated, and the rate of growth of the stimulus–response function was, at least initially, increased in the painful region as compared to the corresponding area (Fig. 30.3).

Patient L.G. This 38-year-old male patient suffered from a painful stump of the third finger on the right hand after a traumatic amputation at the level of the proximal interphalangeal joint 17 years ago. He was pain free at the time of examination but complained of intermittent spontaneous lightning dysesthesias, radiating from the lower arm and hand distally into his stump, as well as a touch-evoked pain or dysesthesia. In addition, a few times a day, he experienced aching pain in his stump with an intensity rated at 100 mm using the VAS. The heat pain threshold was significantly increased on the volar aspect of the proximal phalanx of digit III on the affected side, and the rate of growth of the stimulus–response function was significantly decreased compared to the control region (Fig. 30.3).

Patient E.S. This 37-year-old man had a motorcycle accident a few years ago with a traumatic injury to the right lumbosacral plexus and suffered from subsequent periodic chronic pain in his right foot. At examination, however, he was pain free. In the dorsolateral part of the right foot the heat pain threshold was increased, and the rate of growth of the stimulus–response function was increased compared to the control area (Fig. 30.3)

Patient A.L. This patient, a 37-year-old nurse, suffers from pain in her right leg and foot due to a traumatic S1 rhizopathy caused by epidural anesthesia at labor. At examination she rated the pain intensity at 23 mm using the VAS. The stimulus–response function obtained from the dorsolateral part of her right foot demonstrated an increased heat pain threshold and an increased rate of growth, crossing the curve obtained from the left foot (Fig. 30.3).

Patient A.Å. This is a 43-year-old male who after explorative back surgery experienced excruciating pain in his left leg at removal of the surgical tampons, a pain that still bothers him and clinically resembles an S1 rhizopathy. The intensity of ongoing pain at examination was rated at 18 mm using the VAS. The heat pain threshold was unaltered, but the stimulus–response function had a slightly less steep slope on the dorsolateral part of the painful foot compared to the corresponding region (Fig. 30.3).

Importantly, in all but one of the patients the quality as well as temporal and spatial aspects of the evoked heat pain sensation were identical in both painful and control areas. However, in one patient *(M.V.)* with central neurogenic pain and increased threshold to heat pain as well as a steeper stimulus–response function in the painful area, the evoked pain sometimes was associated with aftersensation of about 10 to 30 sec.

DISCUSSION

This study has described at least five principally different curves representing stimulus–response functions of pain intensity as a function of graded nociceptive heat stimulation in the painful area, compared to the corresponding region, of patients with neurogenic pain (Fig. 30.4): (a) a curve with a steeper slope but unaltered threshold; (b) similar curves in both painful and corresponding areas, including both threshold and slope; (c) curves with increased threshold and steeper slope, eventually crossing the curve obtained on the unaffected side; (d) a curve with unaltered or increased threshold and a less steep slope; (e) a curve with increased threshold but unaltered slope.

According to the current definition of the IASP Subcommittee on Taxonomy (9), hyperalgesia is "an increased response to a stimulus which is normally painful." "Normally painful" probably relates to the magnitude of pain experienced from a stimulus of similar intensity applied for comparison to the homologous unaffected

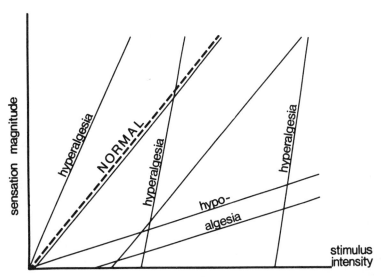

FIG. 30.4. Different schematic stimulus–response curves obtained from the nine examined patients referred to in the text.

region in the same patient or to normal subjects. Our finding of a steeper stimulus–response function in some patients with neurogenic pain and significantly increased thresholds to heat pain in the painful area indicates a pathological gain of the message conveyed in nociceptive pathways, at spinal cord and/or diencephalic or higher levels. An increased threshold is, however, as mentioned earlier, a reasonable finding in such patients. On clinical bedside examination of pain patients, hyperalgesia would thus be present if a painful stimulus, usually a needle or pinch, is reported more intense in the painful area. However, in patients with neurogenic pain and increased threshold to evoked pain as well as a steeper stimulus–response function in the painful area, the stimulus may not produce stronger pain than in the unaffected region if the stimulus used is only slightly suprathreshold. A rapid rate of growth of the stimulus–response function could therefore escape detection, especially in the case of the steep curve located to the right in Fig. 30.4.

Based on our current results, in conjunction with experimental findings in humans (5) showing that the rate of growth of pain intensity as a function of graded nociceptive heat stimulation may not be increased after a standardized skin burn lesion, the following amended alternative definition of hyperalgesia is proposed: "lowered pain threshold due to sensitization of nociceptive afferents or increased rate of growth of pain intensity as a function of graded nociceptive stimulation." Thereby one avoids allusion primarily to pain threshold levels and makes the term hyperalgesia applicable in all three curves labeled "hyperalgesia" in Fig. 30.4. With this definition hyperalgesia not only fits with increased response to nociceptive stimuli in neurogenic pain states but could also be applicable when discussing lowered threshold to nociceptive stimuli in tissues with experimentally induced sensitization of nociceptors, regardless of the profile of the stimulus–response function (1,5). Whether the suggested definition of hyperalgesia is applicable in clinical nociceptive pain has not yet been tested. Campbell et al. (2) have argued against the use of the term allodynia to describe the lowered threshold to heat pain in the sensitized region of an experimental thermal cutaneous injury, and we agree with them that this is hyperalgesia. Hypoalgesia, consequently, should be refined to "unchanged or increased threshold to nociceptive stimulation and decreased rate of growth of pain intensity as a function of graded nociceptive stimulation." Detection and differentiation of hyper- and hypocurves in patients with neurogenic pain require, as mentioned, special attention during bedside examination with various suprathreshold stimuli or, preferably, quantitative sensory testing.

The words "nociceptive stimulation" in our proposed definitions deserve some comments. Here we imply a stimulus strong enough to activate nociceptive afferents. That a particular stimulus activates nociceptive afferents could in clinical practice of course not be confirmed by intraneural recordings but could instead be judged from the stimulus intensity needed to evoke pain in the homologous area, with the exception of painful regions with sensitized nociceptors.

The term allodynia could be reserved for pain evoked by stimuli activating non-nociceptive afferents, as seen in many neurogenic pain patients. An exception is the mechanical and thermal hypersensitivity mediated by sensitized C fibers in a patient with chronic neuropathic pain reported by Cline et al. (3). In addition, it would be adequate to use allodynia to describe the phenomenon of so-called secondary hyperalgesia around acute tissue lesions (1), characterized by pain evoked by mild mechanical stimulation in the absence of sensitized nociceptors.

In conclusion, findings from VAS ratings of pain intensity as a function of graded nociceptive heat stimulation in patients with neurogenic pain form the basis of a proposed refinement of the definition of hyperalgesia, alluding more to pathophysiological mechanisms than the current phenomenological definition.

ACKNOWLEDGMENT

The study was supported by grants from the Karolinska Institute.

REFERENCES

1. Campbell, J. N., and Meyer, R. A. (1986): Primary afferents and hyperalgesia. In: *Spinal afferent processing,* edited by T. L. Yaksh, pp. 59–81. Plenum, New York.
2. Campbell, J. N., Raja, S. N., and Meyer, R. A. (1988): Painful sequelae of nerve injury. In: *Proceedings of the Vth World Congress on Pain. Pain research and clinical management,* edited by R. Dubner, G. F. Gebhart, and M. R. Bond, pp. 135–143. Elsevier, Amsterdam.
3. Cline, M. A., Ochoa, J., and Torebjörk, E. (1989): Chronic hyperalgesia and skin warming caused by sensitized C nociceptors. *Brain,* 112:621–647.
4. Fruhstorfer, H., Lindblom, U., and Schmidt, W. G. (1976): Method for quantitative estimation of thermal thresholds in patients. *J. Neurol. Neurosurg. Psychiatry,* 39:1071–1075.
5. LaMotte, R. H., Thalhammer, J. G., and Robinson, C. J. (1983): Peripheral neural correlates of magnitude of cutaneous pain and hyperalgesia: a comparison of neural events in monkey with sensory judgments in human. *J. Neurophysiol.,* 50:1–26.
6. Lindblom, U. (1985): Assessment of abnormal evoked pains in neurological pain patients and its relation to spontaneous pain: a descriptive and conceptual model with some analytic results. In: *Advances in pain research and therapy,* vol. 9, edited by H. L. Fields, R. Dubner, and F. Cervero, pp. 409–423. Raven Press, New York.
7. Lindblom, U., and Hansson, P. (1991): Sensory dysfunction and pain after clinical nerve injury studied by means of graded mechanical and thermal stimulation. In: *International symposium on lesions of primary afferent fibres as a tool for the study of chronic pain,* edited by J.-M. Besson and G. Guilbaud, pp. 1–18. Elsevier, Amsterdam.
8. Lindblom, U., and Verrillo, R. T. (1979): Sensory functions in chronic neuralgia. *J. Neurol. Neurosurg. Psychiatry,* 42:422–435.
9. Merskey, H., et al. (1986): Classification of chronic pain: description of chronic pain syndromes and definitions of pain terms. *Pain,* Suppl. 3:216–221.
10. Price, D. D., Bennett, G. J., and Rafii, A. (1989): Psychophysical observations on patients with neuropathic pain relieved by a sympathetic block. *Pain,* 36:273–288.
11. Riddoch, G. (1938): The clinical features of central pain. *Lancet,* 1:1093–1098, 1150–1156, 1205–1209.

Hyperalgesia and Allodynia,
edited by W. D. Willis, Jr.
Raven Press, Ltd., New York © 1992.

31

The Treatment of Hyperalgesia Following Neural Injury

Elizabeth Bullitt

*Division of Neurosurgery, Department of Physiology, University of North Carolina,
Chapel Hill, North Carolina 27599*

Hyperalgesia, an increased sensitivity to noxious stimulation, occurs most commonly in inflammatory conditions. Hyperalgesia may also appear following neural injuries, however, and is then almost always found in conjunction with spontaneous, burning pain. Few disease states produce as much suffering. In 1872, Weir Mitchell (49) described wounded civil war soldiers suffering from this symptom complex. "Under such torments," he wrote, "the temper changes, the most amiable grow irritable, the soldier becomes a coward, and the strongest man is scarcely less nervous than the most hysterical girl."

Burning pain and hyperalgesia may appear following injury to sensory pathways at any level of the neuraxis. Regardless of the location of injury, these patients tend to display: (a) constant, burning pain, (b) a variable loss of pinprick discrimination in the affected region, (c) abnormal, often excruciatingly painful sensations induced by light touch or stroking of the skin (allodynia), and, often, (d) abnormal, spreading, burning sensations induced by repetitive stimulation (hyperpathia).

The efficacy of treatment for this type of pain depends partially on the location of the inciting injury. This chapter reviews the therapeutic options available to the patient and focuses on three syndromes: the reflex sympathetic dystrophies, postherpetic neuralgia (PHN), and pain following central nervous system injury.

REFLEX SYMPATHETIC DYSTROPHIES

The reflex sympathetic dystrophies occur following injury to an extremity and produce a symptom complex of allodynia, sympathetic dysfunction, and spontaneous burning pain that is aggravated by emotional factors. Considerable confusion about nomenclature exists in the literature (72,75). At present, most clinicians employ the term "causalgia" when the symptom complex follows direct injury to a major peripheral nerve and the term "reflex sympathetic dystrophy" (RSD) when the symptom complex results from ischemia, infection, or any injury that does not involve a nerve trunk directly. The phrase reflex sympathetic dystrophies is a generic term that refers to both causalgia and RSD (72).

Causalgia complicates 2% to 5% of peripheral nerve injuries (43,68,76,98). RSD follows an unknown but probably lesser percentage of other types of injury to an extremity. The pain usually begins within the first 24 hr of injury but may be delayed in onset by weeks or months (3,66,77,83,86). Initially, the pain is usually located in the distal portion of an extremity but extends proximally over time and may ultimately involve other, uninjured extremities (72,99). Rarely, the syndrome spreads to include the entire body (4). Cutaneous hypersensitivity may be extreme, and the patient will often go to extraordinary lengths to protect the injured limb from any contact. Typically, the pain is also worsened by emotional stress, loud noise, or any stimulus that excites or startles the patient.

Several clinicians believe that the disease can be divided into three phases (7,59,72). In the *acute phase,* both burning pain and allodynia are prominent. The distal extremity exhibits edema and decreased range of motion. Early in this phase, blood flow is increased to the injured extremity, and the skin feels abnormally warm and dry. The *dystrophic phase* begins 3 to 6 months later. There is often spread of pain and edema to adjacent areas, hair loss, cracking of the nails, and joint thickening with further decrease in range of motion. Blood flow is usually decreased to the extremity, which feels abnormally cool. The final, *atrophic phase* begin approximately 6 months after injury. Pain may be less prominent in this phase of the disease. The hair becomes coarse, and the skin smooth and glossy. The muscles atro-

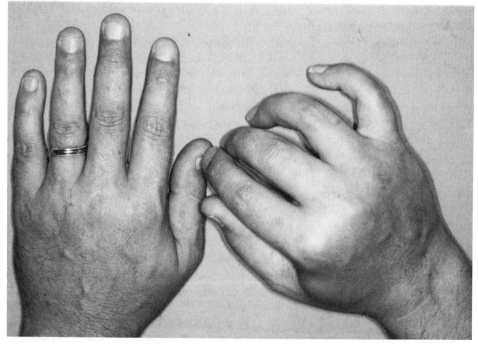

FIG. 31.1. This patient suffered a crush injury to the distal fingers 3 years ago and has the signs and symptoms of reflex sympathetic dystrophy. He has burning pain and severe allodynia that extend proximally to the mid-forearm, well beyond the distribution of his initial injury. Note the edema, the flexion contractures, and the shiny skin of the affected side. He does not bite the nails on that hand.

phy, and the bones exhibit pericapsular fibrosis and demineralization. Flexion contractures appear. The skin is either abnormally cool or of normal temperature. Sweating may be increased or decreased.

It should be noted that the course of the disease is variable. In fortunate patients, the painful symptoms may resolve spontaneously during the acute phase of the disease. For the less fortunate, pain persists throughout the disease course and may persist unabated for years (Fig. 31.1).

TREATMENT OF THE REFLEX SYMPATHETIC DYSTROPHIES

The cornerstone of treatment of the reflex sympathetic dystrophies is interruption of the sympathetic supply to the injured limb early in the course of the disease. Unfortunately for the patient who fails to respond to sympathetic interruption, no other treatment modality has been frequently successful in relieving pain.

Interruption of the Sympathetic Nervous System

As early as 1916, Leriche (35) proposed periarterial sympathectomy as an effective treatment for causalgia. This form of sympathetic interruption has now been abandoned in favor of a number of other approaches, including anesthetic blockade of the paravertebral sympathetic chain, regional blocks with antisympathetic agents, oral delivery of antisympathetic drugs, and sympathetic ganglionectomy. Regardless of the form of treatment, it is important to interrupt the sympathetic supply to the injured extremity early in the course of the disease. Many clinicians have noted that if therapy is delayed, the pain may become refractory to any type of treatment (7,8,19,66,72).

Anesthetic Blockade of the Paravertebral Sympathetic Chain

Anesthetic blockade of the paravertebral sympathetic chain is one of the most common forms of treatment for the reflex sympathetic dystrophies. If blocks are performed early in the course of the disease, the pain disappears in the majority of patients during at least the period of time in which the block is in effect. Some investigators have proposed that the diagnosis of causalgia cannot be made unless sympathetic blockade eliminates the pain (7,43).

The clinical improvement induced by sympathetic blockade is not always transient. In some instances, symptoms remit indefinitely following a single block. For other patients, sequential sympathetic blocks may result in cure. The precise incidence of cure is difficult to determine, however. At one extreme, up to 95% of patients with RSD and up to 50% of patients with causalgia are reported to improve markedly if serial sympathetic blocks are combined with a vigorous physical therapy regimen (7,72,94). At the other extreme, Mayfield (43) found that none of his causalgia patients treated with serial sympathetic blocks demonstrated permanent improvement. Several other clinicians have reported cure rates of approximately 10% following sequential blocks (66,77,80,99). In general, it seems apparent that at least some patients with RSD or causalgia will show permanent benefit when treated with one or more sympathetic nerve blocks, particularly if anesthetic blockade is coupled with physical therapy.

Sympathetic blocks usually relieve both the hyperpathia and the spontaneous burning pain of the reflex sympathetic dystrophies. In their review of a variety of painful conditions treated by sympathetic block, Loh and Nathan (40) concluded that there was a striking relationship between the presence of hyperpathia and the potential for pain relief by block. Sympathetic blocks were unlikely to relieve spontaneous pain in the absence of hyperpathia, but if hyperpathia were present sympathetic blocks usually relieved both the spontaneous pain and the hyperpathia (40). Isolated cases have been described, however, in which sympathetic interruption or differential peripheral nerve blocks relieved the burning pain without affecting allodynia or hyperpathia (3,26,85).

Although the majority of patients with causalgia or RSD demonstrate at least temporary relief of symptoms with sympathetic blocks, some patients fail to respond to sympathetic blockade. Patients who do not respond to sympathetic blocks may be clinically indistinguishable from those in whom pain is relieved temporarily or permanently. The response rate drops when therapy is initiated more than 6 months from the time of symptom onset (7,8,94).

Regional Intravenous Block

An alternative method of producing temporary sympathetic interruption is by regional intravenous block. In this technique, an antisympathetic agent is delivered intravenously distal to a tourniquet placed around the painful extremity.

At the present time, guanethidine is probably the pharmacological agent of choice when regional blocks are used to treat causalgia or RSD. Guanethidine displaces norepinephrine from nerve endings and then blocks transmitter reuptake. RSD patients treated by regional intravenous guanethidine frequently report an initial burning sensation, presumably related to early release of norepinephrine from nerve terminals, followed by pain relief that lasts for hours to days (22,24,41). Because guanethidine blocks norepinephrine reuptake into nerve terminals, guanethidine's duration of action is usually longer than that of local anesthetics injected into the paravertebral ganglia (6,40). Guanethidine also does not interfere with cholinergic portions of the sympathetic nervous system, and so has no effect on sweating (45).

Few long-term data are available on the efficacy of regional intravenous guanethidine in treating the reflex sympathetic dystrophies. In the short and intermediate term, however, regional intravenous guanethidine appears to be equivalent to sympathetic paravertebral block. Pain relief has been reported to persist in some patients after regional guanethidine block during follow-up periods of 4 to 10 months (6,85). For both types of blocks, the results are reportedly better if treatment is begun early in the course of the disease (22,24) and if hyperpathia and allodynia are prominent (24,40).

One disadvantage to guanethidine treatment is that the drug is not currently approved for regional intravenous use in the United States. A small number of case reports have described the regional intravenous use of other drugs, such as reserpine or bretylium. Reserpine, however, does not appear to be a potent sympathetic blocker in normal individuals (45) and is described as less effective than guanethidine in the treatment of the reflex sympathetic dystrophies (24). Bretylium is also considered less advantageous than guanethidine because of its short duration of action (24,41).

Oral Antisympathetic Agents

Several case reports or uncontrolled series have described the successful use of oral antisympathetic agents in the treatment of the reflex sympathetic dystrophies. The alpha blocker guanethidine has been reported to be of benefit in RSD (85). The alpha blocker phenoxybenzamine was used by Ghostine et al. (21) to treat causalgia pain, and all 40 patients in this series were reportedly permanently relieved of pain during the follow-up period of 6 months to 6 years.

Beta blockers are probably less successful in relieving symptoms. Although a few case reports have described treatment of RSD with propranolol (62,79), a double-blind, cross-over study found propranolol to be of no benefit in the treatment of posttraumatic neuralgia (74).

Sympathectomy

Chemical or surgical sympathectomy is indicated when a series of sympathetic blocks produces complete but only transient relief of symptoms. Percutaneous, chemical sympathectomy produces sympathetic denervation for a period of weeks to months (7). This procedure is therefore most often indicated in the elderly or debilitated patient who is unable to tolerate major surgery.

Surgical sympathectomy offers the possibility of cure for many patients. Sympathetic ganglionectomy, first described by Spurling (81) in 1930, produces more complete sympathetic denervation than the periarterial sympathectomy earlier proposed by Leriche (35). In many institutions, sympathetic ganglionectomy has therefore become the treatment of choice for RSD and causalgia when sympathetic blocks produce only temporary relief.

The long-term success rate of sympathectomy has varied greatly from series to series (59). Experience gathered during World War II led many surgeons to believe that almost all causalgia patients could be cured by sympathectomy if the patient responded well to preoperative sympathetic blocks (3,43,80). Postoperative failure of pain relief was often thought to be the result of incomplete sympathetic denervation. However, following an initially successful sympathectomy, up to one-third of patients may develop recurrence of symptoms (99), even when the sympathectomy is apparently clinically complete (31). In some cases, pain in these patients may be mediated by sympathetic ganglia more rostral to those initially resected (26) or even by the sympathetic ganglia of the contralateral side (31).

Other Forms of Therapy

When the pain of causalgia or RSD proves refractory to sympathetic denervation, treatment of the patient becomes much more difficult. No single form of therapy appears to be of consistent value.

Narcotics are of only limited benefit, no matter whether delivered orally (72) or intraspinally (42). Nifedipine, a calcium channel blocker that produces peripheral vasodilation, was reported to relieve pain in seven of 13 patients in one preliminary study (65). A course of oral prednisone may also be helpful in some cases (32).

Stimulation of the peripheral or central nervous system will also sometimes produce pain relief. Meyer and Fields (47) report that transcutaneous nerve stimulation coupled with physical therapy reduced pain in six of eight causalgia patients when the stimulating electrodes were placed directly over the injured nerve proximal to the injury site. Spinal cord stimulation has also been used in the treatment of causalgia, with some groups reporting success rates as high as 70% to 90% (9,70) and others reporting success in only 20% of patients (100).

Physical therapy has been stressed by many clinicians as essential to the rehabilitation process (7,47,72,77). Unfortunately, most patients with severe pain are unable or unwilling to participate in a vigorous physical therapy program unless the pain can be eliminated by sympathetic blocks or other means. Psychiatric support may also be of help in these chronically disabled patients who often become severely depressed.

Recommended Therapy of the Reflex Sympathetic Dystrophies

In general, the optimal treatment of the reflex sympathetic dystrophies includes early treatment by sympathetic ganglion blocks or regional, antisympathetic blocks in conjunction with physical therapy. Oral alpha-blocking agents may be tried in patients who are unable or unwilling to receive repeated blocks. Transcutaneous nerve stimulation is benign and may also be tried, although in my own experience it has not proven very helpful. Surgical sympathectomy is indicated when sympathetic blockade produces definite but only transient relief of symptoms. For those patients who fail to respond to sympathetic interruption, there is no definitive form of therapy. A variety of different medications may be helpful in individual patients, and dorsal column stimulation is worth considering if the pain is refractory to other treatment modalities.

POSTHERPETIC NEURALGIA

PHN is a late sequela of a viral infection. In patients who have contracted chickenpox, the virus may lie latent for many years within dorsal root ganglia. Reactivation of the virus produces herpes zoster, a neurocutaneous syndrome characterized by severe pain and a vesicular rash in a dermatomal distribution. Eruptions occur most commonly in thoracic or trigeminal dermatomes. In the majority of patients, both the rash and the pain resolve within 3 months. Approximately 10% of these patients, however, will develop the severe and persistent pain of PHN. The likelihood of developing PHN is directly related to the patient's age at the time of the zoster eruption. PHN almost never appears in individuals under the age of 40, but 50% of elderly patients will develop PHN (10,38,82).

Like the pain of the reflex sympathetic dystrophies, the underlying pain of PHN is usually described as burning in quality. In addition, patients with PHN often describe stabs of pain lasting seconds to minutes. Allodynia and hyperpathia are prominent features of the syndrome. Allodynia may be so severe that the patient cuts out sections of his shirt in order to prevent the fabric from rubbing against painful regions.

Examination of the patient with PHN generally reveals only the healed scars of the initial zoster eruption (Fig. 31.2). Unlike the reflex sympathetic dystrophies, there is no evidence for sympathetic dysfunction. Also unlike the reflex sympathetic dystrophies, the pain does not spread to contiguous areas but remains confined to the dermatomes in which the eruption occurred.

The pathophysiological changes of an acute zoster infection involve both the skin and the nervous system. Inflammatory changes can be found in all levels of the skin and subcutaneous tissue, in peripheral nerves, in the dorsal root ganglia, in the dorsal and ventral horns of the spinal cord, and in ascending neural pathways (10,20,25,37,102). It is unknown whether the sympathetic ganglia are involved in the disease process. With resolution of the cutaneous eruption, regions of both degeneration and regeneration can be seen in peripheral nerves (38). In one study that evaluated peripheral nerve biopsies in four patients following herpetic eruption, no characteristic differences were found by either light or electron microscopy between patients with PHN and patients without persistent pain (102). Browder and DeVeer (10), however, describe persistent, active inflammatory changes in the skin in patients with PHN.

PHN is most commonly a disease of the elderly. This factor can complicate therapy, as the elderly, debilitated patient with PHN is often unable to tolerate the side effects of medication or the stresses of major surgery.

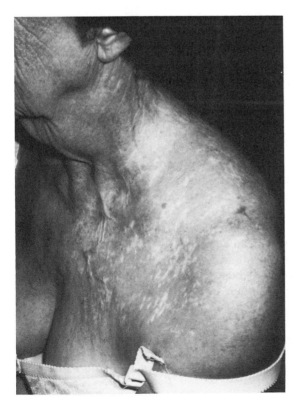

FIG. 31.2. Postherpetic scars in a woman with postherpetic neuralgia. Note the dermatomal distribution.

TREATMENT OF POSTHERPETIC NEURALGIA

Much has been written about the treatment of PHN. However, as noted by Robertson and George (71), the large number of proposed remedies indicates the difficult nature of the problem. In addition, few treatment modalities have been examined by controlled studies, and the majority of published therapeutic victories exist in the form of anecdotal case reports. In general, therefore, there is no single form of therapy that is widely recognized as optimal for the pain of PHN. Some forms of treatment appear to be more frequently beneficial than others, however.

Interruption of the Sympathetic Nervous System

Sympathetic interruption may help some patients with PHN but does not provide reliable amelioration of symptoms. Loh and Nathan (40) report that three of six patients with PHN had temporary relief of pain with sympathetic blocks and that one of these patients was cured by a series of blocks. Another report describes sympathetic blocks as improving pain in 70% of PHN patients followed for 1 month (48). Longer follow-up periods of 6 to 12 months, however, provide evidence that sympathetic blocks are of only doubtful value in the treatment of the postherpetic syndrome (13,14). Similarly, the results of surgical sympathectomy have been disappointing (10,82).

Topical and Local Treatment

In 1901, Mules (51) described a man with such severe pain from herpes zoster that the patient applied carriage varnish and liniment to his scalp, producing a skin slough down to the pericranium. Over the past century, a variety of other, less drastic forms of topical therapy have been recommended for the treatment of PHN. It is not surprising that local denervation should relieve allodynia, as allodynia is, by definition, dependent on neural circuits connecting the periphery with the central nervous system. What is perhaps more surprising is that local therapy can, in some cases, relieve not just the allodynia, but also the constant, burning pain.

Several anecdotal reports have described long-term relief of PHN following infiltration of the painful region with either local anesthetics (10) or steroids (34). Extensive undermining or resection of the involved skin has also been reported as helpful in many cases, although not all patients have been relieved of pain by the procedure (10,98). More recently, the topical application of powdered aspirin suspended in chloroform (30) or lotion (29) has been described as beneficial. Both the spontaneous pain and the allodynia of PHN are reported to respond to this kind of topical therapy (30). Two preliminary studies have also reported that topical capsaicin, a drug that first stimulates and then blocks small-diameter primary afferent fibers, benefits 55% to 75% of PHN patients (5,97). In my own experience, topical capsaicin reduces pain in many patients but is rarely curative. For maximal efficacy the drug should not be applied sporadically but used regularly three or four times a day.

Medical Therapy

Analgesics

Nonsteroidal anti-inflammatory agents are commonly prescribed for the treatment of PHN, but their efficacy is difficult to assess (71). Orally administered narcotics are generally ineffective (38,71). A few case reports have described relief of pain with intraspinally delivered narcotics, however (42,60).

Corticosteroids

A short course of corticosteroids is frequently prescribed during an attack of herpes zoster in the hope of preventing PHN. A recent review of the literature concluded that deficiencies in the published data make it impossible to determine whether or not this practice is actually effective (64). For established PHN, several anecdotal reports describe salutary effects of steroids delivered locally (34) or epidurally (17). Other investigators have failed to discover that epidural steroids are of benefit in any phase of the disease process (61).

Antidepressants

The tricyclic antidepressant amitriptyline is one of the few forms of therapy that controlled studies have demonstrated to be of benefit in the treatment of PHN. Approximately 50% of patients will exhibit good pain relief with amitriptyline or desipramine (95,96). The mechanism by which the drug reduces pain is unknown but is apparently independent of both its antidepressant effect and its effect on central serotonin levels (95,96). The addition of a phenothiazine to the treatment regimen will sometimes increase therapeutic efficacy (89).

Anticonvulsants

Several recent reviews have analyzed the efficacy of anticonvulsants in treating chronic pain states (41,84). In general, the sharp, shooting pain of PHN is likely to respond to anticonvulsant therapy, but both the steady burning pain and the allodynia associated with the condition tend to persist unabated.

Surgical Therapy

No surgical procedure has been reliably effective in treating PHN. A variety of destructive operations have been employed, including undermining or resection of the involved skin, peripheral neurectomy, rhizotomy, anterolateral cordotomy, sympathetic denervation, dorsal root entry zone (DREZ) lesions, thalamotomy, frontal lobotomy, and cortical resection. Although a few patients have improved dramatically with surgical therapy, none of these procedures has met with consistent success (10,18,82,88,98). Cordotomy is sometimes still used in many institutions to treat patients with severe pain refractory to other forms of treatment. As pain may recur after an initially successful operation, however, the procedure is probably best reserved for the elderly, debilitated patient with a short life expectancy. When cordotomy is successful, both the spontaneous burning pain and the allodynia are relieved. DREZ lesions are also sometimes employed to treat severe cases of PHN. The operation relieves or reduces pain in a significant proportion of patients, but lesion placement within the thoracic spinal cord carries a substantial risk of producing motor weakness in the elderly patient (18).

Stimulation of the spinal cord or of various intracranial sites may relieve pain in some patients. The reported success rate varies widely from series to series, however. Siegfried (78) described excellent results in eight of 10 patients with postherpetic facial pain who were treated by stimulation of the somatosensory thalamus and followed for 8 to 17 months postoperatively. Lower success rates of approximately 30% have been reported by other neurosurgeons with stimulation of the same brain site (28,44) or of the spinal cord (46).

Other Forms of Therapy

Transcutaneous nerve stimulation may be of benefit in some cases of PHN (48). This form of therapy is benign and is therefore worth trying, although in my own experience the results have been disappointing. As outlined in a recent review (38), there is no evidence that acupuncture, ultrasound, or diathermy are of any value. Psychiatric support can become important for the many patients with PHN who must learn to live with chronic pain.

Recommended Therapy for Postherpetic Neuralgia

At the present time, there is no course of treatment for PHN that can be recommended as curative. Amitriptyline, given with or without a phenothiazine, is likely to benefit some patients. The topical application of aspirin or capsaicin is a messy but benign form of therapy that may also prove useful. Transcutaneous nerve stimulation is worth trying. Surgical intervention should be restricted to those patients who are disabled by pain despite psychiatric support and medical therapy. DREZ lesions, anterolateral cordotomy, or central stimulation may be considered in these patients with severe, refractory pain; cordotomy is probably best reserved for patients with life expectancies of less than a year.

PAIN FOLLOWING CENTRAL NERVOUS SYSTEM INJURY

In 1906, Déjérine and Roussy (15) examined autopsy specimens in three patients and used the term "thalamic syndrome" to refer to a symptom complex consisting of hemiparesis, hemihypesthesia, hemiataxia, chorea, and pain. The pain in these patients was described as burning or crawling, with paroxysmal exacerbations that could be provoked by any type of cutaneous stimulation of the painful region. Subsequent to this report, many clinicians labeled this type of pain "thalamic pain." In fact, "thalamic pain" is not restricted to patients with lateral thalamic injuries. Similar painful symptoms may appear following damage to afferent sensory pathways at a number of different sites in the central nervous system, including the spinal cord, brain stem, and parietal or insular cortex (58). The onset of pain following injury is immediate in approximately one-third of patients and is delayed by days to years in the remainder (88). As in RSD and PHN, the course of the disease is variable, and symptoms may remit spontaneously or persist unchanged for years.

TREATMENT OF PAIN FOLLOWING CENTRAL NERVOUS SYSTEM INJURY

In their initial description of the thalamic syndrome, Déjérine and Roussy (15) wrote that the intense pain of the condition was refractory to all forms of treatment. Eighty-five years later, a cure remains elusive. In some cases, central pain resulting from spinal injuries can be treated effectively with DREZ lesions. With this exception, the pain that follows central nervous system injury remains notoriously difficult to treat.

Sympathetic Interruption

Surprisingly, sympathetic blockade will temporarily relieve symptoms in some patients with "thalamic pain" (24). Not all patients exhibit even transient relief of symptoms, however (93). In his excellent review of central pain, Pagni (58) wrote that the results of sympathetic blocks and sympathectomy were variable and that pain relief, when obtained, was always brief.

Medical Therapy

No large, controlled series has demonstrated definite benefit of any type of medical therapy for the treatment of pain following central nervous system injury. Analgesics, including narcotics, are usually ineffective (58,88). A few case reports have described symptomatic improvement with diphenylhydantoin (2,11,50). The combination of amitriptyline and a phenothiazine has also been reported as helpful (90).

Surgical Therapy

A wide variety of surgical approaches have been used to treat pain following central nervous system injury. Unfortunately, almost all surgical procedures have resulted in a few successes and a long string of failures. Both Pagni (58) and White and Sweet (98) reviewed the literature and concluded that the results of rhizotomy, anterolateral cordotomy, sympathectomy, and cortical resection were not encouraging. At the present time, the most common operations performed for the treatment of central pain are DREZ lesions, thalamotomy and/or mesencephalotomy, and central stimulation. One intriguing paper described successful treatment of three patients with thalamic pain by chemical hypophysectomy (36), but extensive experience with this technique in patients with central pain has not been reported.

Dorsal Root Entry Zone Lesions

DREZ lesions were first described by Nashold and Ostdahl (55) for the treatment of pain following brachial plexus avulsion injury. The operation is also effective, however, in some patients with pain following spinal injuries (56). In a series of 56 spine-injured patients followed for 6 months to 6 years, DREZ lesions produced long-term pain relief in 80% of those in whom pain was confined to dermatomes just caudal to the level of injury (18). When successful, the operation relieves both spontaneous burning pain and allodynia. The results of operation are less good, however, in patients with posttraumatic sacral pain or with diffuse pain below the level of the lesion (18). DREZ lesions are of particular interest, as this operation appears to be one of very few destructive procedures likely to produce long-term pain relief in a significant proportion of patients.

Thalamotomy and Mesencephalotomy

Medial thalamotomy and mesencephalotomy have been used, both alone and in combination, to treat central pain. Both good results and disappointments have been reported (1,73,87,98). In his review of thalamotomy, Pagni (58) wrote that about 25% of patients were improved but that results were often transient. Consistent with this view, Niizuma et al. (57) described a relatively large series of 18 patients with central pain who were treated by centromedian thalamotomy. About half of these patients improved immediately postoperatively, but pain recurred in all within 1 year. Similarly, in a review of mesencephalotomy, Nashold et al. (54) wrote that approximately 50% of patients with central pain benefit initially from the operation, but that the effect dissipates within 3 to 5 years. These authors noted a 37% complication rate and recommended that central stimulation be tried first.

Stimulation Procedures

Spinal cord stimulation has been used to treat pain associated with spinal cord injury. Although a few good, long-term results have been reported (92), the results have generally been disappointing (12,69,100,101). A recent series evaluated dorsal column stimulation in 15 patients with pain and paraplegia and noted that only 20% of patients responded to stimulation for more than 6 months. Pain relief was incomplete even in the responders, and the authors concluded that spinal cord stimulation was of no clinical benefit in the treatment of central deafferentation pain (46).

It is more difficult to assess the results of deep brain stimulation in the treatment of central pain. Most reported series include relatively few patients with central nervous system injury, and both the length of follow-up and the criteria for determining success vary greatly. Both good results and failures have been described (1,16,27,28,33,44,52,63,67,91,101). It appears from the literature, however, that approximately 50% of patients with central pain will respond to stimulation of the internal capsule or the specific sensory nuclei of the thalamus. Successful pain relief may be maintained for many years in some cases. It should be noted, however, that the definition of "success" varies from series to series, and some of the patients counted as good results have had only partial pain relief.

Recommended Therapy for Pain Following Central Nervous System Injury

Modern medicine can offer only imperfect remedies for the majority of patients with pain following central nervous system injury. When spinal cord injured patients complain of pain in dermatomes just caudal to the level of injury, DREZ lesions may offer an 80% chance of pain relief. For the remainder of patients, there is often no satisfactory solution. Antidepressants and anticonvulsants may benefit some individuals. Deep brain stimulation should be considered in cases of severe, intractable pain. Thalamotomy and mesencephalotomy are probably best reserved as therapies of last resort.

TOWARD BETTER TREATMENT OF HYPERALGESIA FOLLOWING NEURAL INJURY

At the present time, there is no reliable cure for the majority of patients with spontaneous burning pain and hyperalgesia. Until we know more about the anatomical and pathophysiological processes underlying this symptom complex, it is unlikely that better forms of therapy will be developed. The clinical data do suggest a few generalizations, however.

The pathophysiology of the pain that follows neural injury is almost certainly different from that of the pain of peripheral, irritative origin. Some types of peripheral injury, such as burns, produce a symptom complex of burning pain and allodynia similar to that seen following neural injury. If the same central pathways were activated similarly in both conditions, then one would expect the same forms of therapy to be effective in both disease states. Such is not the case. Narcotics are often helpful for the pain of burns but are of little value for the long-standing pain that follows neural injury. Similarly, stimulation of the internal capsule or the sensory thalamus appears to benefit some patients with pain following neural injuries, whereas stimulation of more medial sites does not; the reverse appears to be true in patients with pain of peripheral origin (28,33).

Several additional and often puzzling features characterize the pain that follows neural injury. The timing of pain onset is variable. One-third of patients develop pain immediately following central nervous system injury, for example, whereas symptom onset is delayed by days or even years in the remaining two-thirds (88). The course of the disease is also variable, and symptoms may remit spontaneously or persist unchanged for years. Finally, the development of pain appears to be partially idiosyncratic. Most patients with peripheral nerve injuries, herpes zoster, or central nervous system damage never develop chronic pain states. The factors contributing to an individual's susceptibility to chronic pain are unknown. Although genetic factors may play some role, it should also be noted that children almost never exhibit chronic pain following neural injury.

It is not certain which anatomical pathways or which types of pathophysiological processes are responsible for the development of pain following neural injury. It is possible, however, that central pain may be associated with destruction of neurons contributing to the neospinothalamic tract. Spontaneous pain and allodynia may appear with lesions at almost any point in the afferent sensory pathways. However, the great majority—and perhaps all—of these injuries involve neurons contributing to the neospinothalamic pathway or to its cortical projections (58,98). According to Pagni (58), no case of central pain has been reported in which the lesion was confined to the medially projecting, paleospinothalamic system.

There is also evidence to suggest that central pain states may be associated with abnormal activity in the spinoreticulothalamic pathways terminating in the medial thalamus. Tasker et al. (88) report that stimulation of the medial thalamus and medial midbrain elicits few or no somatosensory responses in patients with pain of peripheral origin. Stimulation of the same regions in patients with central pain, however, reproduces these patients' burning pain (88). Epileptiform activity has been recorded from the medial mesencephalic tegmentum during paroxysms of spontaneous pain in a patient with central pain. Stimulation of the same midbrain site in this patient reproduced the patient's pain, and destruction of this site resulted in pain relief (53). Spontaneous burst discharges have also been recorded from the human spinal cord in a patient with pain and paraplegia (39). It is unknown exactly which neural chains and thalamic nuclei are involved in these pathological changes, which neurotransmitters normally excite or inhibit these neurons, and whether abnormal activity is produced by deafferentation hypersensitivity, ephaptic transmission, loss of inhibition, or by some other factor.

The pathophysiology of the reflex sympathetic dystrophies is probably somewhat different from that of pain following central nervous system injury. As outlined in several recent reviews (8,59), there is good clinical and experimental evidence to suggest that abnormalities in both the peripheral and central nervous systems contribute to the syndrome. It is also possible that peripheral pathology may contribute to the pain of PHN. The anecdotal reports of symptomatic relief with the topical application of agents such as aspirin raise the possibility that irritation or hyperexcitability of peripheral receptors may contribute to the syndrome in some patients.

In the attempted treatment of pain following neural injury, almost every possible pathway in the peripheral or central nervous system has been cut or stimulated. With the possible exceptions of sympathectomy for some patients with RSD and of DREZ lesions for some patients with spinal injuries, no successful form of therapy has been derived. It therefore seems unlikely that further experimentation with lesion or electrode placement will produce a dramatic breakthrough in the therapy of these difficult patients. More successful forms of therapy are likely to be based on a better understanding of the pathophysiological mechanisms involved in the disease process, and, in particular, on the pharmacological manipulation of excitability within particular neuronal pools.

REFERENCES

1. Adams, J. E., Hosobuchi, Y., and Fields, H. L. (1974): Stimulation of internal capsule for relief of chronic pain. *J. Neurosurg.*, 41:740–744.
2. Agnew, D. C. (1976): A brief trial of phenytoin therapy for thalamic pain. *Bull. Los Angeles Neurol. Soc.*, 41:9–12.
3. Barnes, R. (1953): The role of sympathectomy in the treatment of causalgia. *J. Bone Joint Surg.*, 35B:172–180.
4. Bentley, J. B., and Hameroff, S. R. (1980): Diffuse reflex sympathetic dystrophy. *Anesthesiology*, 53:256–257.
5. Bernstein, J. E., Bickers, D. R., Dahl, M. V., and Roshal, J. Y. (1987): Treatment of chronic postherpetic neuralgia with topical capsaicin. A preliminary study. *J. Am. Acad. Dermatol.*, 17:93–96.
6. Bonelli, S., Conoscente, F., Movilia, P. G., Restelli, L., Francucci, B., and Grossi, E. (1983): Regional intravenous guanethidine vs. stellate ganglion block in reflex sympathetic dystrophies: a randomized trial. *Pain*, 16:297–307.
7. Bonica, J. J. (1979): Causalgia and other reflex sympathetic dystrophies. *Adv. Pain Res. Ther.*, 3:141–166.
8. Bonica, J. J. (1990): Causalgia and other reflex sympathetic dystrophies. In: *The management of pain*, edited by J. J. Bonica, pp. 220–243. Lea and Febiger, Philadelphia.
9. Broseta, J., Roldan, P., Gonzalez-Darder, J., Bordes, V., and Barcia-Salorio, J. L. (1982):

Chronic epidural dorsal column stimulation in the treatment of causalgic pain. *Appl. Neurophysiol.*, 45:190–194.

10. Browder, J., and DeVeer, J. A. (1949): Herpes zoster: a surgical procedure for the treatment of postherpetic neuralgia. *Ann. Surg.*, 130:622–636.
11. Cantor, F. K. (1972): Phenytoin treatment of thalamic pain. *B.M.J.*, 4:590.
12. Clark, K. (1975): Electrical stimulation of the nervous system for control of pain. *Surg. Neurol.*, 4:164–166.
13. Colding, A. (1969): The effect of regional sympathetic blocks in the treatment of herpes zoster. A survey of 300 cases. *Acta Anaesthesiol. Scand.*, 13:133–141.
14. Colding, A. (1973): Treatment of pain: organization of a pain clinic: treatment of herpes zoster. *Proc. R. Soc. Med.*, 66:541–543.
15. Déjérine, J., and Roussy, G. (1906): Le syndrome thalamique. *Rev. Neurol. (Paris)*, 14:521–532.
16. Dieckman, G., and Witzman, A. (1982): Initial and long-term results of deep brain stimulation for chronic intractable pain. *Appl. Neurophysiol.*, 45:167–172.
17. Forrest, J. B. (1978): Management of chronic dorsal root pain with epidural steroid. *Can. Anaesth. Soc. J.*, 25:218–225.
18. Friedman, A. H., and Bullitt, E. (1988): Dorsal root entry zone lesions in the treatment of pain following brachial plexus avulsion, spinal cord injury, and herpes zoster. *Appl. Neurophysiol.*, 51:164–169.
19. Gerard, R. W. (1951): The physiology of pain: abnormal neuron states in causalgia and related phenomena. *Am. Soc. Anesthesiol.*, 12:1–13.
20. Ghatak, N. R., and Zimmerman, H. M. (1973): Spinal ganglion in herpes zoster. *Arch. Pathol.*, 95:411–415.
21. Ghostine, S. Y., Comair, Y. G., Turner, D. M., Kassell, N. F., and Azar, C. G. (1984): Phenoxybenzamine in the treatment of causalgia. Report of 40 cases. *J. Neurosurg.*, 60:1263–1268.
22. Hannington-Kiff, J. G. (1977): Relief of Sudeck's atrophy by regional intravenous guanethidine. *Lancet*, 1:1132–1133.
23. Hannington-Kiff, J. G. (1979): Relief of causalgia in limbs by regional intravenous guanethidine. *B.M.J.*, 2:367–368.
24. Hannington-Kiff, J. G. (1982): Hyperadrenergic-effected limb causalgia: relief by IV pharmacologic norepinephrine blockade. *Am. Heart J.*, 103:152–153.
25. Head, H. (1900): The pathology of herpes zoster and its bearing on sensory localisation. *Brain*, 23-3:23–523.
26. Hoffert, M. J., Greenberg, R. P., Wolskee, P. J., et al. (1984): Abnormal and collateral innervations of sympathetic and peripheral sensory fields associated with a case of causalgia. *Pain*, 20:1–12.
27. Hosobuchi, Y. (1980): The current status of analgesic brain stimulation. *Acta Neurochir. Suppl. (Wien)*, 30:219–227.
28. Hosobuchi, Y. (1986): Subcortical electrical stimulation for control of intractable pain in humans. Report of 122 cases (1970–1984) *J. Neurosurg.*, 64:543–533.
29. Kassirer, M. R. (1988): King and Robert, concerning the management of pain associated with herpes zoster and of postherpetic neuralgia, *Pain*, 33: 73–88; 35:368–369.
30. King, R. B. (1988): Concerning the management of pain associated with herpes zoster and of postherpetic neuralgia. *Pain*, 33:73–88.
31. Kleiman, A. (1954): Causalgia. Evidence of the existence of crossed sensory fibers. *Am. J. Surg.*, 87:839–841.
32. Kozin, F., Ryan, L. M., Carerra, G. F., Soin, J. S., and Wortmann, R. L. (1981): The reflex sympathetic dystrophy syndrome (RSDS). III. Scintigraphic studies: further evidence for the therapeutic efficacy of systemic corticosteroids and proposed diagnostic criteria. *Am. J. Med.*, 70:23–30.
33. Kumar, K., Wyant, G. M., and Nath, R. (1990): Deep brain stimulation for control of intractable pain in humans, present and future: a ten-year follow up. *Neurosurgery* 26:774–782.
34. Lefkovits, A. M. (1961): Postherpetic neuralgia. A method of effective treatment. *Neurology*, 11:170–171.
35. Leriche, R. (1916): De la causalgie envisagée comme une névrite du sympathique et son traitement par la denudation et l'excision des plexus nerveux periarteriels. *Presse Med.*, 24:178–180.
36. Levin, A. B., Ramirez, L. F., and Katz, J. (1963): The use of stereotaxic chemical hypophysectomy in the treatment of thalamic pain syndrome. *J. Neurosurg.*, 59:1002–1006.
37. Lhermite, J., and Nicolas. (1924): Les lesions spinales du Zona. La myelite zosterienne. *Rev. Neurol. (Paris)*, 4:361–364.
38. Loeser, J. D. (1986): Herpes zoster and postherpetic neuralgia. *Pain*, 25:149–164.
39. Loeser, J. D., Ward, A. A., and White, L. E. (1968): Chronic deafferentation of human spinal cord neurons. *J. Neurosurg.*, 29:48–50.
40. Loh, L., and Nathan, W. (1978): Painful peripheral states and sympathetic blocks. *J. Neurol. Neurosurg. Psychiatry*, 41:664–671.

41. Maciewicz, R., Bouckoms, A., and Martin, J. B. (1985): Drug therapy of neuropathic pain. *Clin. J. Pain,* 1:39–49.
42. Magora, F., Olshwang, D., Eimerl, D., et al. (1980): Observations on extradural morphine analgesia in various pain conditions. *Br. J. Anaesth.,* 52:247–252.
43. Mayfield, F. H. (1951): *Causalgia.* Charles C. Thomas, Springfield, IL.
44. Mazars, G. J. (1975): Intermittent stimulation of nucleus ventralis posterolateralis for intractable pain. *Surg. Neurol.,* 4:93–95.
45. McKain, C. W., Urban, B. J., and Goldner, J. L. (1983): The effects of intravenous regional guanethidine and reserpine. *J. Bone Joint Surg.,* 65A:808–811.
46. Meglio, M., Cioni, B., and Rossi, G. F. (1989): Spinal cord stimulation in the management of chronic pain. A 9-year experience. *J. Neurosurg.,* 70:519–524.
47. Meyer, G. A., and Fields, H. L. (1972): Causalgia treated by selective large fibre stimulation of peripheral nerve. *Brain,* 95:163–168.
48. Milligan, N. S., and Nash, T. P. (1985): Treatment of post-herpetic neuralgia. A review of 77 consecutive cases. *Pain,* 23:381–386.
49. Mitchell, S. W. (1872): *Injuries of nerves and their consequences.* J. B. Lippincott, Philadelphia.
50. Mladinich, E. K. (1974): Diphenylhydantoin in the Wallenberg syndrome. *J.A.M.A.,* 230: 372–373.
51. Mules, P. H. (1901): Paralysis of third nerve, with unusual complications. *Trans. Ophthal. Soc. U. K.,* 21:292–296.
52. Namba, S., Nakao, Y., Matsumoto, Y., Ohmoto, T., and Nishimoto, A. (1984): Electrical stimulation of the posterior limb of the internal capsule for treatment of thalamic pain. *Appl. Neurophysiol.,* 47:137–148.
53. Nashold, B. S., and Wilson, W. P. (1966): Central pain. Observations on man with chronic implanted electrodes in the midbrain tegmentum. *Confin. Neurol.,* 27:30–44.
54. Nashold, B. S., Slaughter, D. G., Wilson, W. P., and Zorub, D. (1977): Stereotactic mesencephalotomy. *Prog. Neurol. Surg.,* 8:35–49.
55. Nashold, B. S., and Ostdahl, R. H. (1979): Dorsal root entry zone lesions for pain relief. *J. Neurosurg.,* 51:59–69.
56. Nashold, B. S., and Bullitt, E. (1981): Dorsal root entry zone lesions to control pain in paraplegia. *J. Neurosurg.,* 55:414–419.
57. Niizuma, H., Kwak, R., Ikeda, S., Ohyama, H., Suzuki, J., and Saso, S. (1982): Follow-up results of centromedian thalamotomy for central pain. *Appl. Neurophysiol.,* 45:324–325.
58. Pagni, C. A. (1976): Central pain and painful anesthesia. *Prog. Neurol. Surg.,* 8:132–257.
59. Payne, R. (1986): Neuropathic pain syndromes, with special reference to causalgia and reflex sympathetic dystrophy. *Clin. J. Pain,* 2:59–73.
60. Penn, R. D., and Paice, J. A. (1987): Chronic intrathecal morphine for intractable pain. *J. Neurosurg.,* 67:182–186.
61. Perkins, H. M., and Hanlon, P. R. (1978): Epidural injection of local anesthetic and steroids for relief of pain secondary to herpes zoster. *Arch. Surg.,* 113:253–254.
62. Pleet, A. B., Tahmoush, A. J., and Jennings, J. R. (1976): Causalgia: treatment with propranolol. *Neurology,* 26:375.
63. Plotkin, R. (1982): Results in 60 cases of deep brain stimulation for chronic intractable pain. *Appl. Neurophysiol.,* 45:173–178.
64. Post, B. T., and Philbrick, J. T. (1988): Do corticosteroids prevent postherpetic neuralgia? *J. Am. Acad. Dermatol.,* 18:605–610.
65. Prough, D. S., McLeskey, C. H., Poehling, G. G., et al. (1985): Efficacy of oral nifedipine in the treatment of reflex sympathetic dystrophy. *Anesthesiology,* 62:796–799.
66. Rasmussen, T. B., and Freedman, H. (1946): Treatment of causalgia: an analysis of 100 cases. *J. Neurosurg.,* 3:165–173.
67. Ray, C. D., and Burton, C. V. (1980): Deep brain stimulation for severe, chronic pain. *Acta Neurochir. Suppl. (Wien),* 30:289–293.
68. Richards, R. L. (1967): Causalgia. A centennial review. *Arch. Neurol.,* 16:339–350.
69. Richardson, R. R., Siqueira, E. B., and Cerullo, L. J. (1979): Spinal epidural stimulation for treatment of acute and chronic intractable pain: initial and longterm results. *Neurosurgery,* 5:344–348.
70. Robaina, F. J., Dominguez, M., Diaz, M., Rodriguez, J. L., and de Vera, J. A. (1989): Spinal cord stimulation for the relief of chronic pain in vasospastic disorders of the upper limbs. *Neurosurgery,* 24:63–67.
71. Robertson, D. R. C., and George, C. F. (1990): Treatment of post herpetic neuralgia in the elderly. *Br. Med. Bull.,* 46:113–123.
72. Rowlingson, J. C. (1983): The sympathetic dystrophies. *Int. Anesthesiol. Clin.,* 21:117–129.
73. Sano, K. (1977): Intralaminar thalamotomy (thalamolaminotomy) and posteromedial hypothalamotomy in the treatment of intractable pain. *Prog. Neurol. Surg.,* 8:50–103.

74. Scadding, J. W., Wall, P. B., Wynn Parry, C. B., and Brooks, D. M. (1982): Clinical trial of propranolol in post-traumatic neuralgia. *Pain,* 14:283–292.
75. Schwartzman, R. J., and McLellan, T. J. (1987): Reflex sympathetic dystrophy. A review. *Arch. Neurol.,* 44:555–561.
76. Seddon, H. (1975): *Surgical disorders of the peripheral nerves.* Churchill Livingstone, Edinburgh.
77. Shumacker, H. B. (1985): A personal overview of causalgia and other reflex dystrophies. *Ann. Surg.,* 201:278–289.
78. Siegfried, J. (1982): Monopolar electrical stimulation of nucleus ventroposteromedialis thalami for postherpetic facial pain. *Appl. Neurophysiol.,* 45:179–184.
79. Simson, G. (1974): Propranolol for causalgia and Sudek atrophy. *J.A.M.A.,* 227:327.
80. Slessor, A. J. (1948): Causalgia: a review of 22 cases. *Edinburgh Med. J.,* 55:563–571.
81. Spurling, R. G. (1930): Causalgia of the upper extremity. Treatment by dorsal sympathetic ganglionectomy. *Arch. Neurol. Psychiatr.,* 23:784–788.
82. Sugar, O., and Bucy, P. C. (1951): Postherpetic trigeminal neuralgia. *Arch. Neurol. Psychiatr.,* 65:131–145.
83. Sunderland, S., and Kelly, M. (1948): The painful sequelae of injuries to peripheral nerves. *Aust. N. Z. J. Surg.,* 18:75–118.
84. Swerdlow, M. (1984): Anticonvulsant drugs and chronic pain. *Clin. Neuropharmacol.,* 7:51–82.
85. Tabira, T., Shibasaki, H., and Kuroiwa, Y. (1983): Reflex sympathetic dystrophy (causalgia) treatment with guanethidine. *Arch. Neurol.,* 40:430–432.
86. Tahmoush, A. J. (1981): Causalgia: redefinition as a clinical pain syndrome. *Pain,* 10:187–197.
87. Tasker, R. R. (1990): Pain resulting from central nervous system pathology (central pain). In: *The management of pain,* edited by J. J. Bonica, pp. 264–283. Lea and Febiger, Philadelphia.
88. Tasker, R. R., Tsuda, T., and Hawrylyshyn, P. (1983): Clinical neurophysiological investigation of deafferentation pain. *Adv. Pain Res. Ther.,* 5:713–738.
89. Taub, A., (1973): Relief of postherpetic neuralgia with psychotropic drugs. *J. Neurosurg.,* 39:235–239.
90. Taub, A., and Collins, W. F. (1974): Observations on the treatment of 11 denervation dysesthesia with psychotropic drugs: postherpetic neuralgia, anesthesia dolorosa, peripheral neuropathy. *Adv. Neurol.,* 4:309–316.
91. Turnbull, I. M., Shulman, R., and Woodhurst, B. (1980): Thalamic stimulation for neuropathic pain. *J. Neurosurg.,* 52:486–493.
92. Urban, B. J., and Nashold, B. S. (1978): Percutaneous epidural stimulation of the spinal cord for the relief of pain. Long term results. *J. Neurosurg.,* 48:323–328.
93. Waltz, T. A., and Ehni, G. (1966): The thalamic syndrome and its mechanism. Report of two cases, one due to arteriovenous malformation in the thalamus. *J. Neurosurg.,* 24:735–742.
94. Wang, J. K., Johnson, K. A., and Ilstrup, D. M. (1985): Sympathetic blocks for reflex sympathetic dystrophy. *Pain,* 23:13–17.
95. Watson, C. P., Evans, R. J., Reed, K., Merskey, H., Goldsmith, L., and Warsh, J. (1982): Amitriptyline versus placebo in postherpetic neuralgia. *Neurology,* 32:671–673.
96. Watson, C. P. N., and Evans, R. J. (1985): A comparative trial of amitriptyline and zimelidine in post-herpetic neuralgia. *Pain,* 23:387–394.
97. Watson, C. P., Evans, R. J., and Watt, V. R. (1988): Post-herpetic neuralgia and topical capsaicin. *Pain,* 33:333–340.
98. White, J. C., and Sweet, W. H. (1969): *Pain and the neurosurgeon. A forty-year experience.* Charles C. Thomas, Springfield, IL.
99. Wirth, F. P., and Rutherford, R. B. (1970): A civilian experience with causalgia. *Arch. Surg.,* 100:633–638.
100. Young, R. F. (1978): Evaluation of dorsal column stimulation in the treatment of chronic pain. *Neurosurgery,* 3:373–379.
101. Young, R. F. (1987): Brain and spinal stimulation: how and to whom! *Clin. Neurosurg.,* 35: 429–447.
102. Zacks, S. I., Langfitt, T. W., and Elliott, F. A. (1964): Herpetic neuritis. A light and electron microscopic study. *Neurology,* 14:744–750.

Hyperalgesia and Allodynia,
edited by W. D. Willis, Jr.
Raven Press, Ltd., New York © 1992.

32

Hyperalgesia and Allodynia in Patients with CNS Lesions

Jörgen Boivie

Department of Neurology, University Hospital, S-581 85 Linköping, Sweden

Already Head and Holmes (14) pointed out that excessive, often painful, reactions to touch, cold, heat, and various other stimuli are a common feature in patients with central pain. This has been most vividly described in central pain caused by thalamic lesions, i.e., thalamic pain.

Since this is the best known central pain condition, all central pain caused by brain lesions has often been called thalamic pain, thereby giving the impression that such overreactions and central pain are only caused by thalamic lesions. It might seem natural to think so, because of the crucial role of thalamic relays in somatosensory functions. It is nevertheless wrong, because it has been clearly shown by modern imaging techniques that in about half of the patients the lesions do not involve the thalamus. Thus, lesions caudal to the thalamus, mainly in the lower part of the brain stem, and lesions lateral and superior to the thalamus, including cortical ones, can also cause these symptoms (17,21,25).

Most patients with traumatic spinal cord injuries (SCI) have pain. Some of them have central pain, often of a dysesthetic kind (2,11). Sometimes these patients have painful reactions to external stimuli (12,13). But also other lesions in the spinal cord, like those caused by multiple sclerosis (MS), syringomyelia, and vascular malformations, can induce hyperalgesia and central pain (25; below).

The use of the term "hyperalgesia" is discussed in other chapters of this book. Those discussions relate to the occurrence of the phenomenon following events in the peripheral nervous system. In that context one distinguishes primary hyperalgesia, with mainly peripheral mechanisms, from secondary hyperalgesia, with important central mechanisms that are induced by events in the periphery. Hyperalgesias caused by CNS lesions cannot be separated into primary and secondary ones.

Allodynia is closely related to hyperalgesia. The Taxonomy Committee of the International Association for the Study of Pain (IASP) defined allodynia as "pain due to a stimulus which does not normally provoke pain," whereas hyperalgesia was defined as "an increased response to a stimulus which is normally painful" (23).

Both hyperalgesia and allodynia are thus neurological signs that involve pain evoked by stimuli. In this chapter the IASP definitions of the terms will be used. Spontaneous pain, or pain evoked by other events, may or may not be present in regions with hyperalgesia and allodynia. However, as will be evident from this chapter, these signs are mainly found in patients with CNS lesions that have also caused central pain.

FEATURES OF HYPERALGESIA AND ALLODYNIA IN CNS DISEASES

Many questions can be asked about hyperalgesia and allodynia (H/A) in CNS diseases. For instance,

1. Which CNS lesions can induce H/A?
2. Do they only occur in patients with central pain?
3. Is the onset immediate or delayed?
4. Are they constant or intermittent? Do they disappear spontaneously?
5. In which regions are H/A found, i.e., what is their location?
6. To which stimuli do they occur? What determines the character of the overreactions?
7. Are they always accompanied by changes in perception threshold for the stimulus in question?
8. How intense are the overreactions? Is there any relationship between this and the magnitude of other sensory abnormalities?
9. Which are the mechanisms?
10. Is there any treatment for H/A? (This is discussed in the chapter by Bullitt.)

Unfortunately not enough information is available regarding several of these features, so some questions cannot be answered. This chapter reviews the information that can be found in the literature on the subject and reports partly unpublished results from our own studies of patients with stroke and syringomyelia.

CNS LESIONS CAUSING HYPERALGESIA AND ALLODYNIA

A variety of diseases in the brain and spinal cord can induce H/A (Table 32.1). The most common causes are cerebrovascular lesions (CVL), MS, and SCI, but the incidences of H/A are not known. Although the total number of patients with syringomyelia and syringobulbia is low, they may be next in order of frequency with regard to H/A, because they appear to have a particularly high risk of developing central pain and H/A (see below). Details about results from recent studies on patients with CVL and syringomyelia/syringobulbia will be given below, while more brief comments will be made on the other patient groups.

Pain is common in patients with MS. Prevalences of 29% and 55% for patients were found in two recent studies (10,24). Central pain was suspected in about 30% to 40% of the patients studied by Moulin et al. (24). It was mostly of a burning kind ("dysesthetic pain"). No information about H/A was given in the reports. However,

TABLE 32.1. *Diseases in the CNS causing hyperalgesia and allodynia*

Vascular lesions in the brain and spinal cord
  Infarcts
  Hemorrhages
  Vascular malformations
Multiple sclerosis
Traumatic spinal cord injuries
Syringomyelia and syringobulbia
Tumors
Inflammatory diseases other than multiple sclerosis, myelitis by viruses, syphilis

from our own ongoing study we know that these signs are found in some of the MS patients, but they seem to be less common than evoked and spontaneous paresthesias (A. Österberg, J. Boivie, A. Henriksson, and H. Holmgren, *in progress*).

Traumatic SCI are well-known causes of central pain (2,11). In patients with incomplete spinal cord lesions, the pain is usually dysesthetic in character. As in MS, the frequency of H/A has not been studied in SCI patients. An illustrative case was reported by Holmes as early as 1919 [15; cited by Riddoch (26)]. This was a patient with a traumatic SCI in the cervical enlargement. On the first day a "constant, dull, gnawing and aching pain developed in the legs, associated with painful stiffness and numbness. Periodically, violent, shooting pain, like red-hot knives would dart from the patient's foot or knee to his abdomen and down again. Paroxysms of severe burning and tingling of short duration spread over his leg, if it were touched even gently, and the most intense pain was evoked by rubbing or moving his limb" (26).

On examination the patient was completely paralytic in his right leg, completely analgesic and thermoanesthetic on the left side from Th3 down and on the right arm and right side of the chest. On the right leg, light touch was well perceived, but a moving touch stimulus evoked a sensation of cold, followed by tingling and pain, i.e., allodynia to touch. Rubbing with fingers on the leg evoked an awful pain that shot up to the waist. Thermal stimuli also evoked overreactions; water of 24°C was painful and moderate heat felt burning. There was moderate hyperalgesia to pinprick on the right leg, with spread of the sensation up and down. Later the spontaneous pain decreased, but the objective sensory disturbances including the overreactions remained unaltered.

This case shows that SCI can cause central pain as well as H/A to various stimuli, and hyperpathia, i.e., exaggerated painful reactions with a high magnitude. It also shows that these phenomena can start early after an injury.

A condition including painful overreactions to stimuli and central pain sometimes also develops after spinal cordotomies done for relief of intractable pain (25,28). Pagni (25) reports that these patients may develop feelings of "glacial cold, burning pain sometimes with hyperpathia and hyperesthesia." These symptoms can be present in analgesic regions. They may be particularly common after midbrain spinothalamic tractotomies (25).

Tumors in the brain and spinal cord may cause H/A and central pain, but fortunately do so infrequently, possibly with the exception of thalamic tumors, which seem to carry a higher risk (25).

HYPERALGESIA AND ALLODYNIA AFTER CEREBROVASCULAR LESIONS

For some patients with CVL, pain and painful reactions to external stimuli are their major handicap. Many of these patients do not have any of the stroke symptoms that are mainly discussed in texts on stroke, like paresis, dysphasia, ataxia, or visual field defects. Instead they have sensory disturbances and central pain, i.e., pain caused by the CVL itself, although about half of the patients with central poststroke pain (CPSP) have one or more of the other symptoms as well.

Since this chapter deals with H/A, one pertinent question is whether only stroke patients with CPSP have these symptoms. In the only study that gives good information on this issue, allodynia was found only in patients with central pain, but mild hyperalgesia, tested as increased response to pinprick, was found also in two of 20 patients without central pain (18). This kind of hyperalgesia can be considered to be a kind of hyperesthesia, and hyperesthesias are not restricted to central pain patients. However, it appears that allodynia and severe hyperalgesias almost solely occur in patients who also have spontaneous central pain. To learn more about H/A, it is therefore natural to investigate patients with CPSP.

Studies in recent years have provided new knowledge about stroke patients with such symptoms (5,8,16–18,21,22,27). One basic insight relates to which lesions may result in the development of central pain. Contrary to what has previously been thought, it appears that only about half of all patients with CPSP have lesions that involve the thalamus (17,21). In our study, nine of 27 patients with CPSP had thalamic lesions, most of which extended lateral to the thalamus, some considerably so (17). Eight of the patients in that study had low brain stem lesions and six had extrathalamic, subcortical lesions. In the study done with magnetic resonance imaging (MRI), 17 of 36 patients had thalamic lesions (21).

Thus, thalamic lesions are common, but they do not dominate among patients with central pain. Is any particular part of the thalamus crucial for the development of this pain and H/A? In our study, all lesions involved the posterolateral part of the thalamus, i.e., the ventrobasal region where the largest somatosensory relay nuclei are located, but in most patients the lesion extended lateral to the thalamus. More specific information on this question was obtained by Bougosslavsky et al., (3), who studied patients with infarcts restricted to the thalamus. They found that central pain was only induced by lesions in the ventroposterior thalamic region. Three of 16 patients with such lesions developed central pain. This indicates that this region is indeed crucial in this respect, and it is reasonable to deduce that it is also crucial for the development of H/A.

Recently studied patients confirm that extrathalamic, subcortical lesions can also cause central pain and H/A (17,21). A case with a superficially located hemorrhage in the medial part of the right parietal lobe (Fig. 32.1) due to an arteriovenous malformation illustrates this (6). In this patient the lesion was located well above the roof of the lateral ventricle. On the first day after the onset and 2 months later, this

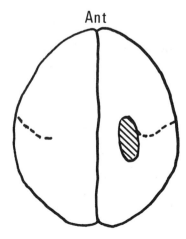

Ant

FIG. 32.1. Reconstruction from computed tomography of a superficial hemorrhage at the central sulcus of the right cerebral hemisphere. (From ref. 6.)

30-year-old man had hyperalgesia to pinprick and allodynia to cold and warmth below Th6 on the left side, where he also had "decreased sensation to light touch." Interestingly he did not have spontaneous central pain.

Stroke lesions in the lower brain stem are of particular interest, because some of these lesions affect the spinothalamic tract without injuring the medial lemniscal pathway. This is usually the case in patients with complete or partial Wallenberg's syndrome (7). The risk of developing central pain and H/A might be as great in patients with this kind of CVL, as in patients with thalamic or subcortical CVL (17). Eight of our 27 patients with CPSP had low brain stem lesions, and three of these had H/A.

There are no indications that there is any relative difference between infarcts and hemorrhages in the incidence of H/A and central pain. Thus, it appears to be the fact that infarcts are about six times more common than hemorrhages that explains why more patients with CPSP have infarcts than hemorrhages.

TEMPORAL AND SPATIAL ASPECTS OF HYPERALGESIA AND ALLODYNIA IN STROKE PATIENTS, AND STIMULUS MODALITY

From available information it appears that H/A, like spontaneous central pain, often develop with a delay after the onset of the stroke. This delay may be as long as 2 to 3 years, but in some patients the onset is immediate (17). In some cases with initial marked loss of sensibility, the H/A and CPSP appear to start when the patient experiences the successive onset of spontaneous paresthesias or dysesthesias.

The question of whether H/A may be intermittent or constant does not appear to have been investigated. From comparisons with CPSP, one would expect that they are constant in most patients. They probably disappear spontaneously with time in some patients but continue for many years in most.

The regions with H/A may be large in stroke patients, sometimes involving the whole left or right side, like the central pain. But in other patients they cover just one extremity or one side of the face (J. Boivie and G. Leijon, *unpublished observations*). We have, for instance, had one patient with Wallenberg's syndrome and central pain who had hyperalgesia to pinprick and allodynia to cold and touch on the left side of the face and right leg and foot. The hyperesthesias are more intense in some parts of the involved regions than in others. It is our impression that the overreactions are more common in the hands and feet than more proximally on the extremities or on the trunk, but we have not systematically studied that.

As in other patient groups, allodynia appears to be more common to cold than to warmth or touch in stroke patients (Table 32.2) (5,18). Contrary to this, overreactions to noxious heat were more commonly observed than to cold in the noxious range. For many of the CPSP patients, a sudden onset of intense heat was the first reaction when the Thermotest stimulator was heated to 45° to 50°C. These patients had lost the sensibility to innoxious heat completely. Many of them had also lost the sensibility to innoxious cold, but deep cooling did not evoke a corresponding sudden onset of cold pain. Instead cold pain would increase successively in a way that appeared to be quite normal, if cold pain was perceived at all. However, we did not systematically examine that with magnitude estimations.

Allodynia to vibration has also been found. Thus, some of our patients experienced increased pain when vibration was tested with the Vibrameter vibrating on

TABLE 32.2. *Portion of CPSP patients with overreactions to somatic stimuli in study by Boivie et al. (5) and with allodynia in study by Leijon and Bowsher (18)*

	BS	TH	SE	UI	All
Hyperesthesia					
Touch	3/7	5/9	2/5	2/4	12/25 (48%)
Cold	4/7	6/9	2/5	2/4	14/25 (56%)
Allodynia					
Touch	0/7	1/8	0/4	0/3	1/22 (5%)
Cold	2/7	3/8	0/4	0/3	5/22 (23%)
Hyperalgesia pinprick	3/7	8/9	3/5	2/4	16/25 (64%)
Allodynia (Leijon-Bowsher, ref. 18)					
Touch					28%
Cold					42%
All					57%

BS, cerebrovascular lesion (CVL) in the brain stem; TH, CVL involving the thalamus; SE, supratentorial, extrathalamic CVL; UI, location of CVL not identified.

bones (metacarpals, metatarsals, tibia). In some instances this stimulus seemed to evoke a pain that was different from their ongoing pain.

It is common that ongoing pain is increased by stimuli and activities. Should that be called H/A? There is as yet no answer to that question. This has been found for touch, cold, and heat, as well as for joint movements, which by themselves are not painful (17). A change in posture was in some patients an aggravating stimulus.

THRESHOLD ABNORMALITIES IN STROKE PATIENTS WITH HYPERALGESIA AND ALLODYNIA

It is not clear whether there can be painful overreactions, i.e., H/A, to a stimulus modality without a concomitant abnormality in perception threshold. We have observed hyperesthesias to touch without threshold changes, but those patients did not have allodynia (5).

The results from our studies on patients with CPSP show that there is a large variation in the pattern of threshold abnormalities to vibration, touch, cold, warmth, and temperature pain among these patients, but they also show that one feature is common to almost all patients, namely, an abnormality in temperature and pain sensibility (Table 32.3) (5,18). The latter is in contrast to the thresholds to vibration and touch, which are normal in about half of the patients.

These results led to the hypothesis that central pain only develops in patients who

TABLE 32.3. *Portion of CPSP patients with threshold abnormalities according to quantitative sensory tests*

	BS	TH	SE	UI	All
Vibration	1/8	7/9	3/6	0/4	11/27 (40%)
Touch	2/8	8/9	2/6	2/4	14/27 (52%)
Innocuous temperature	8/8	9/9	6/6	4/4	27/27 (100%)
Temperature pain	7/8	9/9	5/6	4/4	25/27 (93%)

BS, CVL in the brain stem; TH, CVL involving the thalamus; SE, supratentorial, extrathalamic CVL; UI, location of CVL not identified.
From ref. 5.

have a lesion that involves the spinothalamic pathways, as indicated by abnormal temperature and pain sensibility (4,5).

The conclusion about the abnormal functions in the two major somatosensory pathways in patients with CPSP has also been tested with electrophysiological methods, namely, with the evoked response technique. In the first study the short latency cortical responses to electrical stimuli of the median and tibial nerves were examined (16). The results confirmed previous results showing that stroke patients with abnormal thresholds to touch and vibration have abnormal somatosensory evoked responses (SEP). This SEP does not at all correlate with abnormalities in temperature and pain sensibility. It is dependent on the conduction in the medial lemniscal pathways.

In the second study, stimuli were delivered with a carbon dioxide laser, which stimulates thermoreceptors with afferent fibers in the A-delta range, i.e., slowly conducting afferents that evoke cortical SEPs with long latencies (about 200–300 msec) (8). The abnormalities in this SEP correlated with abnormalities in temperature sensibility, which supports the conclusion that the CPSP patients have abnormally functioning spinothalamic pathways.

HYPERALGESIA AND ALLODYNIA IN SYRINGOMYELIA AND SYRINGOBULBIA

Sensory abnormalities dominate the symptoms and signs in many patients with syringomyelia and syringobulbia. Dissociated sensory loss on the hands and face, respectively, is thought to be the most characteristic sensory abnormality caused by the elongated cavity in the spinal cord and medulla oblongata (1). Some of the patients have hyperalgesia and/or allodynia.

From an ongoing study, results regarding H/A and related symptoms in 25 patients (16 men, 9 women) with syringomyelia will be reported (J. Boivie and A. Österberg, *in progress*). Seven of the patients have an extension of the syrinx into the lower brain stem, as shown by the symptoms, x-ray examinations, or MRI. The median age of the patients at examination was 47 years (range 32–73), with a mean duration of symptoms of 10 years (range 1–39).

At the onset of the symptoms, nine patients noted paresis, 11 sensory disturbances, and nine had pain. At the time of the investigation, the dominating symptom was paresis in 13 patients, sensory abnormalities including H/A in four, and pain in eight.

No less than 15 of the patients appeared to have central pain, i.e., 60%. This is a very high incidence. It was aching in seven, burning in four, pressing in three patients, but several other pain qualities were reported. One side of the thorax or one hand was the most common location of the central pain.

Seven of the patients with central pain were hyperalgesic to pinprick and four were allodynic to touch. Also overreactions to heat, similar to the ones described in patients with CPSP, were shown in a few patients.

The somatic sensibility was extensively tested in 15 of the 25 patients. The tests included quantitative tests of the sensibility to vibration, touch, cold-warmth, and cold pain and heat pain. A Vibrameter was used for vibration, graded von Frey filaments for touch, and the Thermotest device for temperatures, as described by Boivie et al. (5) and in the chapter by Hansson and Lindblom.

TABLE 32.4. *Sensory abnormalities according to
quantitative sensory tests in patients with syringomyelia.
Number of patients with raised thresholds on the
hand with the most pronounced disturbances (n = 15)*

Vibration	11
Touch	8
Cold-warmth	15
Cold pain, heat pain	14
Pinprick	15

Table 32.4 shows that all patients had decreased temperature and pain sensibility and that many of them also had reduced sensibility to vibration and touch. This is roughly in accord with the descriptions in the neurological textbooks. However, in several patients the location of the abnormalities did not correspond to the textbook description, according to which the dissociated sensory loss affects both hands about equally. Instead it was found that the abnormalities were unilateral in several patients, mainly in those with light or moderate neurological symptoms.

The decrease in temperature and pain sensibility was severe in almost all patients, particularly regarding heat pain and cold pain. This explains why many syringomyelia patients have burned their hands without noticing it in time. The abnormalities in vibration and touch were more moderate.

SUMMARY OF CLINICAL OBSERVATIONS REGARDING CENTRALLY INDUCED HYPERALGESIA AND ALLODYNIA

H/A occur with all kinds of lesions that also cause central pain (Table 32.1), but not all patients with central pain experience these overreactions. A few of the patients with these painful overreactions seem to be free from spontaneous central pain. One could then argue that H/A can occur without central pain. However, it appears logical to accept the presence of H/A without spontaneous pain as a criterion for the diagnosis of central pain, provided that the reason for them is a primary lesion or disease in the CNS, in the same way as the presence of spontaneous pain is not a requisite to classify a pain condition as nociceptive.

H/A can occur after lesions anywhere along the neuraxis, from the dorsal horn of the spinal cord to the cerebral cortex. Lesions in the gray matter as well as lesions of fiber tracts can induce H/A and other expressions of central pain. The lesion can be of vascular, traumatic, or inflammatory demyelinating character.

In stroke patients, H/A may, like spontaneous central pain, start at the time of the lesion or with short or long delays of up to 2 to 3 years. In syringomyelia it is more difficult to find out if there is a delay, because the lesion is thought to increase successively during long periods and probably stepwise on other occasions. Central pain can be present early in the disease and can also start several years after other symptoms.

The incidences of H/A are unknown, but they may be as high as 57%, the percentage found in patients with CPSP (18). The intensity varies from patient to patient and may be intense enough to meet the criterion for a hyperpathic reaction.

There is hyperalgesia to both mechanical and thermal noxious stimuli. It has been observed more often to mechanical stimuli, mostly to pinprick, than to heat or cold, but this difference might depend on the fact that pins are more readily available than hot or deep cold objects at the examination of the patient. In quantitative sensory tests on patients with central pain due to CVLs and syringomyelia, it has been observed that some patients who have a severe loss of temperature sensibility experience a momentarily appearing strong burning pain at a particular temperature (hyperpathia), without having otherwise perceived the increasing temperature.

Painful overreactions to innoxious stimuli, i.e., allodynia, appear to be most common to cold, somewhat less common to touch, and least common to warmth. Patients with allodynia to touch usually do not overreact to steady pressure. A light moving stimulus, like a swab of cotton wool, appears to be the worst light mechanical stimulus. It is not yet known if H/A can occur without a concomitant change in perception threshold. If that were the case, it would represent an isolated change in the stimulus–response function, only affecting the magnitude of the percept.

MECHANISMS

In the preceding paragraph it is concluded that centrally induced H/A are features of central pain. From this follows that the mechanisms of these phenomena are those of central pain in general, although it is conceivable that the pathophysiology of the various manifestations of central pain might turn out to differ in some respects.

Based on the results from the studies of patients with CPSP, we have hypothesized that only patients with lesions affecting the spinothalamic pathways develop central pain (4,5), whereas it is not necessary that the lesion involve the medial lemniscal pathways. This hypothesis is contrary to the main previous hypothesis, which stated that central pain develops as a result of lesions affecting the medial lemniscal pathways. This lesion was thought to remove inhibitions that normally control the activity of neurons in the thalamus or cortex, whose activity results in pain. Central pain would thus be a release phenomenon, i.e., the result of disinhibition. Our results from CPSP do not fit with such a role for the medial lemniscal pathways, because many of the patients had normal thresholds to touch and normal cortical SEP after stimulation of these pathways, but the idea that disinhibitions are part of the mechanisms behind central pain is still valid.

According to our hypothesis, central pain is a paradox: a lesion of the "pain pathway" causes pain.

It is reasonable to assume that severe spontaneous central pain is evoked by vigorous activity somewhere in the brain. This supposition is supported by the results from electrophysiological recordings in the thalamus of patients with central pain caused by traumatic SCI. These recordings demonstrated spontaneous vigorous activity in the contralateral ventroposterior thalamic region, where no such activity can be recorded in patients without pain (19). This spike activity had characteristics that indicated that it might be calcium dependent (20).

Evidently such activity in the ventroposterior thalamic region cannot account for central pain in patients with large lesions in this region, as in some of our CPSP patients. In the patients with large thalamic lesions, it seems probable that the abnormal activity is cortically located, but there is no evidence to support this idea.

French investigators have proposed that the reticular and medial thalamic nuclei play an important role for the occurrence of central pain. From experimental studies it is known that these thalamic regions have an inhibitory effect on the activity in the ventroposterior region. Thalamocortical axons from the ventroposterior nuclei give off collaterals to the reticular nucleus, from which projections go to the medial thalamic nuclei. Thus, disappearance of activity in the ventroposterior region could lead to increased activity in the loop via the reticular and medial thalamic nuclei. Results from studies of cerebral blood flow with isotopes and scintigraphic techniques (single-photon emission computed tomography) in patients with CPSP have been interpreted to indicate increased neuronal activity in the medial thalamus on the side opposite the pain (9). The results do not appear to be conclusive, however, because of the poor resolution and low sensitivity of the technique, so far. The hypothesis is interesting and ought to be explored further with techniques that give better spatial and functional resolution, such as positron emission tomography.

Several recent experimental studies of spinal mechanisms behind neurogenic pain induced by peripheral nerve trauma have indicated that excitatory amino acids, particularly glutamate and its effects via *N*-methyl-D-aspartate (NMDA) receptors, play an important role for the development of hyperactive and hyperexcitable neuron pools in the spinal cord (for review, see chapters by Bennett and Laird and by Haley and Wilcox). If the activity of these systems is blocked during the critical period, it looks like the basis for the neurogenic pain can be prevented from developing. It is tempting to guess that similar mechanisms are at play in higher centers in central pain, and it is a fascinating thought that the development of central pain could perhaps be pharmacologically prevented. However, then we have to be able to recognize which patients are at risk of developing central pain, with its accompanying painful overreactions to somatic stimuli. Detailed analyses of the sensory abnormalities, including quantitative sensory testing, appear to be helpful in this endeavor.

ACKNOWLEDGMENTS

The studies from which unpublished results are presented have been supported by grants from the Swedish Medical Research Council (grant no. 9058), the Bank of Sweden Tercentenary Foundation, the Swedish Association of the Neurologically Disabled, 1987 Years Foundation for Stroke Research, and the County Council of Östergötland. The author wishes to express his thanks to Dr. Göran Leijon, Linköping, and Dr. David Bowsher, Liverpool, for information about unpublished results from stroke patients.

REFERENCES

1. Barnett, H. J., Foster, J. B., and Hudgeson, P. (1973): *Syringomyelia*. W. B. Saunders, London.
2. Beric, A., Dimitrijevic, M. A., and Lindblom, U. (1988): Central dysesthesia syndrome in spinal cord injury patients. *Pain*, 34:109–116.
3. Bougosslavsky, J., Regli, F., and Uske, A. (1988): Thalamic infarcts: clinical syndromes, etiology and prognosis. *Neurology*, 38:837–848.
4. Boivie, J., and Leijon, G. (1991): Clinical findings in patients with central poststroke pain. In: *Pain and central nervous system disease: the central pain syndromes*, edited by K. L. Casey, pp. 65–75. Raven Press, New York.
5. Boivie, J., Leijon, G., and Johansson, I. (1989): Central post-stroke pain—a study of the mechanisms through analyses of the sensory abnormalities. *Pain*, 37:173–185.
6. Breuer, A. C., Cuervo, H., and Selkoe, D. J. (1981): Hyperpathia and sensory level due to parietal lobe arteriovenous malformation. *Arch. Neurol.*, 38:722–724.
7. Caplan, L. R. (1986): Vertebrobasilar occlusive disease. In: *Stroke—pathophysiology, diagnosis and management*, vol. 1, edited by H. J. M. Barnett, B. M. Stein, J. P. Mohr, F. M. Yatsu, pp. 549–619. Churchill Livingstone, New York.

8. Casey, K. L., Boivie, J., Leijon, G., Morrow, T. J., Sjölund, B., and Rosén, I. (1990): Laser-evoked cerebral potentials and sensory function in patients with central pain. *Pain,* suppl. 5:204.
9. Cesaro, P., Mann, M. W., Moretti, J. L., et al. (1991): Central pain and thalamic hyperactivity: a single photon emission computerized tomographic study. *Pain,* 47:329–336.
10. Clifford, D. B., and Trotter, J. L. (1984): Pain in multiple sclerosis. *Arch. Neurol.,* 41:1270–1272.
11. Davidoff, G., Guarracini, M., Roth, E., Sliwa, J., and Yarkony, G. (1987): Trazodone hydrochloride in the treatment of dysesthetic pain in traumatic myelopathy: a randomized, double-blind, placebo-controlled study. *Pain,* 29:151–161.
12. Davis, R. (1975): Pain and suffering following spinal cord injury. *Clin. Orthop.,* 112:76–80.
13. Davis, R., and Martin, J. (1947): Studies upon spinal cord injuries. Nature and treatment of pain. *J. Neurosurg.,* 4:483–491.
14. Head, H., and Holmes, G. (1911): Sensory disturbances from cerebral lesions. *Brain,* 34:102–254.
15. Holmes, G. (1919): *Contributions to medical and biological research,* vol. 1. New York.
16. Holmgren, H., Leijon, G., Boivie, J., Johansson, I., and Ilievska, L. (1990): Central post-stroke pain—somatosensory evoked potentials in relation to location of the lesion and sensory signs. *Pain,* 40:43–52.
17. Leijon, G., Boivie, J., and Johansson, I. (1989): Central post-stroke pain—neurological symptoms and pain characteristics. *Pain,* 36:13–25.
18. Leijon, G., and Bowsher, D. (1990): Somatosensory findings in central post-stroke pain (CPSP) and controls. *Pain,* suppl. 5:468.
19. Lenz, F. A., Kwan, H. C., Dostrovsky, J. O., and Tasker, R. R. (1989): Characteristics of bursting pattern of action potentials that occurs in the thalamus of patients with central pain. *Brain Res.,* 496:357–360.
20. Lenz, F. A., Kwan, H. C., Martin, R., Tasker, R., and Dostrovsky, J. O. (1990): Characteristics of spontaneous neuronal activity at different locations in ventrocaudal thalamus of patients with central pain following spinal cord transection. *Pain,* suppl. 5:493.
21. Lewis-Jones, H., Smith, T., Bowsher, D., and Leijon, G. (1990): Magnetic resonance imaging in 36 cases of central post-stroke pain (CPSP). *Pain,* suppl. 5:278.
22. Mauguiere, F., and Desmedt, J. E. (1988): Thalamic pain syndrome of Dejérine-Roussy. Differentiation of four subtypes assisted by somatosensory evoked potentials data. *Arch. Neurol.,* 45:1312–1320.
23. Mersky, H., Lindblom, U., Mumford, J. M., Nathan, P. W., Noordenbos, W., and Sunderland, S. (1986): Pain terms. A current list with definitions and notes on usage. *Pain,* suppl. 3:217–221.
24. Moulin, D. E., Foley, K. M., and Ebers, G. C. (1988): Pain syndromes in multiple sclerosis. *Neurology,* 38:1830–1834.
25. Pagni, C. A. (1989): Central pain due to spinal cord and brainstem damage. In: *Textbook of pain,* edited by P. D. Wall and R. D. Melzack, pp. 634–655. Churchill Livingstone, New York.
26. Riddoch, G. (1938): The clinical features of central pain. *Lancet,* 234:1093–1098, 1150–1156, 1205–1209.
27. Schott, B., Laurent, B., and Maugière, F. (1986): Les douleurs thalamiques: étude critique de 43 cas. *Rev. Neurol. (Paris),* 142:308–315.
28. Sweet, W. H., and Poletti, C. E. (1989): Operations in the brain stem and spinal canal, with an appendix on open cordotomy. In: *Textbook of pain,* edited by P. D. Wall and R. D. Melzack, pp. 811–831. Churchill Livingstone, New York.

Hyperalgesia and Allodynia,
edited by W. D. Willis, Jr.
Raven Press, Ltd., New York © 1992.

33

New Directions for Research on Hyperalgesia

Jean-Marie Besson

*Unité de Physiopharmacologie du Système Nerveux, U161, INSERM,
75014 Paris, France*

This book mainly focuses on various electrophysiological, pharmacological, and clinical aspects of hyperalgesias including those encountered in certain neuropathic states. Various aspects of hyperalgesia are considered, such as the sensitization of nociceptors, the involvement of the sympathetic system, and the respective roles of peripheral and central mechanisms. With the exception of centrally induced hyperalgesia, everybody agrees with the fact that hyperalgesia is a combined process with both peripheral and central components but usually initiated by events at the periphery.

The subject is vast and this brief discussion will be restricted to hyperalgesia either generated by cutaneous injury or nerve injury. Future progress in hyperalgesia research will depend mainly on the improvement of our knowledge of the properties of peripheral nociceptors and of the development of multidisciplinary and more relevant approaches in order to determine precisely the role of the multitude of endogenous compounds entering into the peripheral soup and the respective involvement of peripheral and central mechanisms.

Some of these difficulties, notably those related to the nociceptors, have been repeatedly mentioned for many years (for recent reviews, see refs. 7,8). We will first make a list of the main difficulties encountered in these approaches and then put forward certain propositions for the direction of future research.

THE DIFFICULTIES ENCOUNTERED IN THE STUDY OF HYPERALGESIA

These are many, and the list we will put forward is not exhaustive and in general will cover studies on the peripheral mechanisms.

1. What are the neurochemistry and the pharmacology of different classes of nociceptors in different tissues or species?

a. Differences between species: it is well-known that the type IIA-delta mechanoheat nociceptors that have a thermal threshold similar to those of C-MHs (near 43°C) have only been reported in humans.

b. It must be also emphasized that deep muscular or visceral receptors do not necessarily have the same properties as skin receptors. Two examples can be put forward to illustrate this.

—According to Jänig and Morrison (10) numerous slowly conducting primary afferent fibers innervating the cat's colon or urinary bladder responded to innocuous distention and increased their firing rate according to the stimulus intensity in the noxious range.

—In the cat's knee joint capsule Grigg et al. (5) and Schaible and Schmidt (15) described sleeping nociceptors, which in healthy tissues could not be excited by acute noxious stimuli. Interestingly, they are awakened during pathological tissue alterations (inflammation). This observation gives rise to two major questions: (i) Are these silent nociceptors present in all tissues? (ii) What are the factors that initiate the transition of unresponsive primary afferents into responsive ones?

2. Due to the difficulty in intracellular recording of Aδ and C fibers, the nature of the transduction mechanisms relating noxious stimuli to changes in membrane processes remains difficult to study. Nevertheless it has been shown that activation of sensory neurons occurs by three different major mechanisms: (i) depolarization of the cell through direct interactions with receptor/ion channel complexes (ATP, 5-HT), (ii) depolarization of the cell through the actions of intracellular second messenger (BK), (iii) sensitization of the cell by modifying the intrinsic properties of ion channels to facilitate action potential generation and neurotransmitter release (prostaglandins).

a. Here again several difficulties and unanswered questions can be raised:

—The three proposed modes of action are not mutually exclusive.
—What is the difference between the membrane receptors mediating excitation and the sensitization of nociceptors?
—Do purely mechanical nociceptors exist?

3. Human studies are essential and have provided remarkable information, but which so far, unfortunately, is limited to cutaneous fibers. We do not yet have information on nociceptors in joint, muscle, and visceral tissues.

4. In animals in which most of the pharmacological investigations have been performed, recording from nociceptors requires surgery. Thus, even with the best "microdissector," one is never totally sure about conditions in the microenvironment of the nociceptors (CO_2 and O_2 partial pressures, pH, microcirculation, sympathetic tone, ionic composition of the extracellular fluid). In order to circumvent such difficulties, *in vitro* preparations have been designed. They have the advantage of a better control of the concentration of tested agents, but they are far removed from clinical situations.

5. The microenvironment of the fine terminals in the skin, muscles, and viscera appears to become more and more complex in its pharmacology. This has prompted Handwerker to use the term "peripheral soup." Indeed a myriad of chemical sensitizers and activators has been found at the periphery (see references in ref. 14), and so it is unlikely that a single analgesic substance will affect all types of pain. When faced with the multitude of substances in the peripheral soup or involved in other hyperalgesic states, the pharmacologist has many reasons to be depressed, particularly because:

i. In a given experimental situation (*in vivo* or *in vitro*), one is never completely certain about the conditions in the microenvironment of the nociceptors.
ii. There is a multiplicity of receptors (5-HT, BK).
iii. There are interactions between different agents.
iv. There are undoubtedly more mediators to be discovered.

v. The sensitization by a particular inflammatory mediator is not necessarily due to its direct action on primary afferent neurons. For example, BK induces short-lasting sensitization to heating stimuli, whereas H^+ ions seem to contribute to mechanical sensitization.

6. With some exceptions (see chapters by LaMotte, Guilbaud et al., and Woolf), most of the studies related to hyperalgesia have been performed in the periphery and more information is needed on the central mechanisms involved in hyperalgesia. This point is important since the involvement of central mechanisms seems to differ depending on the type of hyperalgesia (primary versus secondary).

7. Despite the fact that in animals new models of hyperalgesias are more commonly used (1,17; Bennett and Laird, this volume), there is still a need to develop additional models closer to the clinical situations encountered in humans.

NEW DIRECTIONS

We will discuss in turn the studies performed in humans and animals.

In Humans

1. Studies performed in humans have three main advantages over research in animals: (i) the ability to record activity of nociceptors with minimal skin damage; (ii) the ability to correlate neuronal activity with the subject's experience; (iii) the ability to study modifications in peripheral neuronal response properties in relation to well-defined clinical syndromes. There is no doubt that there is a need to extend psychophysiological studies to experimentally induced models of hyperalgesias and in well-defined clinical syndromes such as reflex sympathetic dystrophy, causalgia, and peripheral neuropathies. The systematic development of these studies will lead to a better understanding of various kinds of pains with rational consequences for diagnoses and for the use of analgesics.

2. Do not forget that the modality of the hyperalgesia manifested will vary with the cause of the hyperalgesia. Thus, it is necessary to test systematically mechanical, cooling and heating stimuli and, when possible, chemical stimuli (see Campbell et al., this volume).

3. If technically and ethically possible, it would be essential to have information about the electrophysiological characteristics of muscular, articular, and visceral nociceptors in humans.

4. In humans, it is difficult to detect and to gauge, at the CNS level, the repercussions of the peripheral modifications observed during hyperalgesia. However, the use of magnetic resonance imaging and positron emission tomography, as recently described at the cortical level by Talbot et al. (16), seems highly promising. More interestingly, this technique could possibly be combined with recordings from peripheral afferent fibers.

In Animals

1. With regard to nociceptors (for more details, see refs. 7,8): critical but unfortunately extremely difficult research programs may focus on the various related bio-

physical and biochemical mechanisms of the excitation and sensitization of nociceptive primary afferent fibers. We recommend the following:

—the use of monoclonal antibodies would be useful to identify fiber subpopulations,
—investigating in detail the various mechanisms of peripheral release for activators and sensitizers and measuring their levels,
—design of better antagonists,
—use of combinations of antagonists and antibodies to address cooperative interactions among substances,
—testing the effects of putative analgesics in experimental models of hyperalgesia and not in normal animals.

2. At the level of the CNS:

a. Numerous substances (peptides, excitatory amino acids) are probably released in the spinal cord by the terminals of the various nociceptive primary afferents (see references in ref. 3). Since several compounds are released from the (same) central terminals, the problem is extraordinarily complex. For example, if two compounds are capable of producing excitation alone, then the action of both may need to be blocked to produce transmission failure. Thus, in this condition it is difficult to predict the effect of an antagonist. Here again the same remarks already raised with regard to the periphery are pertinent, notably the design of better antagonists or antibodies and the use of "cocktails" to address cooperative interactions between substances.

b. Dramatic neuronal changes in neuronal responsiveness have been described at the spinal cord, thalamic, and cortical levels (see Guilbaud et al., this volume) and numerous questions remain to be answered:

i. What are the respective central repercussions of hyperalgesia generated either by cutaneous injury or certain neuropathic states?
ii. Are the respective contributions of various spinal *ascending* pathways implicated in pain processes different in normal animals and animals presenting hyperalgesia?
iii. Do sleeping neurons exist in the CNS in the absence of pathological conditions (see ref. 6)?
iv. What modifications occur in the activity of segmental and descending control systems during hyperalgesia? Once again we are faced with complex issues since it has been hypothesized that following nerve injury there is a decrease in segmental controls due to transynaptic degeneration (see Bennett and Laird, this volume), whereas during cutaneous injury (inflammation) the activity of descending controls seems to be enhanced (2; Schaible, this volume).

c. In fact, the issues raised here are but several examples of future research directions; it must be stressed that if we are to increase the value of the studies on hyperalgesic phenomena in different areas of the CNS, in different pain states, one of the major problems to be resolved is the evaluation of the respective roles of peripheral and central mechanisms.

3. The factors relevant to the behavioral tests used:

a. The development of new experimental models is essential not only for the detection of new analgesics but also for our understanding of pain syndromes that are poorly managed clinically. In this context, the use of different inflammatory models (acute or chronic) and peripheral neuropathy accompanied by hyperalgesia will be useful for the ability in most cases to quantify the level of hyperalgesia. However, it is not always obvious how to study pharmacological effects in these models and I present two examples:

i. As far as possible, one should use as many tests as possible comparable to the clinical situation. This is well illustrated by the neuropathic rat model and the effects of morphine (1 mg/kg i.v.) on different behavioral tests. Guilbaud's group in our laboratory has shown an antinociceptive effect of morphine on hyperalgesia to mechanical stimuli, yet the same dose of morphine has no effect on responses to thermal stimuli, either hot (44°C) or cold (10°C).

ii. One cannot always conclude that the clinical signs (e.g., the inflammatory edema) are correlated to the pain threshold. For example, Levine et al. (11,12) have shown that the radiographic and inflammatory signs of arthritis induced by Freund adjuvant can be reduced or partly blocked by chemical and surgical sympathectomy. By contrast, in the same model, hyperalgesia to mechanical stimulation is not modified by chemical sympathectomy (6).

b. From a general point of view, if one considers in humans that in more than 99% of the cases, the relief of pain is based on systemic (mainly oral) administration of analgesics, then we need more direct approaches. So, why not return to simple classical behavioral approaches in freely moving animals with systemic drug administration? Intrathecal and intracerebroventricular injections are not a panacea. In other words, another message for the future is "please be simple."

4. Finally despite the fact that one must be cautious about the interpretation of the proto-oncogene C-fos activation, such as a marker seems to be highly promising. As initially mentioned by Hunt et al. (9) the C-fos is not a specific marker of the activity of nociceptive neurons, but it is clear from a subsequent number of recent studies (see references in ref. 4), it is preferentially induced by noxious stimuli. Interestingly, it has been shown that the fos-like immunoreactivity induced following formalin injection into the paw was significantly reduced by systemic morphine in a dose–response relationship, these effects being antagonized by naloxone (13). In my opinion the cautious use of this new technique using various proto-oncogenes would be extremely well adapted to the study of the various physiological and pharmacological aspects of hyperalgesias.

In conclusion despite the multiplicity of problems encountered, the development of new experimental strategies, and the use of molecular biology should provide a better understanding of hyperalgesia within a few years.

REFERENCES

1. Besson, J. M., and Guilbaud, G. (eds.) (1988): The arthritic rat as a model of clinical pain. *Excerpta Medica*, ICS 837:255.
2. Calvino, B., Villanueva, L., and Le Bars, D. (1987): Dorsal horn (convergent) neurones in the intact anaesthetized arthritic rat. II. Heterotopic inhibitory influences. *Pain*, 31:359–379.
3. Duggan, A. W., and Weihe, E. (1991): Central transmission of impulses in nociceptors: events in the superficial dorsal horn. In: *Towards a new pharmacotherapy of pain*, edited by A. I. Basbaum and J. M. Besson, pp. 35–67. John Wiley, New York.
4. Fitzgerald, M. (1990): C-fos and the changing face of pain. *TINS*, 13:439–440.
5. Grigg, P., Schaible, H. S., and Schmidt, R. F. (1986): Mechanical sensitivity of group III and IV afferents from posterior articular nerve in normal and inflamed cat knee. *J. Neurophysiol.*, 54:635–643.
6. Guilbaud, G., Perrot, S., Attal, N., and Neil, A. Towards animal models for the study of sympa-

thetically maintained pain? In: *International symposium on the pathobiology of the reflex sympathetic dystrophy syndrome (SDR)*, edited by W. Jänig and R. F. Schmidt. (*in press*).

7. Hammond, D. L., et al. (1991): Group report: discussions on the physiological and pharmacological bases of the transmission and control of nociceptive messages. In: *Towards a new pharmacotherapy of pain*, edited by A. I. Basbaum and J. M. Besson, pp. 105–119. John Wiley, New York.

8. Handwerker, H. O. (1991): What peripheral mechanisms contribute to nociceptive transmission and hyperalgesia? In: *Towards a new pharmacotherapy of pain*, edited by A. I. Basbaum and J. M. Besson, pp. 5–19. John Wiley, New York.

9. Hunt, S. P., Pini, A., and Evan, G. (1987): Induction of C-fos-like protein in spinal cord neurons following sensory stimulation. *Nature*, 328:632–634.

10. Jänig, W., and Morrison, J. F. B. (1986): Functional properties of spinal visceral afferents supplying abdominal and pelvic organs with special emphasis on visceral nociception. *Prog. Brain Res.*, 67:87–114.

11. Levine, J. D., Coderre, T. J., Helms, C., and Basbaum, A. I. (1988): Beta 2 adrenergic mechanisms in experimental arthritis. *Proc. Natl. Acad. Sci. USA*, 85:4553–4556.

12. Levine, J. D., Dardick, S. J., Roizen, M. F., Helms, C., and Basbaum, A. I. (1986): Contribution of sensory afferents and sympathetic efferents to joint injury in experimental arthritis. *J. Neurosci.*, 6:3423–3429.

13. Presley, R. W., Menetrey, D., Levine, J. D., and Basbaum, A. I. (1990): Systemic morphine suppresses noxious stimulus-evoked fos protein-like immunoreactivity in the rat spinal cord. *J. Neurosci.*, 10:323–335.

14. Rang, H. P. (1991): The nociceptive afferent neurone as a target for new types of analgesic drug. In: *Proceedings of the VIth World Congress on Pain: Pain research and clinical management*, vol. 4, edited by M. R. Bond, J. E. Charlton, C. J. Woolf, pp. 119–127. Elsevier, Amsterdam.

15. Schaible, H. G., and Schmidt, R. F. (1985): Effects of an experimental arthritis on the sensory properties of fine articular afferent units. *J. Neurophysiol.*, 54:1109–1121.

16. Talbot, J. D., Marrett, S., Evans, A. C., Meyer, E., Bushnell, M. C., and Duncan, G. H. (1991): Multiple representations of pain in human cerebral cortex. *Science*, 251:1355–1358.

17. Vos, B. P., and Maciewicz, R. (1990): Behavioral evidence for the development of trigeminal neuropathic pain following ligation of the infraorbital nerve in the rat. *Soc. Neurosci. Abstr.*, 16:1072.

Hyperalgesia and Allodynia,
edited by W. D. Willis, Jr.
Raven Press, Ltd., New York © 1992.

34

Therapy and Future Directions

Discussion

Kathleen M. Foley, Moderator

Dr. Foley: In starting off this discussion Dr. Chapman will speak to the issues of behavioral and psychological aspects of patients with hyperalgesia and central pain syndromes. He would like to make a few comments related to the more cognitive aspects in this group of patients, and then we'll open up for further discussion.

Dr. Chapman: Dr. Besson has concluded his presentation by saying please be simple, and I think my job here is to attempt to be simple, but it's very hard after these several days of intensive information processing. We have heard so much vast and fascinating material on the transduction, transmission, modulation of information related to hyperpathia and allodynia. Where does all this go? I feel a little bit in looking at all this like that great American philosopher who some 50 years ago (her name is Mae West, by the way) said that too much of a good thing is wonderful. My task here is to bring this around to the behavioral point of view and I think that one can and must be fairly simple in doing that. In listening to many of these presentations, I was reminded of an experience I had in the late 1970s when I taught a class in the evening for the general public on pain at the University of Washington. This was open to whoever wanted to come, and the attendees turned out to be, of course, mainly attorneys, but there was one young woman with facial pain who came to all the sessions and who talked to me extensively. She was one of these people with this terrible problem and she complained that people didn't understand her, nobody would give her any time and this echoed very much in my thoughts as I listened to Dr. Ochoa talking earlier about the least we can do is to listen to these people for 2 or 3 hr. Everyone told her that her problem was fundamentally psychological. Within the year she committed suicide, and I haven't forgotten this young lady.

It's terribly important, I think, for us to remember that these are whole patients and that the care that we give them should be both comprehensive and compassionate, not simply neurologic. If we are going to go about this, how do we look at the behavioral dimensions of all of these complicated problems and phenomena? I've heard so much about these valuable animal models, and I think that's a good point of departure here. If we look at what we're learning from the animal models and we look at the clinical phenomena, there are some rather obvious ways to bring these together, and no one has yet made an attempt to do that. Now of course you can benefit a lot by doing psychologic testing on these patients, by looking at psychophysics and other subjective report-dependent things, but that only enlarges the gulf in understanding and in scientific inference between the laboratory models and the clinical arena. I suggest that, instead, we work at a convergence of these two and that we do so by looking for measures, indicators, that are common to animal models and to the behavioral patterns of patients with hyperpathic or allodynic conditions. There are a number of ways that one could do this. Dr. Bonica has emphasized for decades the nature of the behaviors of these patients, and we could study these fairly effectively by looking at the emotionality of the patients. On one hand, animal researchers have done excellent work on startle as an indicator of emotionality, and human researchers have shown that the eye blink response in humans is virtually a perfect analog of that. That's one area where we can find a convergence. Another would be to look at some indicator of a sympathetic response, like circulating norepinephrine. This is a fairly crude measure, but it still should be useful. There are other neurohumoral indicators that we could get at; we could draw upon the POMC-derived biologically active neuropeptides, ACTH or beta-endorphin, to give us another common ground to look at between the animal and the human arenas. And further we have the glucocorticoids, so there are many areas in which we can compare animals and humans. There are even such things as facial expression. That goes all the way back to Darwin, and there is a rich human literature emerging not only in the pain area, but in the emotion area, which allows us to quantify facial expression either through electromyography in humans or through facial action coding systems. Now all of these approaches suggest that there are some rather concrete ways in which we can work toward a convergence of animal models and human models to help to bridge the gap between what we encounter and deal with in a clinic and what we work with in a laboratory. There are a lot of reasons why I think we should do that, and one of them is obvious—we need to understand these syndromes better—but another reason is that we could identify better therapeutic end-points for controlled trials that we might want to undertake. We don't have a lot of information on something Dr. Black raised awhile ago on the potential value of Tegretol, for example, in certain types of patients. In order to carry out any randomized control trial on that or a neurosurgical intervention or anything else, we need good therapeutic end-points, and the behavioral and the neuroendocrinologic ones are probably the best things that we can use. So I see here ways of being simple, ways of bridging the clinic to the animal models by using behavior as a common ground.

Dr. Foley: Thank you, Dr. Chapman. There are some questions. Yes, if you'd like to start with a question.

Question: Yes, my question is to Dr. Boivie, but before I ask it, I'd like to make a comment like Dr. Ochoa. The most important role of the skin is thermal regulation. This is primitive, as we heard in the initial lectures, to the animal and the effector function in the skin is to maintain core temperature. For 20 years I've looked at all kinds of pain, including viscerocutaneous referral and somatocutaneous referral, and I can tell you that it disturbs thermal regulation. Those spots are hot and Head alluded to this. I would also say to you that thermal regulation of the skin is disturbed in every pain state. As a matter of fact, in syringomyelia, the Japanese have been able to designate by the autonomic change in thermal regulation the configuration of the syrinx, and they have also found that immediately upon the formation of a motor stroke, there is a vasoconstriction in the region of the monoplegia or hemiplegia. I would urge you strongly not only to look at your animal models, but your human models of pain, because you can subclassify the response to the patient's pain. The worst pain of all is the pain of leprosy, which is no pain. Thermal regulation is disturbed in no pain as well as in pain, and if you don't look at thermal regulation in your models, you're missing the most primitive reflex of the spinal cord. Now my question is, have you observed autonomic thermal regulation changes in patients with central pain from either stroke or syringomyelia?

Dr. Boivie: No, we have not specifically looked at that, but there are conflicting reports about this. And there are many difficulties. If you look at stroke, for instance, if you take a body region which is paralytic and therefore one which you don't move very much, that in itself, the inactivity of the extremity, is going to change the temperature in that region. But, I agree, as I pointed out, the autonomic dysfunctions and functions in these patients really need to be studied in detail.

Dr. Foley: Could you please give your name into the microphone just so we have it for the recording?

Dr. Hobbins from Madison, Wisconsin: In comment to your remark, you are absolutely correct that it is the nonmovement of the extremity that causes the coolness and again we've heard of nothing but afferents here and when I stop moving my animated hand, the autonomic system is immediately invoked, wanting to know where the hell my arm went. And if we don't look at the changes in thermal regulation, whether it's a brachial plexus lesion, or whatever, you're going to miss the major influence. Let me just tell you that appendicitis in Romania under the age of 5 is most accurately diagnosed by a hyperthermia at McBurney's point; it's better than a white count, it's better than a physical exam, so look at thermal regulation; it's beautiful and it tells you so much.

Dr. Foley: Now, next question.

Question: I have a question for Dr. Bullitt. I am an anesthesiology pain clinician and I see quite a few postherpetic neuropathy pain patients. Most of the patients I treat are 1 year after a herpetic lesion and consequently my treatment modalities are limited and I was frustrated. We all heard from Dr. Bonica that if you treat by sympathetic block at an early stage, the chance of developing long-term pain is diminished, I was watching yesterday Dr. Basbaum's presentation that peripheral nerve stimulation evokes the expression of c-fos, and I'm speculating that postherpetic pain is largely due to constant noxious stimulation that makes a permanent imprint on the central nervous system. I'm going to admit to the hospital patients with herpes zoster treated with Zovirax, Zostrix, xylocaine jelly in the local area, but I may also provide these patients with continuous sympathetic blockade. My question is, if I do, is it overtreating, knowing that not all herpetic patients go into the permanent pain situation.

Dr. Foley: Dr. Boivie, do you want to comment to that?

Dr. Boivie: No.

Dr. Foley: We weren't sure to whom the question was being addressed. Dr. Bullitt, do you want to start and then Dr. Boivie can comment?

Dr. Bullitt: Yes. At least as far as the question of early sympathetic interruption in patients with herpes zoster, I can say something. There have been several case reports in the literature by anesthesiologists who have said that early treatment with sympathetic interruption can perhaps prevent the pain of postherpetic neuralgia. To my knowledge there has been no controlled study in the literature, and the largest study that I know of that claimed that perhaps early sympathetic interruption could prevent postherpetic neuralgia when he compared his own results to that of the literature in general, his patients had only a 5% to 10% incidence of postherpetic neuralgia, whereas the incidence in the literature is 50%. However, the chance of developing postherpetic neuralgia is very much age related, and the ages of the patients in this particular study were not stated. Now, Dr. Bonica may have a study that's been well-controlled that I don't know about.

Dr. Foley: There is no such study.

Dr. Bullitt: I think this is something that needs to be looked at in a controlled fashion. Finally, one disadvantage of giving steroids in some of these elderly patients who may already be somewhat immunosuppressed is that there may be a slightly increased risk of inducing a more widespread infection. The answer is I don't think anybody knows the answer.

Dr. Foley: But, I think could we get others on the panel to contribute—Dr. Besson, perhaps you'd respond to this. If you have in this kind of a setting a patient with an acute fulminating syndrome that appears to be primarily neuropathic with an inflammatory component, what should be given to these patients. You've suggested a soup; what should be in the soup and where should it be given?

Dr. Besson: Anywhere. Probably at the spinal cord level. Probably glutamate and substance P are the main offenders; ATP is another possibility. My impression is that during 10 years after '77, following the scheme proposed by Jessell and Iversen, the role of substance P was probably overestimated. Recently a lot of people are leaving the substance P field and everybody's for, let's say, glutamate and the excitatory amino acids, but in my opinion, that's a false problem. It's a question of fashion, and the only possibility to answer such a question is to have a clear substance P antagonist. As you know, we have been waiting for substance P antagonists since '77, and we have no substance P antagonist. We have a number of substance P antagonists acting at the periphery, and some of them can induce a relatively good analgesic effect; it's less than perfect but you have an analgesic effect, probably due to its peripheral action, but we have no good antagonists at the central level. The same problem is true for glutamate. For glutamate we have a lot of antagonists, but as mentioned yesterday, we do not have enough good glutamate antagonists. A drug could block the activity of spinal neurons, but it's not necessarily related to analgesia. To give an example, I will mention a paper published by my laboratory in *Pain* on the effect of a muscle relaxant which induces dose-dependent depressant effects on the activity of the dorsal horn neurons. The effect of this drug is much more powerful than morphine, but apparently there are no analgesic effects, so we must be extremely cautious in this situation. But to try to approach, let's say, the soup, we'll need a variety of antagonists, perhaps using monoclonal antibodies. To cure pain we will probably need a cocktail rather than a soup.

Dr. Foley: Do you want to continue that question that we put to the panel?

Dr. Ochoa: Yes. Before the cocktail and the soup, I think I'd like to agree partly with a recommendation Dr. Raja gave us before he left and then I'd like to answer an unfair question I asked Dr. Bullitt earlier. We definitely should not leave this meeting with the idea that the sympathetic system has nothing to do with pain. Of course it has to do with pain. There are very well established situations. For example, if somebody has pain, then the sympathetic system gets engaged in an innocent reflex manner and causes vasoconstriction of the symptomatic part, and sometimes this symptom is misinterpreted. It's misinterpreted in the direction that the sympathetic system is causing the pain. Another situation is where the sympathetic system is severely degenerated or ablated and the symptomatic part develops coolness due to denervation supersensitivity, and that coolness may be an effective adequate stimulus which may trigger pain when the afferent system is abnormal. We have two conditions there. A third possible condition, sensitized nociceptors, polymodal nociceptors which respond to mechanical stimuli and thermal stimuli also respond to chemical stimuli, and it's absolutely unsurprising that Dr. Saito and Dr. Perl have come up with a very beautifully documented animal experiment whereby abnormal nociceptors respond to norepinephrine, and one has to be prepared to concede that in acute "reflex sympathetic dystrophy" it is possible and likely from what we read in the books, that early sympathectomy may improve the symptoms. I am not sure personally because there are no controlled series on this, but I think one has to accept it is possible and likely. Now, what we're talking about, and that was my question to you earlier, and which has to do with my skepticism about the sympathetic system and chronic pain, is that the majority of patients one sees in a clinic where neurological patients with sensory disorders or chronic pain patients come, the majority of patients with symptoms which justify the diagnosis of RSD, the majority of them, chronic patients, have ongoing pain, they have had injury, they have hyperalgesia, they have abnormal temperature of the skin, they respond to sympathetic blocks, but the majority of them do not respond to sympathectomy. My question to you was why? I'll give you the answer. They don't respond to sympathectomy because they do not have a pain which has anything to do with the sympathetic system. They do not. They do respond to blocks because they are placebo responders. Again, 800 patients from Jefferson, 407 from the Mayo Clinic, hundreds from London, hundreds from Freiberg responsive to blocks have not been compared to placebo controls. None of these studies has taken the trouble to do a placebo control for the block. Now, again, two-thirds of these patients with chronic pain that fits the diagnosis of RSD are placebo responders. Now you mention the studies by Dr. Lowe and Dr. Nathan, very interesting papers. Dr. Lowe, I know him well, did not do placebo controls for his sympathetic blocks in the patients that led to the paper in the early '80s. Dr. Nathan is a very good friend of mine; actually I worked in an office adjacent to his for 8 years. He's a very smart neurologist, very witty, and I'll tell you the way he treated most of these patients, and if Dr. Basbaum is here, he's going to be able to confirm what I'm going to say. In the early '70s, I remember when Dr. Nathan asked about this lady who was very grateful because she was so much better with the medication that he was giving her for the chronic pain. The patient left and Dr. Basbaum asked Dr. Nathan, "Peter, how come you're giving this lady vitamin C for her chronic pain?" And Dr. Nathan answered "my dear Allan, for the imaginary symptom, the imaginary treatment." This patient had malignant hypochondriasis.

Dr. Foley: It's all in the diagnosis. Yes.

Dr. Craig, Barrow Neurological Institute: May I offer a possible solution to the riddle, and it's just a conjecture, so I don't present it as any sort of a answer other than a working hypothesis, and that is that a temporary sympathetic block, as Dr. Hobbins has just emphasized, is going to cause a change in thermal regulatory reflexes, that a permanent sympathectomy, after some time, will no longer effect. What that raises is the question of temperature. We all know that in the spinothalamic tract pain and temperature run together, and I don't think there's any real *a priori* reason to understand that conjunction of pain and temperature other than in their relative value for the control of the vasculature in the skin, as Dr. Hobbins has indeed suggested. Both pain and temperature have strong effects on homeostatic control. Now my question to the three clinicians is directly related to that. There's been recent evidence from, in fact, Dr. Ochoa and Dr. Torebjörk's lab, that with a block of cold sensation by a pressure cuff or a pressure block on the nerve, an innocuous thermal stimulus can cause burning pain. Now I wonder if that's the same kind of burning pain that occurs in central pain conditions, whether if on the opposite side in the central pain patient, a nerve block that removes cold input might allow demonstration of a similar kind of pain. The same kind of pain can be experienced, I think, by all of us if we remember the thermal grill illusion that Thunberg published first in 1895. This might support the hypothesis that cold normally inhibits pain sensation, that the two are processed in an integrative fashion at central thalamocortical levels in the control primarily of homeostatic mechanisms. We can test this. The question is that since you describe a difference between end-zone pain and distal burning pain in cases with spinal cord lesions. The distal burning pain is characterized by thermal allodynia, as are most cases of the central pain syndrome. Is the end-zone pain differentiable on the basis of a lack of thermal allodynia?

Dr. Bullitt: Well, a couple of things. First of all, I honestly cannot tell you if the group of patients with end-zone pain and those with diffuse burning pain have different responses to varying temperatures. However, not all patients with this kind of burning pain are alike; some of them may be completely anesthetic over the region, they may have no heat or cold sensitivity at all, or sensitivity to anything at all. In addition, there are patients with central pain on whom you can do a spinal block and block virtually all input from the periphery. In some cases the pain may be relieved during the period of block, even if the source of the initial injury is high, as in a thalamic injury. In other patients the pain will not be affected, so I'm not sure it's quite as simple as the perception of temperature from the outside.

Dr. Foley: I think we're going to have to stop at this point.

Dr. Willis: I know from the standpoint of our local group, and I think of all of those in the audience that I've had a chance to discuss this with, that we've learned a lot. The information is so dense that it's going to take a while to sort it out. We have to worry about even the definitions of hyperalgesia and allodynia, so we start right at a very fundamental point where there is some difference of opinion that needs attention. There are several kinds of hyperalgesia and allodynia due to tissue damage, due to peripheral nerve damage, due to CNS damage and various combinations of those. There are multiple mechanisms at each of these levels that we heard some evidence about. Human disease states and animal models need to be matched up so that we can really address the human mechanisms using animal models in an effective way. We need better conversations between the laboratory scientists and the clinical researchers so that we can do that match. There is an incomplete approximation of those lines of approach. But I think this meeting will help move us in these directions.

Subject Index